AF755788

Advances in REBT

Michael E. Bernard • Windy Dryden
Editors

Advances in REBT

Theory, Practice, Research, Measurement, Prevention and Promotion

Springer

Editors
Michael E. Bernard
Melbourne Graduate School of Education
University of Melbourne
Melbourne, VIC, Australia

Windy Dryden
Goldsmiths University of London
London, UK

ISBN 978-3-319-93117-3 ISBN 978-3-319-93118-0 (eBook)
https://doi.org/10.1007/978-3-319-93118-0

Library of Congress Control Number: 2019933301

© Springer Nature Switzerland AG 2019
This work is subject to copyright. All rights are reserved by the Publisher, whether the whole or part of the material is concerned, specifically the rights of translation, reprinting, reuse of illustrations, recitation, broadcasting, reproduction on microfilms or in any other physical way, and transmission or information storage and retrieval, electronic adaptation, computer software, or by similar or dissimilar methodology now known or hereafter developed.
The use of general descriptive names, registered names, trademarks, service marks, etc. in this publication does not imply, even in the absence of a specific statement, that such names are exempt from the relevant protective laws and regulations and therefore free for general use.
The publisher, the authors, and the editors are safe to assume that the advice and information in this book are believed to be true and accurate at the date of publication. Neither the publisher nor the authors or the editors give a warranty, express or implied, with respect to the material contained herein or for any errors or omissions that may have been made. The publisher remains neutral with regard to jurisdictional claims in published maps and institutional affiliations.

This Springer imprint is published by the registered company Springer Nature Switzerland AG
The registered company address is: Gewerbestrasse 11, 6330 Cham, Switzerland

Preface

At the 2nd International Congress on Cognitive Behavioral Coaching held in Athens in June, 2016, Windy and I agreed that it was timely for current REBT theory, practice, research, measurement, and applications to be written about by leading REBT scholar-practitioners throughout the world. Sharon Panulla, Executive Editor at Springer whom we have worked with over two decades, agreed to support the project. In discussing the range of global REBT professional activity, we arrived at 36 topics for chapters, and the project with Sharon's support became two books.

Windy and I first met in 1980 while attending the REBT Supervisor's Practicum at the Institute for Rational Emotive Therapy in New York that was conducted by Richard Wessler. 1980 was an important year for REBT as four books were published on the theory and practice of REBT by authors other than Ellis (Wessler/Wessler, Bard/Fisher, Grieger/Boyd, Hauck). It was an exciting time for both of us as we had the opportunity to work directly with Albert Ellis, sat in on his group therapy sessions, and became close to an amazing array of REBTers including but not limited to Ray DiGiuseppe, Janet Wolfe, Dom Dimattia, and Ann Vernon. Subsequently, we became serial editors of the *Journal of Rational-Emotive & Cognitive-Behavior Therapy.*

Albert Ellis was a genius (we know he scored in the top 99% of the Army Alpha IQ test). As a result of his superior aptitude, his extensive reading of philosophy and psychology, and his 150,000+ hours of clinical practice, he discovered something about the human psyche that is quite unique. This discovery and its derivative clinical, counselling, educational, and coaching practices continue to stand the test of time and form a major part of his legacy. Ellis discovered *rationality* as a mental strength that helps people overcome adversity and self-manage negative emotions and self-defeating behaviors and as a self-actualizing force that assists people to live fulfilled, goal-achieving lives. Of course, Ellis also shed light on an oppositional force within the human psyche, *irrationality*, that, as he so eloquently discussed and wrote about, is more important as a contributor to people's mental health problems than their surrounding environment or their early childhood experiences.

Ellis expressed his view that the goal of REBT, when practiced in its most elegant and powerful form, is to educate people to become more rational in order to achieve their goals (and dreams) largely through changes in their philosophy of life. Ellis considered that all people construct personal beliefs that together form a *belief system* that ideally helps them to achieve their goals of living a long, self-actualized, and happy life and which leads to achievement, love, and an absence of stress. Unfortunately, because of people's largely biological propensity, rational beliefs ("I very much want to be successful, loved and stress free") are made into rigid, irrational shoulds, oughts, musts, and needs ("I need to be successful, loved and comfortable"). This is how people's belief system can prevent them from achieving their goals, leading to emotional misery. Much of REBT is devoted to helping strengthen people's rational beliefs. At the same time, and deriving from his self-confessed *gene for efficiency*, Ellis and REBT methods help people through the use of his renowned ABC model to become great problem-solvers in the emotional domain – further developing their mental faculty of rationality.

We think the chapters in this book on REBT measurement and REBT empirical status by Professor Daniel David, Department of Clinical Psychology and Psychotherapy/International Institute for Psychotherapy, "Babeş-Bolyai" University of Cluj-Napoca, and his colleagues deserve special mention. In the early days, REBT was unfavorably compared with Beck's cognitive therapy because the scientific rigor and evaluation studies were not up to the best standards. Through Professor David's research, meta-analyses of REBT research, and thoughtful discussion of how current REBT assessment surveys exemplify best measurement practice, REBT can now be viewed better through the lens of science and research.

Thirty-eight years later, Windy and I are as excited about REBT's contribution to our own work and the mental health and well-being of everyone as we were in the 1980s. And this view is shared by the contributors to these two books and the many, many mental health practitioners using REBT today. The contributors know and practice REBT very well. They share Ellis' views on the empowering aspects of rationality and how REBT methods achieve this end. We have no doubt that you will share in the excitement we have about how REBT continues to make a difference to the lives of many.

Melbourne, VIC, Australia Michael E. Bernard
London, UK Windy Dryden

Contents

Chapter 1
Early Theories and Practices of Rational Emotive Behavior Therapy and How They Have Been Augmented and Revised During the Last Three Decades

Albert Ellis

Theories and Practices of REBT to Which I Still Subscribe

A large number of Rational-Emotive Therapy theories and practices that I wrote about in the mid-1950s and early-1960s and that I largely summarized in my book, *Reason and Emotion in Psychotherapy* (Ellis, 1962), are still central tenets of REBT. These include the following:

1. Active-Directive Therapy is significantly more helpful to more people than is passive, less active therapy. Effective therapists not only listen carefully to their clients and not only unconditionally accept them with their problems and with their ineffective, and sometimes antisocial, behavior but also teach them what they did and still are doing to disturb themselves and how they can think, feel, and act differently to ameliorate their emotional and practical difficulties. Whenever obnoxious or unpleasant activating events occur in people's lives, they have a choice of making themselves feel healthily and self-helpingly sorry, disappointed, frustrated, and annoyed, or making themselves feel unhealthily and self-defeatingly horrified, terrified, panicked, depressed, self-hating, and self-pitying. They usually, though not always, create and construct healthy feelings by believing rational or functional beliefs, and they usually, though not always, create self-defeating feelings and behaviors by constructing and creating irrational or self-defeating beliefs. When people take their strong preferences or desires for success, love, or comfort and define them as absolutist musts, needs, and commands, they tend to make themselves grandiosely anxious, depressed, hostile, and self-pitying. People

A. Ellis (✉)
Albert Ellis Institute, New York, NY, USA
e-mail: info@rebt.org

© Springer Nature Switzerland AG 2019

M. E. Bernard, W. Dryden (eds.), *Advances in REBT*,
https://doi.org/10.1007/978-3-319-93118-0_1

who feel inadequate and worthless learn and create definitional premises or philosophies by which they tend to make themselves disturbed.

2. When people accept the fact that they largely control their own emotional and behavioral destiny, and that they can make themselves undisturbed or less disturbed mainly by acquiring realistic and sensible attitudes about the undesirable things that occur or that they make occur in their lives, they then usually have the ability and power of changing their belief system, making it more functional, and helping themselves to feel and to behave in a significantly less disturbed fashion.
3. When people understand or have insight into how they needlessly disturb themselves and create unhealthy and dysfunctional feelings and behaviors, that insight often will help them change and make themselves less disturbed. But understanding and insight are not enough. In order to significantly change themselves, they almost always have to pinpoint their irrational philosophies and work at changing them to more functional and self-helping attitudes. They can do this in a number of cognitive, emotive-evocative, and behavioral ways.
4. Humans, unlike just about all the other animals on earth, create fairly sophisticated languages that not only enable them to think about their feeling, and their actions, and the results they get from doing and not doing certain things, but they also are able to think about their thinking and even think about thinking about their thinking. Because of their self-consciousness and their ability to think about their thinking, they can very easily disturb themselves about their disturbances and can also disturb themselves about their ineffective attempts to overcome their emotional disturbances.
5. Practically all humans are born very gullible or teachable, especially in the course of their childhood, and consequently they accept many kinds of ideas, feelings, and actions that their parents and other caretakers tell them are beneficial and often reward them for believing, feeling, and behaving. They can also accept from their parents and other caretakers dysfunctional and self-defeating ideas that help them disturb themselves.
6. Even when they accept such dysfunctional beliefs from others, they tend to reconstruct them and actively carry them on; and they are not merely affected years later by the fact that they accepted these beliefs but by their continuing to promulgate them and to act on them.
7. When people acknowledge that they are now needlessly upsetting themselves with their own absolutist musts, and their own necessitizing about themselves, about others, and about the world, they can almost always dispute and challenge their dysfunctional philosophies, act against them, and return to their non-disturbing preferences and desires.
8. When people keep challenging and questioning their self-disturbing core philosophies, after a while they tend to automatically, and even in advance, bring new, rational, self-helping attitudes to their life problems and thereby make themselves significantly less upsett*able*, sometimes for the rest of their lives.
9. REBT assumes that human thinking, emotion, and action are not really separate or disparate processes but that they all significantly overlap and are rarely

experienced in a pure state. Much of what we call emotion is nothing more nor less than a certain kind—a biased, prejudiced, or strongly evaluative kind—of thought. But emotions and behaviors significantly influence and affect thinking, just as thinking significantly influences what we call emotions and behaviors.

10. Evaluating is a fundamental characteristic of human organisms and seems to work in a kind of closed circuit with a feedback mechanism: Because perception biases response and then response tends to subsequent perception. Also, prior perceptions appear to bias subsequent perceptions, and prior responses to bias subsequent responses. What we call feelings almost always have a pronounced evaluating or appraisal element.
11. Although emotions may sometimes exist without thought, it appears to be almost impossible to *sustain* an emotional outburst without bolstering it by repeated ideas.
12. Human thinking may be done by imaging, by using mathematical signs, by dream symbols, and by other forms of communication, but it is usually experienced in the form of words, phrases, and sentences. Therefore, much but hardly all of our emoting takes the form or follows self-talk or internalized conversation. Because of this, people may control their emotions by changing the internalized sentences or self-talk, with which they largely create these emotions.
13. Human emotions are very valuable and probably essential to human existence, and although we may help ourselves by controlling or changing them, it would be folly to try to get rid of them or even to reduce them to a bare minimum.
14. There are a number of very common irrational, unrealistic, grandiose, self-defeating beliefs that people in our culture and in most other cultures have; and when they strongly believe these ideas they frequently, though not always, produce dysfunctional emotions and behaviors. The goal of REBT is not only to show clients what their specific irrational philosophies are, but how they construct these ideas and how they can think more rationally, thereby unupset themselves, and thereby create fewer dysfunctional beliefs in the future.
15. People's irrational and self-defeating ideas are unrealistic, illogical, and absolutist. They can then be logically and empirically challenged, and individuals who hold them can be shown that if they continue to subscribe to them, they will often bring about obsessions, compulsions, disturbed feelings, and other self-sabotaging behaviors. Disturbed people can be taught by a Rational Emotive Behavior therapist to challenge and dispute these dysfunctional ideas and can learn how to do this for themselves.
16. On the surface, it looks like children acquire feelings of inadequacy and worthlessness because they are severely criticized and excoriated by their parents when they are quite young. This is partly true, because almost all children are so gullible and influenceable that they will take negative views from their parents about themselves and make them their own. A small percentage of children, however, will not choose to do so and will not blame their parents or the world for their shortcomings. Or they may even take responsibilities for their failures, but not conclude that they themselves are bad children. Even

when children do accept bad ideas about themselves from their parents or caretakers, it is their forcefully carrying on these ideas in their adolescence and adulthood, rather than their early imbibing of such philosophies, that largely makes them neurotic.

17. Some of the irrational ideas of children, such as the idea that they must be approved or loved by all the significant people in their lives, are not entirely inappropriate to their childhood state, because children really have to be taken care of by others if they are to survive. But when these ideas are maintained in adolescence and adulthood, as they frequently are, they become very self-defeating. It is their maintenance in the present, then, and not their early acquiring of these ideas, that is most important when they are treated as adolescents or adults.
18. An effective REBT practitioner uses the general techniques of therapy, such as relationship, expressive-emotive, supportive, and insight interpretive techniques, but he or she never stops there but goes on to directly contradict and undermine the self-defeating irrationalities that clients may have originally learned but are now instilling in themselves. The Rational Emotive Behavior therapist may first approach clients in a cautious, supportive, permissive, and warm manner and may encourage them to ventilate their feelings and to use a number of expressive techniques. However, it is assumed that the clients may thereby see that they are behaving illogically and self-defeatingly, but that they also have so strongly habituated themselves to dysfunctional thoughts and actions that their knowing exactly how they have been disturbing themselves is far from enough. In addition, the therapist had better actively show the clients how they are still forcefully upsetting themselves and how they can think and act their way out of their self-defeating philosophies and bring themselves to a point where they acquire basic new philosophies of living that will largely prevent them from disturbing themselves again in the present and future.
19. The therapist not only shows clients how they now are irrationally condemning themselves, other people, and the world, but how they have a lifelong pattern of doing this, and shows them how they can make a basic philosophic change so that they uproot this pattern and think much more functionally in the present and future.
20. The Rational Emotive Behavior therapist strongly believes in a rigorous application of the rules of logic, straight thinking, and of scientific method to everyday life. He or she ruthlessly uncovers the most important elements of irrational thinking in the client's experience and energetically encourages these clients to take more reasonable channels of feeling and behaving. The clients' emotions are not ignored or eradicated, but they are helped to change them when they are disordered and self-defeating. They are helped to do this through the same means by which they commonly initiated these dysfunctional behaviors in the first place—that is, by changing their thinking and acting in self-sabotaging ways.
21. Humans are born with strong tendencies to be both rational and irrational, both self-helping and self-defeating. In both these ways, they are innately

constructivist. Because they largely upset themselves with their beliefs, they can be helped to examine, to question, to think about these beliefs and thereby to develop a more workable, more self-helping set of constructs than they possess when they come to therapy.

22. Freud believed that virtually all clients have to be approached in the course of an intense, highly emotionalized, supportive, and transference relationship, but in REBT it is found that though this is true of some exceptionally disturbed, and especially psychotic and personality disordered clients, most neurotic clients take quite well to the Rational Emotive Behavior active-directive approach, and have no need of an intensely emotionalized transference relationship, including a transference neurosis, with the therapist. Although reasoning and philosophizing have their distinct limitations in helping people with their problems, humans are uniquely rational, as well as irrational, and therefore the use of logic and rationality in therapy, as well as in the lives of people who are not in therapy, can often bring about unusually good results in helping people adjust to the difficult problems of everyday living.
23. Many therapists, such as Carl Rogers, Sigmund Freud, Otto Rank, Wilhelm Reich, and Harry Stack Sullivan, have insisted that there are certain requisites that must be met in therapy if clients are to make basic personality changes. It seems obvious that many individuals over the centuries have changed themselves considerably without undergoing the kinds of therapeutic processes that these therapists have insisted must be undergone. REBT would suggest that although basic constructive personality change, as opposed to temporary symptom removal, seems to require fundamental modifications in the ideologies and value systems of the disturbed individual, there is probably *no* single condition that is absolutely necessary for the inducement of such changed attitudes and behavior patterns. It is hypothesized that an active-directive, Rational Emotive Behavioral approach will help people make basic personality changes more than will any of the other therapeutic approaches. But there are many other change procedures, some of which are instituted by clients themselves without any psychotherapy, that also lead to basic personality modification. Humans have an innate constructive tendency to be self-changing and self-actualizing and can use this tendency both inside and outside of regular psychotherapy.
24. REBT is much more than didactic, rational, and philosophic. In addition to verbal discussion between clients and therapists, it strongly emphasizes that logical parsing and rational persuasion on the part of both therapists and clients be employed to help the clients *act* and *work* against their neurotic attitudes and their self-defeating habit patterns. Clients are shown that they had better *fight*, in practice as well as in theory, against their acquired and invented irrational ideas *and* the dysfunctional behavior patterns that accompany these ideas. Unless therapists somehow induce their clients to un*do*, as well as to un*think*, their self-defeating philosophies, no thoroughgoing reversal of the client's neurotic process is expected to occur.
25. Rational Emotive Behavior therapists not only teach their clients how to think logically, empirically, and self-helpingly, but also tend to encourage an

existentialist and humanist point of view. They favor many of the existentialist philosophies of Martin Buber, Jean Paul Sartre, Martin Heidigger, and Paul Tillich. They believe that humans have a considerable degree of choice in regard to what they think, feel, and act upon, but that it requires a great deal of effort and practice, as well as scientific thinking, for them to achieve any amount of individual freedom and social democracy.

26. REBT agrees that humans often act incompetently and immorally and that their behavior had better be assessed and changed when it is individually and socially destructive. But it is opposed to people making themselves feel depressed and guilty about their poor behavior. It teaches people to condemn many of their and others' *acts* and *performances*, but never to condemn or rate themselves as *humans*. It holds that when people accept or give themselves a sense of sin, guilt, or self-blame, they tend to act more ineffectively and immorally. So it encourages them to evaluate their deeds, acts, performances, feelings, and thoughts, but not to create a *self*-rating and not to see themselves as globally good or bad people. It accepts the reality that people usually have extrinsic value to others as well as intrinsic value to themselves, but that they easily confuse the two and *define* themselves as good or worthwhile, mainly in terms of their assumed value to others.
27. REBT holds that ideas and feelings about self-worth are largely definitional and are not empirically confirmable or falsifiable. We really *choose* to accept or denigrate our "selves" and falsely assume that because we can fairly accurately measure our deeds and performances, as good or bad, once we establish goals and purposes to measure them against, that we can also measure our "self" or our "being." People's intrinsic value or worth cannot really be measured accurately because their *being* includes their *becoming*. They are a *process* with an ever-changing present and future. Therefore, they can never really be accurately rated as people while they are still alive and changing.
28. REBT can show people that they are only worthless by definition—because they *think* they are. Therefore, they'd better choose to define themselves as worthwhile, because that will lead to much better emotional and behavior results than if they *choose* to define themselves as worthless. By measuring only their deeds and acts, but *not* measuring their "self" or their "being" by how well they do or by how much they are approved by others, people can *unconditionally* accept themselves or gain what Carl Rogers calls unconditional positive regard.
29. Lack of self-acceptance comes not only from believing, "I am no good when I have done bad things," but also from putting oneself down as a result of this self-damnation and then putting oneself down *again*, on a secondary level, by telling oneself "I am not good for being depressed." So, by attaching one's worth as a person to one's good and bad performances, one frequently creates a *double* dose of self-worthlessness.
30. To help people gain unconditional self-acceptance and to believe that they *are okay* or are good just because they exist had better be taught to all children in the course of their schooling, from early childhood onward.

31. Taking one's preferences for success and approval and making them into musts and demands often leads to feelings of worthlessness since people easily falsely conclude, "Because I must do well and actually am doing poorly, my *behavior* is not only no good, but *I* am no good." If they change their musts and needs back into preferences and believe, "I very much *want* to do well, but I never *have to* do so," they will eliminate most of their self-rating and self-downing that almost always goes with their self-rating.
32. People naturally have conscious and unconscious thoughts and processes and create their neurotic feelings and behavior with unconscious as well as conscious irrational beliefs, "iBs." Instead of their irrational beliefs being deeply hidden or repressed, as psychoanalytic theory alleges, these irrational beliefs are almost always just below the level of consciousness, in what Freud originally called their preconscious thinking, and can fairly easily be brought to light if one uses REBT theory to look for and reveal them.
33. Although early traumatic events and feelings about them may be unconsciously repressed, this seems to be much rarer than psychoanalysis assumes. The disturbed feelings that accompany these traumatic feelings are not automatically kept alive by early conditioning. Instead, the disturbed philosophies or irrational beliefs that originally accompanied these traumatic feelings and that were *constructed* by the dysfunctional individuals who had these feelings, are actively kept alive today by these traumatized persons. It is the *current* philosophic and behavioral re-traumatizing that keeps the early disturbance alive in the present. Much of the re-traumatizing may be unconscious but it is just below the surface of consciousness and rarely deeply repressed.
34. Digging up and making conscious people's early traumas and the disturbed thoughts and feelings that went with them may be somewhat helpful in some cases but it may also be harmful unless people bring to consciousness the core irrational and musturbatory, rather than preferential, beliefs they held about the original traumas and that they still tend to strongly hold. Making these irrational beliefs fully conscious and then actively and consciously disputing them and strongly and persistently acting against them rather than merely seeing them will alleviate them and undo them and relieve people of their cognitive-emotional disturbances.
35. When unconscious thoughts and feelings, such as hating one's mother, are repressed, the repressor feels ashamed about having them and therefore unconsciously forgets them and consciously denies them. By using REBT to help repressors refuse to blame or damn their *self* or *being* for anything, but only to condemn their wrong or stupid *behaviors*, and by helping them to see that their early traumas were bad and unfortunate, but *not* "awful" or "terrible," REBT often enables them to look at what really happened and may still be happening and to unrepress their repressed thoughts and feeling and then to unupset themselves by *changing* their disturbing ideas and actions.
36. Instead of merely passively listening to their clients, and through free-association revealing their unconscious, presumably repressed traumas, thoughts, and feelings, REBT practitioners can uncover and alleviate client's

unconscious, as well as their conscious, disturbances by using active, directive methods of confrontation, deindoctrination, and re-education and by teaching clients to actively look for and to vigorously dispute their irrational beliefs and their dysfunctional feelings and behaviors.

37. REBT takes a forthright stand in favor of intensive *activity* on the part of both the client and the therapist. The therapist helps convince the clients that they definitely can change their thoughts, feelings, and behaviors just as millions of other people have changed them over the years, but that they can only do so by considerable work and practice.
38. REBT assumes, along with Kurt Goldstein, Abe Maslow, and Carl Rogers, that humans have a considerable potential for changing and actualizing themselves, but that existential encounters alone will rarely help them do this. They had better, instead, be taught to specifically see what their irrational philosophies are and actively and constructively dispute them and force themselves to feel and act against them.
39. REBT assumes that clients often resist psychological treatment and that they frequently do so because they have a biological tendency to keep habituated to their dysfunctional thoughts, feelings, and behaviors. They also have a great deal of low frustration tolerance, which makes it difficult for them to work at changing themselves even when they see the desirability of doing so. Therefore, their therapist had usually better be exceptionally active-directive and keep showing them the benefits of change and the disadvantage of staying the way they are. The therapist had also better actively push and encourage them to make the changes that would be helpful to them. Although the REBT practitioner invariably fully accepts the client with his or her self-defeating, and often anti-social behavior, the therapist also unpamperingly shows clients that they are behaving dysfunctionally and actively pushes them to behave more functionally. REBT theory says that if clients are persuaded and induced to act differently they frequently at first are very uncomfortable but then become comfortable and even may enjoy their new behaviors.
40. Because humans become habituated to their dysfunctional thoughts, feelings, behaviors, they often find it very difficult to unlearn them and change them. And therefore they had better steadily, persistently, and forcefully act against them, as well as feel and think against them. Consequently, REBT is exceptionally behavioral and encourages clients to engage in a good deal of in vivo desensitization. Almost all clients are persuaded to do a good many activity homework assignments that tend to counterattack their irrational beliefs and their self-defeating feelings. Both in REBT sessions and in the course of clients' homework assignments, clients had better be induced to do vigorous rethinking, which will often lead them to change their motor and behavioral actions and also induced to forcefully repattern their sensori-motor activity that will often lead to their changing their ideation. The quickest and most deep rooted behavioral modification will usually follow from a *combined* verbal and sensory-motor attack on the old, dysfunctional ways of thinking and doing. REBT therefore tries to help people powerfully and forcefully dispute *and* act against their self-defeating thoughts and behaviors.

Revisions in the Theory and Practice of REBT Since 1962

Early Childhood Conditioning

REBT now holds that although people largely learn their goals, values, and desires from their parents and their culture, and that although the standards that they learn often get them into problems and difficulties if they follow them or if they refuse to follow them, just about all people in all parts of the world frequently take their socially imbibed preferences and standards and *create* and *construct* absolutist, unrealistic shoulds, oughts, musts, and demands about these goals. They thereby largely *make* themselves disturbed and also then disturb themselves about their disturbances. Their self-disturbing demands are both conditioned by their environment *and* are self-taught. They construct them *on top of* and *far beyond* the disturbed (conditioning) that they pick up from their environment. In other words, humans often learn that it is bad or wrong for them to fail and to be rejected by other people, but then they *naturally* and *easily* add, "I *absolutely must not* ever behave improperly and if I behave as I *must not* I am a rotten person." The absolutist musts and overgeneralizations that they add to their desires to perform well and to be approved by others, are (a) unrealistic (b) exaggerated conclusions, and (c) definitional. Because they are language prone and communicate with language to themselves as well as to others, humans can be much more unrealistic, overgeneralizing, and definitional about their disturbed concepts and feelings than can the rest of the members of the animal kingdom.

Basic Core Musturbatory Philosophies and Their Derived Attributions and Inferences

People are born and reared with the ability to look at the data of their lives, particularly the negative things that happen to them against their goals and interests, and to make inaccurate inferences and attributions about these data. Thus, when they see someone frown at them, they easily and often wrongly conclude, "He hates me, and thinks that I am a bad person and he is right about this." Because such attributions and inferences are often false and because they lead to disturbed feelings and behaviors, they had better be questioned and disputed and significantly changed. REBT originally pointed out these mistaken inferences and showed clients how to question and challenge their catastrophizing, their awfulizing, their overgeneralizations, their personalizing, their mind-reading and their other attributions. A number of years later, other cognitive-behavior therapists, such as Aaron Beck, Maxie Maultsby, Donald Meichenbaum, and David Burns, also began to show clients how to dispute their self-defeating attributions. Most of these therapists, however, place dysfunctional attributions on the same level as people's shoulds and the musts, which they also include as *one* of the disturbed forms of thinking with which people upset themselves. From the start, and even more so later, REBT has held that the absolutist musts that people add to their strong preferences and dislikes are more basic to their disturbances than the negative inferences that they largely derive from these musts. Thus, if people rigorously stayed only with their preferences, and had fundamental philosophies such as, "I very much would like significant others to approve of me, but they never *have* to," they would rarely infer, when significant others did not presumably like them, that it would be awful, that they couldn't stand it, that they are worthless as individuals, that they will never be approved by decent people, etc. As soon, however, as they strongly believe that they absolutely *must* be approved by significant others, then they find it almost impossible not to invent self-defeating inferences and attributions that logically seem to stem from these musts. Unlike the other Cognitive-Behavior therapies, therefore, the main disputational rule of REBT consists of showing clients, when they are emotionally and behaviorally disturbed, that they almost invariably have conscious or unconscious demand, commands, and musts, and that they had better quickly find these and actively and strongly question and challenge them; and then they had better *also* go on to ferret out the dysfunctional inferences and attributions that they derive from these musts and give them up too. REBT holds that showing disturbed people that they are profound musturbators is most probably the most important thing that a therapist can do to help them, and that showing them that their dogmatic and imperative musts are just about always illegitimate and self-sabotaging and that they can be directly and indirectly challenged and given up is probably the most beneficial aspect of Cognitive-Behavior therapy (Bernard, 1991; Ellis, 1998a, 1998b; Ellis & Blau, 1998; Ellis & Dryden, 1997; Ellis & Harper, 1997; Ellis & MacLaren, 1998).

Verbalization and Self-Talk

REBT pioneered in showing disturbed people that their emotional problems almost always stem from verbalizing and talking to themselves about the reality problems they encounter or might encounter in the world. And it pioneered in showing them how to change their disruptive self-talk. It also showed them that they often created secondary symptoms of disturbance by negatively talking to themselves about their original negative self-talk and about the emotional and behavioral symptoms that this original self-talk largely created. REBT today is still very much concerned with the specific self-verbalizations that people use to upset themselves, to upset themselves about their upsetness, and to keep upsetting themselves all throughout their lives. But it now is more interested in the explicit and implicit *meanings* and *philosophies* that people use to upset themselves. These meanings and philosophies are very frequently created and used in the form of self-sentences and self-phrases. They are, however, often held implicitly, tacitly, or unconsciously as core philosophies of life, which can be translated into self-talk, but which also arise and are held in other kinds of cognition, such as imaging, fantasizing, symbolizing, and other forms of intercommunication and intracommunication. Although REBT is usually done today mainly by the form of teaching clients how to look at their self-verbalizations, as well as their communication with others, and to see how they disturb themselves by their talking to themselves, it also emphasizes imagery and visualization technique and other forms of symbolic thinking that people consciously or unconsciously use to disturb themselves and that they can also use to reduce disturbances.

Secondary Disturbances or Symptom Stress

REBT was one of the pioneer systems of therapy that clearly pointed out that people frequently disturb themselves about their disturbances and that they believe that they *must not* think crookedly, *must not* have disturbed feelings, *must not* have dysfunctional behaviors. They thereby create secondary symptoms or symptom stresses that are frequently worse than their original disturbances and that often block them from seeing exactly what their original disturbances are and from unraveling them. This is particularly true of people who experience panic and then tell themselves, "I must not panic! I must not panic!" and who thereby create panic about their panic, which exacerbates their emotional problems mightily. A fundamental therapeutic principal of REBT today is that seriously neurotic and personality disordered individuals very often have severe secondary symptoms of their disturbance and that an effective REBT practitioner had better investigate to see if these secondary symptoms exist, and if they do, had better help the clients see them and often work at giving up their secondary symptoms before they seriously work at giving up their primary disturbances. Because of its concern with people's thinking about their thinking and thinking about their feelings and dysfunctional behaviors, REBT often specializes in ferreting out and ameliorating secondary disturbances. It also assumes that when people go to psychotherapy they often bring about a tertiary disturbance about the therapeutic process. Thus, they believe "I *must* do well at therapy and my goddamned therapist must significantly help me in a brief period of time!" and they thereby disturb themselves significantly about the therapeutic process. If so, this tertiary symptom had better be importantly discovered and dealt with while the client and the therapist are working on the primary and the secondary symptoms (Ellis & Dryden, 1997; Ellis, Gordon, Neenan, & Palmer, 1998; Ellis & MacLaren, 1998).

Emotive Methods of REBT

REBT has always been very forceful, confrontative, and opposed to namby-pamby methods of therapy. It has particularly encouraged therapists to take the risks of quickly showing clients how they defeat themselves, rather than taking a long time to get to this point and rather than allowing clients to be evasive and defensive. REBT practitioners, therefore, model risk-taking, show that they are not disturbed when clients resist therapy, and are willing, if necessary, to antagonize and to lose some of their clients. REBT practitioners, also, frequently directly answer clients' questions and reveal some of their own problems and their own personal lives while trying to help the clients. As the years have gone by, REBT has seen more clearly than it originally did, that clients very powerfully hold on to their self-disturbing thoughts, feelings, and behaviors and that when they do light, instead of forceful, disputing of their irrationalities, they only temporarily or mildly give them up and then tend to return to them. It seems to be the human condition that people can lightly believe sensible ideas, such as "I would prefer that significant other people approve of me, but they really don't have to," while at the same time, they strongly believe self-defeating ideas, such as "I *absolutely need* the approval of significant others and I *can't stand it* when I don't get it!" REBT over the years has therefore increasingly used a number of evocative-emotive techniques of therapy such as Rational Emotive Imagery, shame attacking exercises, role playing, reverse role playing, forceful coping statements, unconditional acceptance of clients, and other emotive methods. It has devised rational-encounter marathons, 9 hour intensives, affective group and work-shop exercises, and other emotive methods of encouraging clients and group members to get in touch with some of their unrevealed feelings, to express themselves in a risk-taking manner, to work at increasing their relationship and their sex pleasures, and to use various other emotional methods of undermining their disturbances and increasing their happiness (Ellis & Dryden, 1997; Ellis & Velten, 1998).

The Increased Use of Behavioral Methods in REBT

REBT has always been quite behavioral and is still more behavioral than most of the other cognitive therapies, because instead of using Wolpe's (1958) systematic desensitization to help people overcome their destructive fears and panic states it favors the use of in vivo desensitization and exposure. It also encourages people to stay in a bad situation, such as working for a disturbed boss or living with an angry mate, until they first overcome their feelings of rage and inadequacy, and then decide whether or not to leave the situation. REBT often uses reinforcement, but it also favors penalties, such as encouraging people to burn a fifty or a hundred dollar bill when they fail to do the homework that they have promised themselves to do to change themselves (Ellis, 1998a, 1998b; Ellis & Dryden, 1997). It has pioneered in assertion training since 1963 and often includes a great deal of other kinds of skill training (Ellis & Tafrate, 1997; Wolfe, 1980). It is also a double-systems therapy in that it helps people unupset themselves while they are still in a bad system, such as a bad family, or a bad work system, and then it helps them go back to point A, the activating events or the adversity in their lives and work out practical and problem-solving solutions to these realistic problems. But again it usually encourages people to stop upsetting themselves when they are within a disordered system and then at the same time to work at changing the system. It does not encourage them to only change the system, without also changing their own disturbed thoughts, feelings, and behaviors, which the system may *contribute to* but does not solely *cause* (Ellis, 1996a, 1996b, 1997).

Evolutionary Origin of Grandiose Musts and Other Irrational Beliefs

If, as REBT now hypothesizes, absolutist shoulds, oughts, musts, and their many derivative unrealistic and overgeneralized inferences and attributions are not only acquired from early upbringing but are also part of the human biological tendency to think crookedly and self-defeatingly, the question may be asked as to why people have this biological tendency. One answer is that self-defeating feelings of depression, anxiety, and self-hatred, as well as phobias and obsessions, still have some life-preserving values even though they help people to feel quite miserable. Thus, if one is phobic about driving on the highway, or panicked about acquiring an illness, one will be super-cautious and may preserve one's life, even at the expense of overly restricting it. REBT tends to go along with evolutionary psychologists who believe that tens of thousands of years ago, when humans lived under serious threats to their lives from animals and other humans, and when they were thin skinned animals who were vulnerable to a great deal of hurt and death, they may have been practically forced to acquire musturbatory ways of thinking in order to flee rapidly from potential destroyers. Also, in a competitive world, they may have had to insist that they must do well and must be approved by other people, or else they may not have survived without these musts. Children, even today, may well be required to have the ideas that they must be taken care of and must be rescued from pain, else they might not call attention to their painful straits, and again might not survive. So people who raise their strong preferences to absolutist musts, may have in the past, or even in the present, acquire survival value, even though they thereby create for themselves a great deal of "needless" anxiety and depression. Nature seems to be mainly interested in the survival of a species and not in how happy the species is while it survives.

REBT and the Scientific Method

When I wrote *Reason and Emotion in Psychotherapy* in 1962, I said that "Science is intrinsically empirical, and scientific knowledge must, at least in principal be confirmable by some form of human experience." This is the position of logical positivism, but I have no longer been a logical positivist since 1976, when I read Mike Mahoney's (1975) book, *Scientist as Subject*. Since then I have subscribed to the philosophy of William Bartley and Karl Popper, which is called Critical Rationalism or Critical Realism. REBT is not just interested in proving beyond a shadow of doubt that rational ideas work better than irrational ideas, but it is more interested in showing that when people think irrationally, and particularly when they raise their strong preferences to absolutist musts, they tend to disturb themselves and can be shown how to uproot a great deal of their disturbances by falsifying these musts. REBT always was opposed to any kind of absolutism and is now more strongly opposed to this view. It holds that dogmatic, rigid, and absolutist thinking is one of the main essences of human neurosis and that openness, flexibility, and acceptance of human diversity is one of the main essences of nondisturbance. It consequently specializes in showing people what their own basic theories about themselves and the world are and how these hypotheses often lead to destructive feelings and actions, how they can be forcefully falsified and replaced with more workable philosophies. It uses reason, empiricism, logic, and flexible, alternative-seeking ways of thinking. But it also stresses the use of metaphor, hermeneutics, philosophy, narrative, drama, humor, and other presumably non-rational and non-logical means of understanding and alleviating human disturbance. It partly subscribes to some elements of postmodern philosophy, which shows that nothing, including science, is sacred (Ellis, 1994, 1997, 1998a).

Biological Aspects of Human Disturbance

REBT has always held that humans are biologically prone to think, feel, and behave in a self-destructive manner, and especially that people with personality disorders and psychoses are strongly biologically predisposed to think and behave as they do. But I strongly stressed in my early writings that neurosis is partly caused by irrational and dysfunctional beliefs. In some ways, this may be the case, but some severe neurotics, such as those afflicted with panic states and with serious disturbance, seem to have strong endogenous elements in their upsetability. Endogenous depressives, for example, may indeed have irrational views about themselves, others, and the world, but it is probable that some of these views did not merely originate in their basic philosophy of life, but also are sparked by deficiencies in their neurotransmitters and other aspects of their nervous system. Once they feel severely depressed, even if the depression suddenly overtakes them without any activating experiences or disturbed beliefs about these experiences, they then can easily tell themselves that they *must not* be depressed and that it's *awful* for them to feel the way they do, and therefore they may seriously exacerbate their depression. So it is likely that endogenously depressed individuals often think disturbedly because of some biochemical deficiencies, and that then they also think disturbedly about their depressed symptoms. Irrational and dysfunctional beliefs, then, are almost always involved in seriously disturbed feelings and actions. But these beliefs may be set off by biological processes, and then may also exacerbate these processes. Biological processes may also encourage disturbed feelings and behaviors that, once again, influence and help to create musturbatory and other dysfunctional beliefs. Consequently, although in 1962 I rarely sent my disturbed clients for medication I, and other REBT-ers, now frequently recommend that our clients try various kinds of medications, especially anti-depressants, when they feel severely disturbed and when their feelings seem to be partly endogenous as well as sparked by irrational cognitions (Ellis, 1997).

Cool, Warm, and Hot Beliefs in REBT

Robert Abelson in 1962 distinguished cool from hot beliefs. REBT distinguishes among cool, warm, and hot beliefs. A cool belief is "this is a table" or "this is a round table." A warm belief is an evaluation, such as "I like or dislike this table." A hot belief is a very strong evaluation, such as "I hate this table very much, and I think that it shouldn't exist and should be destroyed!" REBT rarely argues with people's cool beliefs and also rarely argues with warm beliefs or their preferences. It mainly teaches clients to dispute their hot beliefs, particularly when these contain a demand, such as, "Because I dislike this table, it absolutely must not exist and should be completely destroyed." REBT, once again, encourages people to feel quite warmly and even hotly about many things that happen to them or that they make happen to them in their lives. But it discourages them from having hot beliefs that are also inflexible, dogmatic, and absolutist. It holds that a warm belief, as long as it is a preference, consists of a statement such as, "I like this table very much, *but* I can live without it and I can be happy even if I use another kind of table." A hot musturbatory belief, such as, "Because I like this table very much, I absolutely must be able to use it and will not be happy at all with any other table," is a belief that usually brings on emotional and behavioral disturbance. In *Reason and Emotion in Psychotherapy* (1962), I listed eleven irrational beliefs and showed why they were irrational and how they could be disputed by therapists and clients and changed into self-helping preferences. I still hold that these eleven ideas, which are very common among humans all over the world, are dysfunctional, but I would reword several of them so that they clearly include an absolutist should, ought, or must. I now put all eleven of them and several other important ones under three major headings:

1. "I must be thoroughly competent, adequate, achieving, and lovable at all times, or else I am an incompetent worthless person." This belief usually leads to feelings of anxiety, panic, depression, despair, and worthlessness.
2. "Other significant people in my life, must treat me kindly and fairly at all times, or else I can't stand it, and they are bad, rotten, and evil persons who should be severely blamed, damned, and vindictively punished for their horrible treatment of me." This leads to feelings of anger, rage, fury, and vindictiveness and to actions like feuds, wars, fights, genocide, and ultimately, an atomic holocaust.
3. "Things and conditions absolutely must be the way I want them to be and must never be too difficult or frustrating. Otherwise, life is awful, terrible, horrible, catastrophic and unbearable." This leads to low-frustration tolerance, self-pity, anger, depression, and to behaviors such as procrastination, avoidance, and inaction.

Once people accept these irrational beliefs from their parents or culture and once they create some of them largely on their own, they almost always derive self-defeating and society-defeating inferences from them such as awfulizing, I-can't-stand-it-itis, self-deprecation, damnation of others, personalizing, overgeneralizing, phonyism, etc. When people experience or expect to experience unfortunate events, they quickly have a number of negative "automatic" thoughts that seem to stem from the events themselves, but actually are derived from or are "conditioned" to underlying core musturbatory philosophies that they consciously or implicitly hold.

The Social and Environmental Origin of Neurotic Disturbances

I said in *Reason and Emotion in Psychotherapy* (1962) that "Ours is a generally neuroticizing civilization in which most people are more or less emotionally disturbed because they are brought up to believe, and then to internalize and to keep reinfecting themselves with, arrant nonsense which must inevitably lead them to become ineffective, self-defeating, and unhappy." I still believe that this is partly true, because people in our and other societies are often reared to believe many silly rules, especially sex and loves rules, that help them be miserable for the rest of their lives. Thus, they may be helped to believe that romantic love lives forever and that good sex relations largely consists of intercourse. However, even silly rules that people learn and that they foolishly follow do not by any means necessarily disturb them. They largely disturb themselves by creating absolutist musts about these rules. Thus, they convince themselves, "I *must* be romantically loved by my mate forever!" and "I *must* always have successful intercourse with my mate leading to both of us achieving a terrific orgasm!" It is their musts, far more than their adherence to societally inculcated goals and standards, that make them emotionally disturbed.

Importantizing and Sacredizing in REBT

I wrongly implied in *Reason and Emotion in Psychotherapy* that it is not terribly important if one fails at a task or loses the approval of a significant person. In today's REBT, I distinguish clearly between importantizing and sacredizing. Anyone is entitled to make anything in his or her life quite important and to value it considerably or even value it more than he or she values anything else in the world. This kind of importantizing does not make people disturbed unless they add to it, "Because I find love or success at work terribly important, I therefore *have to* succeed at it and *must* get exactly what I want in connection with it." As soon as an absolutistic must is added to importantizing, it becomes sacredizing; and what we call neurosis largely results from making something quite important to oneself and/or others and then foolishly sacredizing it and insisting that its importance makes it imperative that it *absolutely must* be achieved. So REBT often encourages people to importantize many things and events in their lives as long as they do not sacredize these things and insist that success at them is completely imperative (Ellis, 1998b; Ellis & Blau, 1998; Ellis & MacLaren, 1998).

The Use of REBT with Children

In *Reason and Emotion in Psychotherapy* I took a dim view of using REBT successfully with young children. A few years later, however, I reversed this stand and the Institute for Rational-Emotive Therapy in New York actually ran a school for 5 years that taught children from the ages of six to fourteen the elements of rational thinking that they could apply to their home, school, and to their other life. In 1974, William Knaus published a book on Rational-Emotive Education, and since that time, REBT has been successfully used with young and older children (Knaus, 1974). In doing REBT with young children, they are shown how some of their ideas and feelings and behaviors will often create needless difficulties and that they can change their self-defeating thoughts, feelings, and actions. But instead of using a good deal of active disputing of irrational beliefs, which is done with adolescents and adults, the children are shown how to use rational coping self-statements that will help them in the difficult situations that they encounter. They are also taught the elements of REBT in the forms of stories, fables, plays, films, and other media that they can easily understand. Parents are also taught how to use REBT methods with their children and how to teach the children some of the elements of Rational Emotive Behavior Therapy (Bernard & Joyce, 1984).

REBT and Morality

In *Reason and Emotion in Psychotherapy* (1962), I indicate how REBT accepts the usual moral rules of any society or culture and shows clients how they are wrong and immoral if they act against these rules. But it particularly tries to help them to *only* criticize and regret their dysfunctional behavior and not to put themselves down, as total humans, for engaging in immoral behavior. I wrongly state, however, "Blaming is the essence of virtually all emotional disturbances and, as I tell my patients on many occasions, if I can induce them never, under any circumstances, to blame or punish anyone, including and especially themselves, it will be virtually impossible for them ever to become serious disturbed." I now find this to be an exaggeration, because some seriously disturbed people, especially narcissists and psychopaths, have strong biological tendencies to be disturbed even if they don't blame themselves, and some psychotics are quite disturbed without having strong blaming tendencies. Moreover, in addition to damning oneself and other people, innumerable individuals have low-frustration tolerance, in the course of which they demand that conditions and things be exactly the way they want them to be and suffer from self-pity and depression when the world is not exactly giving them what they "must" have. We could say that they are still blaming, in the sense that they are damning the world and society, but not in the sense that they are necessarily damning themselves and other specific people. In 1978, I created the terms Discomfort Anxiety, Discomfort Depression, and Discomfort Disturbance. These are other terms for low-frustration tolerance and mean that when people experience what they consider extreme discomfort, they frequently insist that the conditions under which they experience this discomfort absolutely *must not* exist and it is *awful* and *unbearable* that they do exist. They therefore create neurotic disturbances, in addition to those they create by self-denigration. Moreover, when they create self-downing *and* low frustration tolerance, these two neurotic behaviors, and the core philosophies often interact with and exacerbate each other, thereby considerably enhancing their disturbances (Bernard & Ellis, 1998).

REBT and Personal Worth

I still largely go along with the views on self-rating and personal worth that I explained in Chap. 8 of *Reason and Emotion in Psychotherapy*. In this chapter, however, I largely offer people the solution of unconditionally accepting themselves, and never damning themselves for any of their thoughts, feelings, or behaviors, just because they *choose* to accept themselves, because they *decide* that they are okay, and because they *define themselves* as good persons. I still tell my clients that they can use this practical or pragmatic solution to the problem of personal worth, instead of using the utterly self-defeating notion of hating themselves for their presumably bad or wrong acts. However, I now stress more than I did in 1962, the more elegant solution to the problem of self-worth. This more elegant solution consists of having people refuse to give a global or total rating to their self or their being or their essence at all, and to *only* rating their deeds, acts, performances, thoughts, and feelings. In other words, people can set themselves goals, values, and purposes and then rate as good or satisfactory those behaviors that aid and abet these goals, and they can rate as bad or unsatisfactory those deeds and acts that sabotage these goals. Ideally, they never have to give themselves a global rating or a self rating at all, although this is very difficult for most people to do. They seem to be born with a strong tendency to rate both their acts and feelings and their total self or being for experiencing these acts and feelings. But they can teach themselves, with the help of REBT, to never or at least rarely, rate themselves at all and only rate what they do. If they find it too difficult to do this, they can go back to the practical or pragmatic solution of saying "I am a good person just because I exist or because I choose to see myself as a good person." This is a definitional proposition that cannot be falsified, but it is much more practical and realistic than the belief, "I am a bad person because I do bad and wrong things."

I wrongly state in *Reason and Emotion in Psychotherapy* that a person "originally learns that he is no damn good because his parents think that he is when he doesn't do things their way." This is of course sometimes true because children easily take the negative views of their parents about themselves and make them their own. But most parents only yell at and defame their children a small percentage of the time, while they accept them the rest of the time. So the children have a good deal of empirical data that the parents really don't think that *they* are no good, but merely that they think that some of their *behaviors* are not good. Nonetheless, most children often tend to condemn themselves and their poor behaviors, because that is the way they naturally think. They believe that because it is good for them to do well and please their parents, they absolutely *must* do so and that they are *worthless individuals* when they don't. So although self-deprecation can be learned, it would exist on a tremendous scale among the human race if parents never thoroughly condemned the children but only condemned their poor thoughts, acts, and feelings (Bernard & Ellis, 1998; Ellis, 1999; Ellis & Blau, 1998; Ellis & Harper, 1997).

I say on page 166 of *Reason and Emotion in Psychotherapy* (1962) that my client's sentences and her self-deprecating words, phrases, and paragraphs about herself made her feel worthless, I now see that it was not just her words, phrases and paragraphs, but her *basic meaning* or her *core philosophy* that largely created her general feelings of worthlessness. So attributing her self-downing to internalized sentences is partly correct, but this loses much of the cognitive and philosophic complexity of the *meanings* we create about ourselves that we use to denigrate our entire being.

The Major Insights of REBT

On page 187 of *Reason and Emotion in Psychotherapy* (1962), I list three major insights of REBT, but I would considerably revise them today. I now would state them as follows:

1. People seeing and accepting the reality that their emotional disturbances at point C do *not* stem from the activating events or adversities at point A that precede C. Although A contributes to C, and although strong negative A's (such as being assaulted or raped) are much more likely to be followed by disturbed C's (such as feelings of panic and depression) than they are to be followed by weak A's (such as being disliked by a stranger), the main or more direct cores of emotional disturbances (C's) are people's irrational beliefs—the absolutistic musts and their accompanying inferences and attributions that people strongly believe about their undesirable activating events.
2. No matter how, when, and why people acquire self-defeating, irrational beliefs that mainly lead to their dysfunctional, emotional-behavioral consequences, if they are disturbed today, they tend to *keep* holding these irrational beliefs and upsetting themselves by them not because they held them in the past but because they are still actively, though often unconsciously, reaffirming them and acting as if they are still valid. They still *follow*, in their minds and in their hearts, the core musturbatory philosophies that they may have taken over or invented years ago, or that they have more recently accepted or constructed for themselves.
3. No matter how well they have achieved insight #1 and insight #2, insight alone will rarely enable people to undo their emotional disturbances. They may *feel* better when they know, or think they know, how they became disturbed and are

still making themselves upset largely because they believe these insights to be useful and curative. It is unlikely, however, that they will really *get better* and *stay* better unless they accept insights #1 and 2 and also go on to #3: There is usually no way but work and practice—yes, work and practice—to keep looking for and finding one's core irrational beliefs; to actively, energetically, and scientifically dispute them; to replace one's absolutist musts with flexible preferences; to change one's unhealthy feelings to healthy, self-helping emotions; and to firmly act against one's dysfunctional fears and compulsions. Only by a combined cognitive, emotive, and behavioral, as well as a quite persistent and forceful, attack on one's serious emotional problems is one likely to significantly ameliorate or remove them—and *keep* them removed (Bernard, 1991; Ellis, 1998a, 1998b, 1999; Ellis & MacLaren, 1998).

References

Bernard, M. E. (Ed.). (1991). *Using rational-emotive therapy effectively: A practitioner's guide*. New York, NY: Plenum.

Bernard, M. E., & Ellis, A. (1998). Albert Ellis at 85: Professional reflections. *Journal of Rational-Emotive and Cognitive Behavior Therapy, 16*, 151–181.

Bernard, M. E., & Joyce, M. R. (1984). *Rational-emotive therapy with children and adolescents* (2nd ed.). New York, NY: Wiley.

Ellis, A. (1962). *Reason and emotion in psychotherapy*. Secaucus, NJ: Citadel.

Ellis, A. (1994). *Reason and emotion in psychotherapy*. Revised and updated. Secaucus, NJ: Carol Publishing Group.

Ellis, A. (1996a). *Better, deeper and more enduring brief therapy*. New York, NY: Brunner/Mazel.

Ellis, A. (1996b). *How to maintain and enhance your rational emotive behavior therapy gains* (Rev. ed.). New York, NY: Institute for Rational-Emotive Therapy.

Ellis, A. (1997). Postmodern ethics for active-directive counseling and psychotherapy. *Journal of Mental Health Counseling, 18*, 211–225.

Ellis, A. (1998a). How rational emotive behavior therapy belongs in a constructivist camp. In M. F. Hoyt (Ed.), *The handbook of constructivist therapies* (pp. 83–99). San Francisco, CA: Jossey-Bass.

Ellis, A. (1998b). *How to control your anxiety before it controls you*. Secaucus, NJ: Carol Publishing Group.

Ellis, A. (1999). *How to make yourself happy and remarkably less disturbable*. San Luis Obispo, CA: Impact Publishers.

Ellis, A., & Blau, S. (Eds.). (1998). *The Albert Ellis reader*. Secaucus, NJ: Carol Publishing Group.

Ellis, A., & Dryden, W. (1997). *The practice of rational-emotive behavior therapy*. New York, NY: Springer.

Ellis, A., Gordon, J., Neenan, M., & Palmer, S. (1998). *Stress counseling*. New York, NY: Springer.

Ellis, A., & Harper, R. A. (1997). *A guide to rational living*. North Hollywood, CA: Melvin Powers.

Ellis, A., & MacLaren, C. (1998). *Rational-emotive behavior therapy: A therapist's guide*. San Luis Obispo, CA: Impact Publishers.

Ellis, A., & Tafrate, C. (1997). *How to control your anger before it controls you*. Secaucus, NJ: Birch Lane Press.

Ellis, A., & Velten, E. (1998). *Optimal aging: Get over getting older*. Chicago, IL: Open Court Publishing.

Knaus, W. (1974). *Rational emotive education*. New York, NY: Albert Ellis Institute.
Mahoney, M. (1975). *Scientist as subject*. Cambridge, MA: Ballinger.
Wolfe, J. L. (Speaker). (1980). *Woman—assert yourself*. Cassette recording. New York, NY: Institute for Rational-Emotive Therapy.
Wolpe, J. (1958). *Psychotherapy by reciprocal inhibition*. Stanford, CA: Stanford University Press.

Chapter 2
The Distinctive Features of Rational Emotive Behavior Therapy

Windy Dryden

Introduction

Rational emotive behavior therapy (REBT) was originated by Albert Ellis in 1955 and, as such, it can be regarded as the first approach within the cognitive behaviour therapy (CBT) tradition. People often ask what the differences are between REBT and CBT, but this is not a fair question as it would involve a comparison between a therapy approach (specific) with a therapy tradition (general), a bit like asking what the difference is between an apple (a specific fruit) and fruit (the general category). A fairer question would be: 'What are the features of REBT that make it distinctive within the CBT tradition and within the wider field of psychotherapy?' This chapter is devoted to answering this question. A word before we start. While some of the features discussed here are unique to REBT, others are not; but all these features *taken together* represent the distinctiveness of REBT.

The Distinctive Theoretical Features of REBT

In this section, I will briefly outline the distinctive theoretical features of REBT, while in the following section of the chapter, I will discuss the distinctive practical features of this approach.

W. Dryden (✉)
Goldsmiths University of London, London, UK

© Springer Nature Switzerland AG 2019

M. E. Bernard, W. Dryden (eds.), *Advances in REBT*,
https://doi.org/10.1007/978-3-319-93118-0_2

Post-modern Relativism

REBT theory is based on a theoretical proposition that I have called 'post-modern relativism' (Dryden, 2015). This proposition argues that phenomena cannot at present be logically or empirically regarded in fixed and unchanging ways and that there, is in all probability (rather than definitely), no absolute way of determining reality. Thus, while REBT puts forward certain criteria to differentiate what are currently known as irrational (i.e. rigid and extreme) beliefs from (i.e. flexible and non-extreme) beliefs, it holds that these criteria are relative rather than absolute (Dryden, 2015).

REBT's Position on Human Nature

REBT theory has a distinctive position on human nature. This viewpoint was put forward by Daniel Ziegler (2000) who helped to pioneer a "basic assumptions" approach in personality theory (Hjelle & Ziegler, 1992). Each of the proposed nine basic assumptions can be placed on a seven point continuum with strong (7/1), moderate (6/2) or slight (5/3) leanings towards one end of each continuum or the other with a mid-point of 4. The following ratings are provided by Ziegler (2000).

- Freedom (6) – Determinism: REBT holds that people have a moderate amount of freedom to choose the way they respond to external and internal factors.
- Rationality – Irrationality. REBT holds that people occupy the mid-point (4) between these two ends of the continuum. Thus, they are prone to irrationality, but capable of rationality.[1]
- Holism (6) – Elementalism. While REBT holds that people can be understood by considering their thinking, behaving and emoting as separate processes, they are better understood when these processes are more accurately considered to be interdependent.
- Constitutionalism (7) – Environmentalism. While most CBT approaches adopt an environmental-focused social learning approach to human disturbance, REBT argues that humans are biologically disposed to disturb themselves about life's adversities. (see Ellis, 1976 for a full discussion of this point).[2]
- Changeability (6) – Unchangeability. Despite the above, REBT holds that with committed work, humans are moderately capable of fundamental change over time.
- Subjectivity (7) – Objectivity. REBT has a strong phenomenological emphasis and holds that humans are much more influenced by subjective factors than

[1] Other REBT scholars may give a higher rating towards the irrationality end of the continuum given the ease in which people think irrationally.

[2] Other REBT scholars may give a '6' towards the constitutionalism end of the continuum (rather than a '7' in recognitition of there being a learned-cultural component to irrational beliefs.

external, objective factors. Thus, when they do face objective negative events they more frequently disturb themselves about subjective, inferential features of these events more than about the events themselves.

- Proactivity (7) – Reactivity. REBT holds that people are strongly proactive in generating their responses to events. They are not seen as passive responders to external stimuli.
- Homeostasis – Heterostasis. REBT holds that people occupy the mid-point (4) between being motivated to (a) reduce tensions and maintain an inner homeostasis and (b) to actualize themselves. Practically, they are helped more effectively with the latter area when they are first helped with the former.
- Knowability – (2) Unknowability. REBT holds that while we can learn much about human affairs, much of human nature is not fully knowable. As Ziegler (2000) notes, this assumption explains why Ellis did not devote much time to formulating an REBT-based personality theory.

REBT's Distinctive "ABC" Model

While an "ABC" model for understanding psychological problems can be found in different CBT approaches, REBT uses a distinctive "ABC" model in this respect. In this model, the person is deemed to disturb themself at "C" about an aspect of the situation that they are in (known as the adversity at "A") largely because they hold a set of rigid and extreme beliefs at "B" (Dryden, 2016). This is outlined and exemplified in Table 2.1.

While Table 2.1 outlines REBT's ABC model of psychological disturbance, Table 2.2 outlines REBT's ABC model of a psychologically healthy response to the same adversity at "A". Here, the person is deemed to respond healthily at "C" to the same adversity at "A" largely because they hold a set of flexible and non-extreme beliefs at "B" (Dryden, 2016).

These two models have several distinctive features:

1. They hold that 'A' is often inferential in nature. Inferences are deemed to go beyond the data at hand and may be accurate or inaccurate, In the absence of

Table 2.1 The 'ABC' of psychological disturbance

Situation	My colleague walked past me in the street without acknowledging me
"A" (*Adversity*)	I have upset my colleague
"B" (*irrational Belief*)	(*Rigid belief*) = "I must not upset my colleague" (*Extreme self-devaluation belief* = "I am a bad person for upsetting my colleague"
"C" (*disturbed Consequences*)	(*Emotional*) = Guilt (*Behavioural*) = Going out of my way to please my colleague (Cognitive) = If I don't appease my colleague they will make my life a misery

Table 2.2 The ABC model of psychological health

Situation	My colleague walked past me in the street without acknowledging me
"A" (*Adversity*)	I have upset my colleague
"B" (*rational Belief*)	(*Flexible belief*) = I don't want to upset my colleague, but that does not mean that I must not do so (*Non-extreme unconditional self-acceptance belief*) = "I am not a bad person for upsetting my colleague. Rather, I am a fallible human being who acted in a way that led to his upset"
"C" (*healthy Consequences*)	(*Emotional*) = Remorse (*Behavioural*) = Checking to see if I have upset him and if so, making amends (*Cognitive*) = If my colleague is still upset after I have spoken to him, it is unlikely that he will make my life a misery, but if he does then I will respond in a healthy way to that situation

finding out the 'truth' about what happened, the person may be encouraged to make the 'best bet' given the available data. As will be shown later, to identify rigid and extreme beliefs at 'B', practitioners of REBT first encourage their clients to *assume temporarily* that 'A' is true and will work with distorted inferences at 'A' *after* the clients have made progress at changing 'Bs' to their flexible and non-extreme alternatives. This contrasts with other approaches to CBT which are more likely to encourage clients to respond to these distorted inferences at an earlier juncture.

2. As shown above, these models show that beliefs at 'B' are the central determining factor of functional and dysfunctional responses at 'C' to adversities at 'A'.
3. These models argue that 'C' can be emotive, behavioural and cognitive.
4. These models also stress that 'ABCs' are best understood within a situational context.

Rigid Beliefs[3] *Are at the Very Core of Psychological Disturbance*

Perhaps the central tenet of REBT theory is that rigid beliefs are at the very core of psychological disturbance.[4] Ellis (1994) argued that while what he called irrational beliefs can be rigid or extreme, of the two it is rigid beliefs that are at the very core of disturbance. Rigid beliefs are often based on preferences, but are then transformed into absolutes. Thus, if I hold that it is important for me to do well, then this is my preference. When I make this preference rigid, I transform it into a demand, thus: "I want to do well and therefore I must do so". It is important to note that rigid beliefs are often expressed without the preference being made explicit. Thus: "I must do well".

[3] While Ellis more frequently referred to rigid beliefs as absolute, he also used the term 'rigid to refer to these primary irrational beliefs (Ellis & Joffe Ellis, 2011).

[4] For research evidence on this and other points made in this chapter, see Chap. 5, this volume.

The view that rigid beliefs are at the very core of psychological disturbance is unique to REBT and can be regarded as a transdiagnostic theoretical construct (Frank & Davidson, 2014), meaning that it occurs across diagnoses of psychological disturbance.

Extreme Beliefs Are Derived from Rigid Beliefs

REBT theory argues that extreme beliefs are derived from rigid beliefs (Ellis, 1994). Since the theory posits that rigid beliefs are at the very core of psychological disturbance, it follows that other dysfunctional beliefs and highly distorted cognitions are derived from this rigid core. Extreme belief derivatives are the closest derivatives to this core. REBT theory argues that there are three extreme belief derivatives from rigid beliefs. In the material that follows I will list and define each extreme belief and show that it is derived from the person's rigid belief. These extreme beliefs are known as:

1. *Awfulising beliefs*. Here, a person believes, at the time, that something is so bad that it couldn't get any worse. For example: "I must do well and it would be absolutely awful if I don't"
2. *Discomfort intolerance beliefs*. Here, a person believes, at the time, that they cannot tolerate the adversity that they are facing or about to face. For example: "I must do well and I couldn't bear it if I don't".
3. *Devaluation beliefs*. Here, a person, at the time, gives themself, others or life a global negative evaluation which, at the time, they think defines self, others or life. For example, "I must do well and if I don't, I'm valueless".

Flexible Beliefs Are at the Very Core of Psychological Health

The corollary of the point that rigid beliefs are at the very core of psychological disturbance is that flexible beliefs are at the very core of psychological health. Ellis (1994) argued that while what he called rational beliefs can be flexible or non-extreme, of the two it is flexible beliefs that are at the very core of psychological health. Flexible beliefs, like rigid beliefs, are often based on preferences, but they are flexible because the person is explicit that they are not rigid. Thus, if I hold that it is important for me to do well, then this is again my preference. When I keep this preference flexible, I negate the demand, thus: "I want to do well, but I don't have to do so".

The view that flexible beliefs are at the very core of psychological health is unique to REBT and can again be regarded as a transdiagnostic theoretical construct (Frank & Davidson, 2014), meaning that it occurs across all forms of psychological health.

Non-extreme Beliefs Are Derived from Flexible Beliefs

REBT theory also argues that non-extreme beliefs are derived from flexible beliefs (Ellis, 1994). Since the theory posits that flexible beliefs are at the very core of psychological health, it follows that other functional beliefs and realistic cognitions are derived from this flexible core. Non-extreme belief derivatives are the closest derivatives to this core. REBT theory argues that there are three non-extreme belief derivatives from flexible beliefs. In the material that follows, I will list and define each non-extreme belief and show that it is derived from the person's flexible belief. These non-extreme beliefs are known as:

1. *Non-awfulising beliefs*. Here, a person believes, at the time, that something is bad, but not the end of the world. For example: "I want to do well, but I don't have to do so. It's bad if I don't do well, but not awful".
2. *Discomfort tolerance beliefs*. Here, a person believes, at the time, that it is difficult tolerating the adversity that they are facing or about to face, but that they can tolerate it and that it is worth it for them to do so. In addition, they assert that they are willing to tolerate the adversity and commit themself to doing so. For example: "I want to do well, but I don't have to do so. It would be difficult for me to tolerate not doing well, but I can tolerate it and it's worth doing so. I am willing to tolerate not doing well and will commit myself to do so by doing the task at hand and risk not doing well".
3. *Unconditional acceptance beliefs*. Here, a person acknowledges that they, others or life are far too complex to merit a global negative evaluation and that such an evaluation does not define self, others or life. For example, "I want to do well, but I don't have to do so. I am the same fallible person whether I do well or not".

REBT's Position on Negative Emotions

REBT theory distinguishes between unhealthy (dysfunctional) negative emotions (UNEs) and healthy (functional) negative emotions (HNEs) and this distinction is unique to REBT. The theory argues that UNEs and HNEs are qualitatively different from one another as UNEs stem from rigid and extreme beliefs about adversity and HNEs stem from flexible and non-extreme beliefs about the same adversity (see Dryden, 2016). As such these distinguishable emotions exist on two separate continua rather than on one single continuum.

For example, anxiety about a threat is underpinned by a rigid and extreme belief about the adversity and its healthy alternative about that same threat is concern which is underpinned by a flexible and non-extreme belief. The goal in REBT is not to reduce the intensity of anxiety about a threat; rather it is to help the person to feel concerned rather than anxious about the threat.

How Clients Create Highly Distorted Inferences: An REBT Perspective

When clients discuss their problems with their REB therapists, it sometimes occurs that they report highly distorted inferences. Given the available evidence, it is usually apparent to the therapist that such inferences are negatively biased in a highly skewed manner. However, these inferences seem very real to clients. Examples of such inferences are: "I am going to have a heart attack"; "Nobody will ever talk to me again" and "I will always fail and will end up as a bag lady"

REBT theory argues that such inferences are cognitive consequences (at 'C') of rigid and extreme beliefs (e.g. Bond & Dryden, 2000). Such inferences are highly distorted because prior related and usually less distorted inferences at 'A' have been processed by the person using their rigid and extreme beliefs at 'B'. However, the client is usually only aware of the highly distorted inference at 'C' as it is very compelling and related to their disturbed emotion and the client is usually unaware of both their inference at 'A' and their rigid and/or extreme belief at 'B'. Here are three examples of this process. Note how the rigid and the extreme processing of 'A' leads to the highly distorted the inference at 'C'. Thus:

'A' = I am feeling out of control
'B' = I must gain control immediately
'C' (cognitive) = If I don't I will have a heart attack

'A' = My friends are not talking to me
'B' = My friends must talk to me and it is terrible that they are not
'C' (cognitive) = Nobody will ever talk to me again

'A' = I may fail a crucial forthcoming exam
'B' = I must pass this exam and it will be the end of the world if I do not
'C' (cognitive) = If I fail, I will always fail and will end up as a bag lady

REBT's Position on Human Worth

REBT theory has a unique position on human worth. Actually. it has two positions on this subject, a preferred position and a back-up position. It holds that unchangeable aspects of humans are our:

(i) Humanness (we are human till we die)
(ii) Complexity (we are too complex to justify a single defining global rating)
(iii) Uniqueness (there will never be another you)
(iv) Fallibility (we have an incurable error-making tendency)
(v) Changeability (we are constantly in flux)

REBT's preferred position on human worth is that we are neither worthwhile or worthless; rather we just *are* and we can either choose to accept ourselves as human and as having the above unchangeable aspects or choose not to do so. When we do make this affirmative choice, we can be said to be operationalising a philosophy of unconditional self-acceptance (USA) which encapsulates REBT's preferred position on human worth.

When clients do not resonate with this position and prefer to regard themselves as having worth, then the best way that they can do this is without making themselves vulnerable to ego disturbance (see below) is to opt for unconditional self-worth. This back-up position states that I am worthwhile because I am human, complex, unique, fallible and changeable. I could, of course, state that I am worthless because I have these aspects, and this is equally valid for I can neither prove that I am worthwhile nor worthless. However, if I want to live healthily and happily, then unconditional self-worth position will facilitate this far more than the unconditional worthlessness position.

According to REBT, the real culprit (apart from unconditional worthlessness) when it comes to ego disturbance is conditional self-worth. Thus, when I say that I am worthwhile when I am loved, successful, popular and wealthy for example, then I disturb myself when I lose any of these factors and I am vulnerable to self-disturbance when I have these factors because I can always lose them.

REBT Distinguishes Between Ego and Discomfort Disturbance (and Health)

REBT theory argues that we have two major domains in which we function as humans: ego and non-ego (here referred to as comfort/discomfort). It, therefore distinguishes between ego disturbance and discomfort disturbance, on the one hand, and ego health and discomfort health on the other.

Ego Disturbance and Health

Ego disturbance in the face of adversity is marked by a rigid belief and a self-devaluation belief that is derived from it. For example: "I must pass my exam and I am a failure if I don't". By contrast, ego health in the face of the same adversity is marked by a flexible belief and an unconditional self-acceptance belief that is derived from it. For example: "I would like to pass my exam, but I don't have to do so. If I don't, I'm not a failure. I am an unrateable human being who has failed in this respect".

Discomfort Disturbance and Health

Discomfort disturbance in the face of adversity is marked by a rigid belief and a discomfort intolerance belief that is derived from it (Ellis, 1979, 1980a). For example: "I must have the benefits that I will get if I pass my exam and I couldn't bear to be derived of these benefits should I fail". By contrast, discomfort health in the face of the same adversity is marked by a flexible belief and a discomfort tolerance belief that is derived from it. For example: "I would like to have the benefits that I will get if I pass my exam, but I do not need these benefits. If I fail the exam and am thus deprived of these benefits, then it would be a struggle for me to tolerate this deprivation. But I could tolerate it, it is worth it to me to do so, I am willing to do so and I commit myself to so doing by...."

There are two other important points worth noting about ego and discomfort disturbance. First, a rigid belief on its own does not make clear the type of disturbance a person is experiencing (Dryden, 1994). The extreme belief derivative helps to make this clear. Thus, if my rigid belief is: "I must retain my autonomy", this belief, on its own, does not indicate ego or discomfort disturbance. However, if my major extreme belief derivative is: "...and I am a pathetic person if I lose my autonomy" then I am experiencing ego disturbance, whereas if it is: "...and I can't bear the resultant conditions if I lose of my autonomy" then I am experiencing discomfort disturbance.

The second important point is that ego disturbance and discomfort disturbance frequently interact. Thus, I may begin by experiencing ego disturbance and create a disturbed negative emotion such as shame and then I may focus on the pain of this emotion and tell myself that I can't bear this emotional pain (discomfort disturbance).

Focus on Meta-disturbance

REBT recognises that once a person disturbs themself, it often happens that they disturb themself about this original disturbance. This is known as meta-disturbance (literally disturbance about disturbance). So, REBT has a decided focus on meta-disturbance and has done so for many years. It also distinguishes between different types of meta-disturbance. Thus, it argues that a person can disturb themself about:

- **Disturbed emotions at 'C'.** A person may disturb themself either because of the pain of the emotional experience (e.g. "I can't stand the pain of feeling depressed") or because of the meaning the disturbed emotion has for the person (e.g. "Feeling depressed is a weakness and proves that I am a weak person")
- **Dysfunctional behaviour or action tendencies at 'C'.** Here, a person focuses on what they did or what they felt like doing, but did not do and disturbs themself about one or the other, largely because of the meaning the behaviour or action tendency has for the person (e.g. "I felt like punching her lights out which is really nasty and proves that I am a nasty person").

- **Distorted cognitions at 'C'.** Here, a person may focus on a distorted cognition, which becomes their new 'A' and disturbs themself about the meaning that such a thought has for them. Thus, suppose the person disturbs themself about finding a young person attractive and thinks that they may abuse the person (their distorted cognitive consequence at 'C'). They may then disturb themself about this thought because they infer that is shameful and that they are a disgusting person for having it.

Biological Basis of Human Irrationality

Most approaches to CBT are based on social learning principles whereby it is held that people learn to disturb themselves. REBT also argues that human disturbance is partly learned, but it is unique among the CBT approaches in claiming that the biological basis of human irrationality and related disturbance is often more influential than its social learning basis. Thus, in a seminal paper, Ellis (1976) put forward a number of arguments in favour of the 'biological hypothesis' as it is known in REBT circles. Here are a few of Ellis's arguments

1. People easily transform their strong preferences into rigid demands and have a difficult time giving up these demands and remain with their strong flexible preferences.
2. People are rarely taught to procrastinate and live self-undisciplined lives, but millions do.
3. People easily fall back into self-defeating patterns after they have made progress in dealing constructively with these patterns.
4. People can easily give people sound advice in dealing with their problems, but find it difficult to apply this advice consistently to themselves when they experience the same problems.

REBT's Position on the Origin and Maintenance of Psychological Problems

We have seen that one of the key theoretical principles of REBT is that summarized in the maxim that: "People are not disturbed by events but by their rigid and extreme beliefs about these events". This means that while adversities contribute to the development of psychological disturbance, particularly when these events are highly aversive, disturbance occurs when people bring their tendencies to hold rigid and extreme beliefs about these events.

REBT does not, therefore, have an elaborate view of the origin of disturbance. Having said this, it does acknowledge that it is very easy for humans, when they are young, to disturb themselves about highly aversive events. However, it argues that even under these conditions people react differently to the same event and thus we need to understand what a person brings to and takes from an adversity. People learn their standards and goals from their culture, but disturbance occurs when they bring their rigid and extreme beliefs to circumstances where their standards are not met and their pursuit of their goals is blocked.

By contrast, REBT has a more elaborate view of how psychological disturbance is maintained. It argues that people perpetuate their disturbance for several reasons including the following:

- They lack the insight that their psychological disturbance is underpinned by their rigid and extreme beliefs and think instead that it is caused by events.
- They think that once they understand that their problems are underpinned by rigid and extreme beliefs, this understanding alone will lead to change.
- They do not work persistently to change their rigid and extreme beliefs and to integrate the flexible and non-extreme alternatives to these beliefs into their belief system.
- They continue to act in ways that are consistent with their rigid and extreme beliefs
- They disturb themselves about their original disturbances
- They lack or are deficient in important social skills, communication skills, problem-solving skills and other life skills.
- They think that their disturbance has pay-offs that outweigh the advantages of the healthy alternatives to their disturbed feelings and/or behaviour.
- They live in environments which support the rigid and extreme beliefs that underpin their problems.

As will be seen below, REBT's view on the perpetuation of psychological disturbance informs its position on psychological change

REBT's Position on Psychological Change

REB therapists consider that the core facilitative conditions of empathy, unconditional acceptance and genuineness are often desirable, but neither necessary nor sufficient for constructive therapeutic change. For such change to take place, clients need to be helped to:

- Realize that they largely create their own psychological problems and that while situations contribute to these problems, they are, in general, of lesser importance in the change process.
- Fully recognize that they can address and overcome these problems.
- Understand that their problems stem largely from rigid and extreme beliefs.
- Detect their rigid and extreme beliefs and discriminate between them and their flexible and non-extreme beliefs.

- Dispute their rigid and extreme beliefs and their flexible and non-extreme beliefs until they see clearly that the former are false, illogical and unconstructive while the latter are true, sensible and constructive.
- Work towards the internalization of their new flexible and non-extreme beliefs by using a variety of cognitive (including imaginal), emotive and behavioral change methods. In particular, act in ways that are consistent with the flexible and non-extreme beliefs that they wish to develop and refrain from acting in ways that are consistent with their old rigid and extreme beliefs.
- Extend this process of disputing beliefs and using multimodal methods of change into other areas of their lives and committing to doing so for as long as necessary.

REBT Advocates Choice-Based Constructivism and a "Going Against the Grain" View of Change

REBT favours what might be called choice-based constructivism in that it argues that humans have choices when their hold preferences (e.g. I want to do well"). Thus, they can construct a rigid belief from this preference ("I want to do well…and therefore I have to do so") or a flexible belief from the same preference (e.g. "I want you to do well…but I don't have to do so"). Although a person may have a biologically-based tendency to construct a rigid belief when their preference is strong, they do not have to do this and can choose to construct a flexible belief instead. The extent to which the person does this in a meaningful way depends on the extent to which they are prepared to "go against the grain" and think and act according to the less powerful flexible belief and refrain from thinking and acting according to their more powerful rigid belief.

REBT's Position on Good Mental Health

REBT has a clear position on what constitutes good mental health with flexibility and non-extremeness at its heart. Here is a partial list of such criteria which is self-explanatory: personal responsibility; flexibility and non-extremeness; scientific thinking and non-utopian in outlook; enlightened self-interest; social interest; self-direction; high tolerance of uncertainty; strong commitment to meaningful pursuits; calculated risk-taking and long-range hedonism.

The Distinctive Practical Features of REBT

In this section, I will consider REBT's major distinctive practical features.

REBT's View on the Importance of the Therapeutic Relationship

The therapeutic relationship in REBT is deemed to be important, but not curative and draws fully on working alliance theory (Bordin, 1979) as a way of understanding the importance of bonds, views, goals and tasks in REBT.[5] In brief, effectiveness in REBT is enhanced when therapist and client:

- Have a well-*bond*ed relationship in which the client experiences the therapist as understanding both their feelings and the beliefs that underpin these feelings, as accepting them as fallible human beings and as being genuine in the therapeutic encounter. In this respect Ellis (in Dryden, 1997) cautioned REB therapists against being overly warm with clients so as not to reinforce the latter's needs for love and approval. In general, REB therapists consider that client experience of these therapist offered "core conditions" (Rogers, 1957) are deemed to be important, but neither necessary, nor sufficient for enduring client change (Ellis, 1959).
- Share common *views* on such matters as problem assessment, 'case' formulation, treatment and practical issues concerning therapy.
- Agree on the client's treatment *goals*.
- Understand one another's *tasks* concerning what needs to be done for the client's goals to be met and are able to and commit to carrying out their respective tasks.

REBT's Position on Case Formulation

REBT takes a flexible approach to case formulation using this to guide interventions, particularly in complex cases. However, it argues that one can do good therapy based on problem assessment without making such a formulation and holds that frequently this formulation can be developed during therapy rather than fully at its outset. However, when a "case" is deemed to be complex or a client is not making expected progress, then doing a more formal extensive case formulation may be indicated (see Dryden, 1998, for a full discussion on the REBT approach to case formulation which is outside the scope of this chapter).

REBT Has a Decided Psycho-educational Emphasis

REBT has a decided psycho-educational emphasis and argues that its theory of disturbance and change as well as its core concepts can actively be taught to and learned and implemented by clients. This principle is underpinned by the idea that REB therapists are very explicit about the REBT model and actively teach it to

[5] See Chap. 7 on 'REBT and the Working Alliance', this volume.

clients at an early stage so that the latter can give their informed consent before proceeding with this form of therapy.

While REBT can be practised in several ways, its skills of assessing and addressing problems can be directly taught to clients so that they can learn to be their own therapists almost from the outset. Indeed, some of the material that have been devised to help clients to learn REBT self-help skills can also be used by people who wish to help themselves without formal therapy (e.g. Dryden, 2001). In addition there are a number of REBT self-helps books based on particular themes that also serve the same purpose (e.g. Ellis, 2000).

Skilled REBT therapists will work explicitly with clients so that together they can choose whether and when to take a skills teaching and learning approach to REBT therapy.

REBT's Preferred Treatment Order

REBT recommends a preferred order of treatment and argues that client problems should ideally be dealt with in the following order: (a) disturbance, (b) dissatisfaction, and (c) development. Disturbance is deemed to be present when the client is facing an adversity and holds a set of rigid and extreme beliefs about that adversity. The resultant dysfunctional ways of responding (emotionally, behaviourally and cognitively) means that the client is ill equipped to deal with the adversity while they are in a disturbed frame of mind. When they deal successfully with their disturbance, they are then ready to deal with the dissatisfaction of facing the adversity since at this point the client holds a set of flexible and non-extreme beliefs about the adversity which has now become a focus for dissatisfaction rather than disturbance. Development issues, as the name implies, concern the client exploring ways of developing themself so that they can get the most out of their potential. They will not be able to do this as effectively as they could until they have dealt with the dissatisfaction of having an adversity in their life. Thus, their REBT therapist would encourage them to take steps to change the adversity if it can be changed or adjust constructively to the adversity if it can't be changed – while holding flexible and non-extreme beliefs rather than rigid and extreme beliefs – before focusing their attention on development issues, if the client is seeking help in this area. Such work might be better described as REB coaching rather than REB therapy (Dryden, 2018).

While this is the preferred REBT order and a clear rationale will be given to and discussed with the client for using this order, if the latter is adamant that they want to use a different order, then the therapist will be mindful of the working alliance (see above) and encourage the client to proceed according to their preferences and review the results of doing so at a later date. There is little to be gained, and much to be lost, by the therapist attempting to force a client to use the preferred REBT order when they are very reluctant to do so. Indeed, an REBT therapist who does this is likely to hold rigid ideas about how REBT must be practised and is thus being unhelpfully dogmatic!

A second area where REBT has views on treatment order concerns whether to deal with meta-disturbance issues before disturbance issues or vice versa. The preferred order is to deal with a meta-disturbance issue first if (a) its presence interferes with the client working on the disturbance issue in or out of the session, (b) it is clinically the most important issue of the two and centrally, from a working alliance perspective, (c) if the client sees the sense of doing so.

A final area where REBT has a preferred order of treatment is where this is suggested by a case formulation (for more information about doing an REBT-based case formulation see Dryden, 1998).

REBT Advocates an Early Focus on Clients' Rigid and Extreme Beliefs

As outlined in the theoretical section above, REBT theory hypothesises that a client's rigid and extreme beliefs largely determine their psychological problems and of the two, rigid beliefs are at the very core of such disturbance.

It follows from this that REB therapists target for change their clients' rigid and extreme beliefs and particularly the former as early in therapy as is feasible. Other approaches in the CBT tradition (see Wills, 2015) argue that to focus on such underlying beliefs early on therapy will engender resistance, but REBT therapists argue differently. They hold that as long as clients understand the role that such rigid and extreme beliefs play in determining and maintaining their problems and appreciate that they need to examine and change these beliefs if they are to effectively address their problems, then such resistance is kept to a minimum. It is important, therefore to realise that skilful REB therapists minimise resistance on this issue because the work that they are doing with their clients is based firmly on a strong working alliance between the two (see Chap. 7, this volume).

Helping Clients to Change Their Rigid and Extreme Beliefs to Flexible and Non-extreme Beliefs

Perhaps the most distinctive feature about REBT practice is the efforts that REB therapists make to help their clients change their rigid and extreme beliefs to flexible and non-extreme beliefs, once they have identified the former and helped their clients construct the latter. This process involves a number of steps.

Helping Clients to Detect Their Rigid and Extreme Beliefs

The first step in helping clients to change their rigid and extreme beliefs to their flexible and non-extreme beliefs is to assist them to detect the former. In the first instance, this involves teaching clients about these irrational beliefs and their nature. These are characterised by rigidity and by being extreme. Rigid beliefs occur most frequently in the form of demands and musts and extreme beliefs which are derived from these rigid beliefs take the form of awfulising beliefs, discomfort intolerance beliefs and devaluation (of self, others and life conditions) beliefs. REB therapists use a number of ways to teach clients about this vital aspect of REBT theory and help them to apply this knowledge in the assessment process to detect the irrational beliefs that underpin their emotional problems.

Helping Clients to Construct Flexible and Non-extreme Beliefs

Helping clients to examine and change their rigid and extreme beliefs is a key task of the REB therapist. To expedite the belief change process, the therapist first needs to help a client to construct alternative flexible and non-extreme beliefs and encourage them to understand that these beliefs will help them to achieve their therapeutic goals.

As guided by REBT theory, if the therapist is targeting a rigid belief for change (e.g. "I must do well"), they first need to help the client to construct a flexible belief (e.g. "I want to do well, but I don't have to do so") and if they are targeting an extreme belief (i.e. an awfulising belief, a discomfort intolerance belief or a devaluation belief) they first need to help the client construct a non-extreme belief (i.e. a non-awfulising belief, a discomfort tolerance belief or an unconditional acceptance belief). Thus, if the therapist is targeting an extreme, awfulising belief (e.g. "It would be awful if I don't do well"), they would first help the client to construct an alternative non-extreme, non –awfulising belief (e.g. "It would be bad if I don't do well, but it would not be awful") If the therapist fails to help the client to construct a flexible and/or non-extreme belief alternative to their rigid and/or extreme belief, then they will impede the change process as the client will be in a belief vacuum, being encouraged to give up their irrational belief, but without anything to replace it with.

Helping Clients to Discriminate Their Rigid and Extreme Beliefs from Their Flexible and Non-extreme Alternatives

REBT theory holds that if REB therapists are going to help their clients overcome their problems most effectively, then they need to help them to think flexibly and in a non-extreme way about life's adversities. As part of this process, an important task is helping clients to discriminate their rigid and extreme beliefs from their constructed flexible and non-extreme beliefs. In the same way that REB therapists educate their clients to understand what irrational beliefs are and the forms that they take, they also teach them to understand what rational beliefs are and the forms that they take.

A very important part of this process is helping clients to understand keenly the differences between irrational and rational beliefs. For example, it is not sufficient to show a client that the rational alternative to their rigid belief, "I must impress my new boss straightaway" is the belief "I'd like to impress my boss straightaway". The latter may not be rigid, but it is not fully flexible. While it asserts the client's preference, it does not negate their demand. The flexible alternative to the person's rigid belief is: "I'd like to impress my new boss straightaway, but I do not have to do so", which incorporates both components of the flexible belief. Table 2.3 outlines clearly the full differences between rigid and extreme beliefs, on the one hand and flexible and non-extreme beliefs, on the other.

Disputing Clients' Rigid and Extreme Beliefs and Flexible and Non-extreme Beliefs

After REB therapists have helped their clients to see the differences between their irrational and rational beliefs, they move on to help their clients to question or examine these beliefs. Albert Ellis (1994) referred to this process as "disputing". This is done after clients understand the relationship between their rigid and extreme beliefs and their emotional problems and their flexible and non-extreme beliefs and their goals. What follows applies both to clients' specific beliefs and their more general beliefs.

Table 2.3 Irrational and rational beliefs in REBT theory

Irrational belief	Rational belief
<u>Rigid belief</u>	<u>Flexible belief</u>
X must (or must not happen)	I would like X to happen (or not happen), but it does not have to be the way I want it to be
<u>Awfulising belief</u>	<u>Non-awfulising belief</u>
It would be terrible if X happens (or does not happen)	It would be bad, but not terrible if X happens (or does not happen)
<u>Discomfort intolerance belief</u>	<u>Discomfort tolerance belief</u>
I could not bear it if X happens (or does not happen)	It would be difficult to bear if X happens (or does not happen). But I could bear it, it would be worth it to me to do so, I am willing to bear it and I am going to do so
<u>Devaluation belief</u>	<u>Unconditional acceptance belief</u>
If X happens (or does not happen) I am no good/you are no good/life is no good	If X happens (or does not happen), it does not prove that I am no good/, you are no good/life is no good. Rather, I am/you are am a fallible human being and life is a complex/mixture of good bad and neutral

As DiGiuseppe (1991) has shown, "disputing" involves questioning both clients' rigid and extreme beliefs and flexible and non-extreme beliefs to the point where they see the reasons for the irrationality of the former (i.e. they are false, illogical and lead largely to poor results) and for the rationality of the latter (i.e. they are true, logical and lead largely to good results). In addition, short didactic explanations are given until clients reach the same insight. These questions/explanations are directed to clients' rigid and flexible beliefs as well as to their extreme and non-extreme beliefs and this is done using a variety of styles (see below).

The use of logical arguments in questioning/disputing beliefs In common with other CB therapists, REB therapists ask clients questions about the empirical status and the pragmatic status of their beliefs. However, they also ask them about the logical status of their beliefs, which other CB therapists do less frequently and thus, this is a distinctive feature of REBT. It may be that empirical and pragmatic arguments are more persuasive to clients than logical arguments. We do not know because the relevant research has not been done. Even if this is the case, in general, REBT therapists would still use logical questioning/disputing of beliefs for two reasons. First, they do not know, on a priori grounds, which clients will find which arguments most persuasive in changing their rigid and extreme beliefs to their flexible and non-extreme alternatives. Just because the majority of clients may find logical arguments unpersuasive, it does not follow that all will do so and to withhold such arguments from those who might find them persuasive would not be good practice. So, REB therapists tend to use all three arguments to see, as I said above, which arguments will be most persuasive with which clients.

Second, REB therapists use empirical, pragmatic and logical arguments while questioning/disputing beliefs in order to be comprehensive. This comprehensiveness may itself be effective. Thus, even if clients find empirical and pragmatic arguments more persuasive than logical arguments, it may still be worthwhile employing such arguments in that they may add value to the overall effectiveness of the questioning/disputing process. Some clients may find it persuasive that their irrational beliefs are false, unhealthy and logical even if they find the logical argument weak on its own.

REBT Advocates the Use of a Variety of Therapeutic Styles

While REBT advocates therapists taking an active-directive stance in therapy, particularly at its outset, it is not prescriptive about how its therapists implement that stance in terms of therapeutic style Thus, it is possible for REB therapists to be informal or formal, humorous or serious, self-disclosing or non self-disclosing, Socratic or didactic and using metaphors, parables and stories or refraining from their use. Skilful REBT therapists vary their therapeutic style according to the client that are working with and the stage of therapy that they have reached.

REBT Encourages Clients to Seek Adversity When Carrying Out Homework Assignments, but Does so Sensibly

There are basically three ways of tackling emotional problems. To face problems head on fully, to take steps to face them in a way that is challenging, but not overwhelming (Dryden, 1985) or to go gradually. REBT discourages clients from going gradually, if at all possible, because doing so tends to reinforce their discomfort intolerance beliefs – e.g. "I must avoid feeling uncomfortable as I tackle my problems" (Ellis, 1983). In my experience, clients will only face their problems head on if they have powerful motivation to do so. Most clients can be encouraged to take the 'challenging, but not overwhelming' route. However, it is better to allow clients to go gradually than to threaten the working alliance. They can always be encouraged to challenge their discomfort intolerance ideas and "speed up" later.

REBT's Realistic View of Psychotherapeutic Change

REBT has a realistic view of change that takes in therapy and encourages clients to accept that such change is hard work and consequently it urges therapists to be forceful, energetic and persistent as long as doing so does not threaten the therapeutic alliance (Dryden & Neenan, 2004). It gives clients direct guidance with respect to understanding and implementing the REBT change process as follows:

1. Understand that your problems are underpinned by rigid and extreme beliefs
2. Set goals
3. Construct flexible and non-extreme alternatives to these beliefs and see that they will help you to achieve your goals
4. Examine both your rigid and extreme beliefs and their flexible and non-extreme alternatives and see that the former are false, illogical and unhelpful and the latter are true, logical and helpful
5. Commit yourself to developing and strengthening your flexible and non-extreme beliefs
6. Act in ways that are consistent with your flexible and non-extreme beliefs while rehearsing them and continue to do this until you truly believe them.
7. Identify and deal with obstacles to change
8. Implement relapse prevention procedures
9. Generalise change to other relevant situations
10. Accept yourself for backsliding and continue to use REBT change techniques

REBT Recommends Teaching General Flexible and Non-extreme Philosophies to Clients Whenever Feasible

While REB therapists will, as a matter of course, encourage their clients to acquire, develop and maintain specific flexible and non-extreme beliefs, they will also, whenever possible, offer to teach them general flexible and non-extreme philosophies and encourage them to make a "profound philosophic change" (changing general rigid beliefs, such as "I must be liked by significant people" to general flexible beliefs such as "I want to be liked by significant people, but they don't have to like me") if they are capable of doing so and interested in doing so. Not all clients, will be so capable and/or interested, but if therapists do not offer to do this they may be depriving a significant minority of their clients of getting the most out of REBT.

Compromises in REBT

REBT therapists have a preferred strategy and, as we have seen, this involves encouraging clients to achieve belief change. However, it recognises that clients may not be able or willing to change their rigid and extreme beliefs and, in such cases, it recommends making compromises with the ideal of belief change (Dryden, 1987). Thus, when a client is not able or willing change their dysfunctional beliefs, the REBT practitioner can help them to:

(a) Change their distorted inferences
(b) Change their behaviour
(c) Learn new skills
(d) Change or leave the situation which provides the context for their problem

When to Use a Change-Based Focus (CBF) and When to Use an Acceptance-Based Focus (ABF)

One the major recent developments within the CBT tradition has been the growth of those CBT approaches which recommend that clients mindfully accept the presence of dysfunctional cognitions and troublesome feelings without engaging with them. This may be thought of as an acceptance-based focus (ABF) in CBT and is typical of what has become known as 'third-wave CBT'. REBT (which would be regarded as a 'second-wave' CBT approach), on the other hand, generally recommends that clients identify, challenge and change rigid and extreme basic belierfs (at 'B') in the ABC framework, and respond, usually afterwards, to distorted inferences (either at 'A' or at 'C'). In short, REBT recommends that clients mindfully engage with troublesome cognitions (i.e. beliefs and inferences) with the purpose of changing them. This may be known as a change-based focus (CBF) in CBT.

While it may be thought that these two foci could not both be utilized in REBT, I believe they can. Here is how I make use of both a change-based focus (CBF), where beliefs and inferences are targeted for change and an acceptance-based focus (ABF) where these cognitions are mindfully accepted.

- I use a change-based focus (CBF) when encouraging clients to examine or question their rigid and extreme beliefs in the first instance. When clients consider that they have got enough out of this focus as they can on any particularly occasion, I encourage them to shift to an acceptance-based focus (ABF) if the irrational beliefs are still in their mind. It is unrealistic to expect a person to be convinced fully of their CBF interventions in any single questioning episode. I use a gym analogy to explain this to clients. When you go to a gym, it is for a work out which adds to your level of fitness and then you rest. You do not expect the work-out to lead to full fitness. In the same way, an episode of disputing adds to the person's level of conviction in their rational belief. It does not lead to full conviction. The rest period involves using acceptance-based methods as the person takes a break from disputing.
- With highly distorted cognitive consequences of rigid and extreme beliefs, I initially teach clients to understand why these thoughts are so distorted (i.e. they are the product of irrational beliefs. I then help them to use the presence of these thoughts to identify the rigid and extreme beliefs that have spawned them and then to use a change-based focus (CBF) with these irrational beliefs. I may then help them to use the same change-based methods to respond to these cognitive Cs, but to recognize that these thoughts may still reverberate in their mind, at which point I encourage them to switch to an acceptance-based focus (ABF). Such reverberation is a natural process as the mind does not switch off from such thoughts just because CBF methods have been successfully used on any one occasion.

As third wave CBT therapists note, little productive change can be gained when clients get enmeshed and entwined with their irrational (i.e. rigid and extreme) beliefs and distorted inferences and it is then when I advocate the use of an acceptance-based focus (ABF). However, from an REBT perspective, little can be gained by failing to encourage clients to respond constructively to these cognitions by employing a change-based focus (CBF) when they are able to do so.

It should be noted that this is one REBT therapist's perspective concerning when to encourage clients to respond to problematic beliefs and inferences and when to accept them mindfully. However, it shows that REBT practitioners are open to consider what newer CBT approaches can offer the theory and practice of REBT.

Dealing with Clients' Doubts, Reservations and Objections to REBT

Like other therapists, REBT practitioners address client obstacles to change. However, since REB therapists endeavour to teach clients salient REBT concepts it often transpires that such obstacles are rooted in clients' doubts and reservations about or objections to these concepts.[6] It frequently happens that these DROs are based on client misconceptions of these concepts. If the REB therapist does not elicit clients' DROs, then these clients will still have them and be influenced by them and they will thus resist making changes. However, as the therapist has not elicited their clients' DROs, they will not know why the clients are resisting change. For example, a client sometimes thinks that their rigid beliefs in the form of 'musts' are helpful in the sense that they are motivating and without them, the client would not strive towards their goals. In this case, the REB therapist would help the client understand that it is their preference (common to both their rigid and flexible belief) that is motivational, but when this preference is made rigid it creates psychological disturbance which does not happen when the preference is kept flexible.

Emphasis on Therapeutic Efficiency

All therapeutic approaches are (or should be) concerned with matters of therapeutic effectiveness. REBT is also concerned with the principle therapeutic efficiency – bringing about changing in the briefest time possible (Ellis, 1980b). This is why Ellis counsels REBT therapists to adopt an early focus on clients' rigid and extreme beliefs (see above) and to encourage their clients to tackle their problems full on, if possible. Ellis's concern with therapeutic efficiency had its roots in his early experiences as a therapist of carrying out lengthy diagnostic procedures with clients who dropped out before the treatment phase began which he regarded as a waste of a clinician's time and thus therapeutically inefficient (Ellis, 1962).

REBT Is an Eclectic Therapy

Although REBT is clearly placed in the tradition of CBT, it can also be regarded as an eclectic therapy. Indeed, I have called REBT a form of 'theoretically-consistent eclecticism' – advocating the broad use of techniques, from wherever, but to achieve goals in keeping with REBT theory (Dryden, 1987). However, it sometimes will use techniques that are not in keeping with REBT theory when theoretically-consistent techniques bear no therapeutic fruit (see Ellis, 2002). Ultimately, REBT therapists' primary concern is to help their clients rather than to practise REBT!

[6] I refer to these doubts, reservations and objections here as DROs.

References

Bond, F. W., & Dryden, W. (2000). How rational beliefs and irrational beliefs affect people's inferences: An experimental investigation. *Behavioural and Cognitive Psychotherapy, 28*(1), 33–43.

Bordin, E. S. (1979). The generalizability of the psychoanalytic concept of the working alliance. *Psychotherapy: Theory, Research and Practice, 16*, 252–260.

DiGiuseppe, R. (1991) Comprehensive cognitive disputing in rational-emotive therapy. In M. Bernard (Ed.), *Using rational-emotive therapy effectively* (pp. 173–195). New York: Plenum Press.

Dryden, W. (1985). Challenging but not overwhelming: A compromise in negotiating homework assignments. *British Journal of Cognitive Psychotherapy, 3*(1), 77–80.

Dryden, W. (1987). *Current issues in rational-emotive therapy*. London, UK: Croom Helm.

Dryden, W. (1994). When musts are not enough: A note on determining the type of your client's disturbance by referring to her secondary irrational beliefs. *The Rational Emotive Behaviour Therapist, 2*(2), 59–60.

Dryden, W. (1997). *Therapists' dilemmas. Revised edition*. London, UK: Sage.

Dryden, W. (1998). Understanding persons in the context of their problems: A rational emotive behaviour therapy perspective. In M. Bruch & F. W. Bond (Eds.), *Beyond diagnosis: Case formulation approaches in CBT* (pp. 43–64). Chichester, UK: Wiley.

Dryden, W. (2001). *Reason to change: A rational emotive behaviour therapy (REBT) workbook*. Hove, UK: Brunner-Routledge.

Dryden, W. (2015). *Rational emotive behaviour therapy: Distinctive features* (2nd ed.). Hove, UK: Routledge.

Dryden, W. (2016). *Attitudes in rational emotive behaviour therapy: Components, characteristics and adversity related consequences*. London, UK: Rationality Publications.

Dryden, W. (2018). *Rational emotive behavioural coaching: Distinctive features*. Abingdon, UK: Routledge.

Dryden, W., & Neenan, M. (2004). *The rational emotive behavioural approach to therapeutic change*. London, UK: Sage.

Ellis, A. (1959). Requisite conditions for basic personality change. *Journal of Consulting Psychology, 23*, 538–540.

Ellis, A. (1962). *Reason and emotion in psychotherapy*. Secaucus, NJ: Lyle Stuart.

Ellis, A. (1976). The biological basis of human irrationality. *Journal of Individual Psychology, 32*, 145–168.

Ellis, A. (1979). Discomfort anxiety: A new cognitive-behavioral construct (Part I). *Rational Living, 14*(2), 3–8.

Ellis, A. (1980a). Discomfort anxiety: A new cognitive-behavioral construct (Part II). *Rational Living, 15*(1), 25–30.

Ellis, A. (1980b). The value of efficiency in psychotherapy. *Psychotherapy: Theory Research and Practice, 17*, 414–418.

Ellis, A. (1983). The philosophic implications and dangers of some popular behavior therapy techniques. In M. Rosenbaum, C. M. Franks, & Y. Jaffe (Eds.), *Perspectives in behavior therapy in the eighties* (pp. 138–151). New York, NY: Springer.

Ellis, A. (1994). *Reason and emotion in psychotherapy. Revised and updated edition*. New York, NY: Birch Lane Press.

Ellis, A. (2000). *How to control your anxiety before it controls you*. New York, NY: Citadel.

Ellis, A. (2002). *Overcoming resistance: A rational emotive behavior therapy integrated approach*. New York, NY: Springer.

Ellis, A., & Joffe Ellis, D. (2011). *Rational emotive behaviour therapy*. Washington, DC: American Psychological Association.

Frank, R. I., & Davidson, J. (2014). *The transdiagnostic road map so case formulation and treatment planning: Practical guidance for clinical decision making*. Oakland, CA: New Harbinger Publications.

Hjelle, L. A., & Ziegler, D. J. (1992). *Personality theories: Basic assumptions, research and applications*. New York, NY: McGraw-Hill.

Rogers, C. R. (1957). The necessary and sufficient conditions of therapeutic personality change. *Journal of Consulting Psychology, 21*, 95–103.

Wills, F. (2015). *Skills in cognitive behaviour therapy* (2nd ed.). London, UK: Sage.

Ziegler, D. J. (2000). Basic assumptions concerning human nature underlying rational emotive behaviour therapy (REBT) personality theory. *Journal of Rational-Emotive and Cognitive-Behavior Therapy, 18*, 67–85.

Chapter 3
A Comparison of REBT with Other Cognitive Behavior Therapies

Walter Matweychuk, Raymond DiGiuseppe, and Olga Gulyayeva

In a paradigm shifting presentation at the American Psychological Association's conference in Chicago in 1956, Albert Ellis argued for addressing the important role cognition plays in the creation and maintenance of emotional and behavioral disturbance. This presentation then appeared in a 1958 article in the *Journal of General Psychology* titled "Rational Therapy". This marked his official departure from psychoanalysis and earned Ellis the distinction of being the field's first cognitive behavior therapist. His work welded ancient and modern philosophy, especially Stoicism, with clinical strategies and techniques from behavior therapy. Ellis proposed that attitudes, beliefs, and philosophical ideas, what we now commonly refer to as cognitions, were at the core of emotional and behavioral disturbance. Over the next 60 years, Ellis developed, refined, and disseminated the theory and practice of Rational Emotive Behavior Therapy (REBT: Ellis, 1962, 1994). Subsequent to and independent of Ellis's work, Aaron T. Beck published "Thinking and Depression" in the *Archives of General Psychiatry* in 1963. By this time, he also had come to appreciate the important role thinking played in clinical depression. Due to Ellis's pioneering work and Beck's subsequent empirical research, it is fair to consider Ellis and Beck the founding fathers of cognitive behavior therapy (CBT).

This chapter discusses the important differences between REBT and subsequent CBT systems as they are currently portrayed by their originators. In the case of Ellis who is deceased, REBT is discussed from what we believe is the classic version of REBT as depicted in some of his final and major works (e.g., Ellis, 1962, 1994:

W. Matweychuk (✉)
Department of Psychiatry, Perelman School of Medicine,
University of Pennsylvania Health System, Philadelphia, PA, USA
e-mail: walterma@pennmedicine.upenn.edu

R. DiGiuseppe · O. Gulyayeva
Department of Psychology, St. John's University, Queens, NY, USA
e-mail: digiuser@stjohns.edu; olga.gulyayeva16@stjohns.edu

© Springer Nature Switzerland AG 2019

M. E. Bernard, W. Dryden (eds.), *Advances in REBT*,
https://doi.org/10.1007/978-3-319-93118-0_3

Ellis & Dryden, 1997). We compare REBT with Beck's Cognitive Therapy first (CT: Beck, 1976; Beck & Haigh, 2014) because REBT and CT are foundational to CBT. Then, we examine two popular, more recent therapies, Hayes's Acceptance and Commitment Therapy (ACT: Flaxman, Blackledge, & Bond, 2011; Hayes, Strosahl, & Wilson, 1999) and Linehan's Dialectical Behavior Therapy (DBT: Linehan, 1993; Swales & Heard, 2017). To help the readers understand the similarities and differences between these models, we present three tables. Table 3.1 presents the position of the four models on the goals of therapy. Table 3.2 present the core, primary interventions of each of the four models. Table 3.3 presents the positions of each model on the use of some important therapeutic strategies.

Before proceeding, it is helpful to discuss the names of the therapies being examined. What is now referred to as REBT was initially referred to by Ellis as Rational Therapy (Ellis, 1958), which he later called Rational Emotive Therapy (Ellis, 1962), before eventually settling on Rational Emotive Behavior Therapy (Ellis, 1993). Beck's approach was initially called Cognitive Therapy (Beck, 1976) and more recently he and his daughter, the standard bearers of the approach, refer to it as Cognitive Behavior Therapy. However, the term CBT is presently used as an overriding term to incorporate many approaches along with ACT and DBT in the cognitive behavioral therapeutic tradition in so far as they all theorize how cognition relates to psychopathology. To avoid confusion, when we speak of Beck's model, we will refer to it by its original name Cognitive Therapy, to make clear it is one of several cognitive behavior therapies.

CBT addresses thoughts (i.e. cognitions), and these different models of psychotherapy postulate different types of thoughts and cognitions such as automatic thoughts and deeper level beliefs. When we use the term automatic thoughts, which can be negative or positive, we mean cognitions, which are quick, inferential and evaluative thoughts and images that are situation specific. These cognitions are very much like hypotheses that naturally and often tacitly occur as we make observations that may or may not be true (Ellis & Dryden, 1997). Most importantly, patients might not be aware of these thoughts and the influence they have on their mood. Furthermore, when we refer to beliefs, we wish to denote a particular kind of deeper level cognition that is either an imperative demand that the world, other people, and ourselves must or must not be a certain way, or an extreme evaluative stance a person has about an adversity that leads to self-defeating emotional and behavioral consequences.

Recently, some in the REBT community have argued for the use of the word *attitude* instead of *belief* and maintain it more clearly denotes the fundamental imperative demands and evaluations which REBT draws particular attention to in theory and practice (Dryden, 2016). Nevertheless, beliefs are the traditional term Ellis used and which is more widely found throughout the REBT literature, and therefore throughout this chapter we will use beliefs to refer to these fundamental imperative demands and evaluations.

Over the last decade or more, debates have occurred at professional conferences on the nature of CBT. ACT and DBT (Follette & Hazlett-Stevens, 2016) have declared these models to represent a new third wave of CBT, which are very

Table 3.1 A comparison of the therapeutic goals of, acceptance and commitment therapy, cognitive therapy, dialectic behavior therapy, and rational emotive behavior therapy

Issue	Shared	REBT	ACT	CT	DBT
Specification of goals of therapy	All models emphasize clear articulation of the therapeutic goals	Goals are set by the client and usually represent symptom reduction but can involve improving wellbeing. Therapist can recommend goals consistent with REBT's 12 aspects of healthy human adjustment. While this is true, it has not traditionally defined the practice of REBT.	Behavioral goals are stated in positive terms. What the client will do, not what the client will not do or stop doing. Changes in emotions are not acceptable goals. What behaviors clients can do when they experience the emotions are the goals. Live a valued life.	Goals are logically related to presenting symptoms (e.g., reduction of anxiety, depression), and are individualized based on the patient's specific symptoms.	Initial goals include the reduction of therapy interfering behaviors. Reduction of serious symptoms such as suicidal behavior. Learning to solve problems and tolerate distress in a healthy way. Living a life worth living.
Symptom reduction	All models allow for symptom reduction when it can be achieved	Symptom reduction is an explicit aim, as is the improvement of well-being.	Symptom reduction for decrease in thoughts and emotions per se are not the explicit aim; the therapy focuses on what behaviors clients do when they experience the symptoms.	Symptom reduction is an explicit aim.	Primarily aims at symptom reduction as this model was created for severe disorders.
Quality of life	All modes target improvements in quality of life, which will include success in major life domains	Increasing the quality of life is achieved by a set of behaviors and beliefs that represent 12 aspects of psychological adjustment and adaptive functioning.	Quality of life is a product of the degree to which someone is living a life consistent with his/her values.	Freedom from bothersome thoughts, feelings, and other symptoms is an important component of quality of life.	It aims to reduce symptoms to achieve a life worth living.

Table 3.2 Core interventions used in REBT, acceptance and commitment therapy, cognitive therapy, and dialectic behavior therapy

Shared aspect across therapies	Relationship-building interventions such as empathy, validation, and reflection Setting specific goals for therapy and for sessions Didactic instruction of skills Experiential learning Summary statements Behavioral interventions, especially exposure to feared stimuli, behavioral activation, problem solving, role playing, and modeling of adaptive behavior Between session homework to rehearse new behaviors
Rational emotive behavioral therapy	Presentation of the A-B-C model (activating event/adversity → inferences → beliefs → affective, behavioral, subsequent inferential and evaluative cognitive consequences) Distinguishing healthy negative emotions from unhealthy negative emotions Setting a goal to replace unhealthy negative emotions with healthy adaptive negative emotions Emphasize and model precision in the use of language linked to general semantic theory. Identification of absolutistic and extreme beliefs Distinguishing irrational from rational beliefs Identification of the presence of demandingness and the derivative irrational beliefs Modification of the rigid and extreme beliefs such as demandingness, awfulizing, discomfort intolerance, and global evaluations of human worth (self or others) Replacing the above irrational beliefs with rational alternatives such as a non-demanding acceptance of self, others, and life, non-awfulizing evaluations of events, belief in the ability to tolerate frustration, and acceptance of the worth of self and others despite flaws and misbehavior Behavioral homework such as behavioral exposure for targeting shame, anxiety, behavioral activation for targeting depression, and assertiveness training and relaxation for targeting anger. Use of humor, force, metaphors, parables, and energy in facilitating attitudinal change Developing the frustration and discomfort tolerance to pursue vitally absorbing interests to provide satisfaction and meaning in life
Cognitive therapy	Presentation of the A-B-C-model (situation → cognitions (inferences and core schema) → affective and behavioral consequences) Identification of negative automatic thoughts Labeling thought errors and cognitive distortions Identification of core beliefs, schemas, and attributional styles Cognitive conceptualization recognizing that early experiences shape core beliefs which, in turn, determine conditional assumptions, intermediary rules, automatic thoughts, and compensatory strategies Modification of dysfunctional cognitions; generation of alternative responses Behavioral experiments to test clients' thoughts/beliefs
Acceptance and commitment therapy	Presentation of the idea that attempts to control internal experiences is more of a problem than a solution Induce a necessary state of hopelessness toward doing "more of the same" (i.e., attempts to control) Increase acceptance of internal experiences (thoughts, feelings, images, sensations, urges) Increase awareness of present moment experiences Increase *diffusion*, – the ability to step back from thoughts and other internal experiences to allow seeing them as "just thoughts" that are not necessarily true Decrease attachment to *conceptualized self* (i.e., one's personal narrative) Clarification of core life values Increased commitment toward values-consistent behavior and a willingness to have difficult internal experiences for the sake of moving toward life values

Table 3.2 (continued)

Dialectical behavior therapy	Dialectical principles with validation of the patients suffering and negative disturbed emotions while encouraging change Explicitly validating patients' emotional suffering when it is expressed Accepting discomfort and disturbed emotions Discussions concerning change occurs after validation of the patients' psychological pain Emphasis on the primacy of affect Biosocial theory of etiology Use of Zen Principles Acceptance of internal affect experiences Targeting any behavior that interferes with therapy (such as lateness, avoidance of topics, anger at the therapists) first before targeting symptoms Integrative multiple CBT treatments Skills based groups Coaching the client on the telephone to facilitate generalization of coping skills to home environment avert a crisis Providing a forum for psychotherapists to discuss their frustrations and emotions about the patients' progresses and provocative behaviors

different from the second generation of CBT that includes the models of Ellis and Beck. A major criticism that the third-wave therapies have against the second-generation forms of CBT is the challenging of negative thoughts. We propose that many of these discussions have been aimed at the limitations of the challenging of negative automatic, inferential thoughts and cognitive errors that is at the heart of the cognitive model proposed by Beck's CT. REBT is similar to both ACT and DBT in initially avoiding targeting negative, automatic inferential thoughts and cognitive errors, for different reasons. REBT initially avoids challenging these thoughts because they might not be distorted, that is inconsistent with empirical data, and therefore these thoughts could very well be true. Later in the therapeutic process, the empirical data for or against their validity is considered in REBT, but this is secondary to REBT's initial stance in the therapeutic process which is to accept them as true and to focus on theoretically more critical cognitions, namely, underlying beliefs.

However, ACT avoids challenging automatic thoughts not only because they might be true, but because they are thoughts rather than the things the thoughts are about. ACT avoids interventions focused on thoughts and, instead, directly changes behaviors. DBT avoids challenging automatic thoughts because they could be interpreted by patients as a failure to validate the their negative life experiences.

Differences Among the Theorists

The personality of the theorist has a great influence on the nature of a theory. Each of the four psychotherapies discussed here was formulated by a person whose values and personality influenced the theoretical underpinnings and structure of the approach.

Table 3.3 A comparison of rational emotive behavior therapy, acceptance & commitment therapy, cognitive therapy, and dialectic behavior therapy on therapeutic strategies

Issue	Shared	REBT	ACT	CT	DBT
Role of meta-disturbance	All models acknowledge that internal experience can trigger more emotional and behavioral disturbance.	Theorizes that disturbance about internal experiences is often present, and therapists always assess the presence of this. However, meta disturbance is not always present. It is targeted first when it is present.	Changing ones disturbed reactions to thoughts, emotions, and images is the primary mechanism of change.	Acknowledges that internal experiences are a possible activating event, however, this idea is not empathized.	Changing ones disturbed reactions to thoughts, emotions, and images is the primary mechanism of change.
The dual nature of human thoughts and emotions.	All models acknowledge that humans have two types of cognitive processes as identified by Kahneman. We can think and behave rationally and irrationally.	Acknowledges that humans experience both irrational and rational beliefs and that rational beliefs can overcome irrational ones.	Acknowledges that humans are prone to distorted negative thinking that be countered by empirical, rational thoughts.	Acknowledges that humans have negative distorted thoughts and dysfunctional beliefs, and people can choose to act in their best interest against these experiences.	The dialectical philosophy acknowledges that one can hold two contradictory ideas. Acknowledging adversity can help one behave adaptively
Role of disputation	All are averse to attempts to directly "control" thoughts. That is to just not have the thoughts.	Disputation, challenging, and examining beliefs is a core strategy. Uses functional, empirical, and logical challenges to dysfunctional beliefs.	Skeptical of disputation and challenging strategies and avoids them. Relies on functional arguments that dysfunctional thoughts do not help one accomplish goals.	Disputation, challenging, and examining thoughts is a core strategy of CT. Primarily relies on empirical tests of the veracity of the clients' thoughts	Disputation is one of several strategies that might be integrated to treatment.

Characteristic treatment of techniques	All interventions focus on the present and future events and experiences.	Uses Socratic questioning, didactic teaching, use of metaphors and humor, role-playing and psychoeducation.	Uses diffusion as the primary intervention. Liberally uses metaphors and experiential exercises.	Socratic questioning is the primary strategy to empirically test negative thoughts.	Uses Socratic questioning, didactic teaching, and experiential exercises.
Therapeutic focus on changing the content of cognitions versus changing the connection between cognitions or emotions and behaviors	All models emphasize the importance of private experiences (thoughts, feelings, memories, etc.) in triggering adaptive and maladaptive behavior.	Focuses mainly on changing the content of private events as precursor to emotional and behavioral change. However, behavioral change can be a goal itself.	Focuses on disentangling private experience from behavior and increasing clients' willingness to experience distressing thoughts/feelings to engage in valued behavior.	Focuses on changing content of private experience as precursor to emotional and behavior change.	Integrates both interventions. Changes the content of cognitions and increases the willingness to experience distressing thoughts/feelings to engage in valued behavior
Role of diffusion	All view cognitions as observable by the self.	Diffusion is a byproduct of cognitive restructuring, but not a primary strategy. Distancing oneself form thoughts can make it easy to see irrationality of the thought.	Diffusion is a core strategy to enhance willingness to promote action.	Diffusion is a byproduct of cognitive restructuring, but not a primary strategy.	Diffusion is a core strategy to enhance willingness and promote action
Identification of alternative adaptive responses	All models identify some new skill or behavior that clients do	Developing alternative rational beliefs are strongly encouraged. They are based on Stoic and other ancient and modern philosophies. Develop healthy negative emotions to replace unhealthy negative emotions	Content of thoughts are not targeted. Clients learn to have a new flexible connection between thoughts and emotions with behaviors consistent with one's values	Encourages the construction of adaptive automatic thoughts that are consistent with empirical reality and adaptive schema that are flexible.	Uses and integrates approaches that include changing discomfort tolerance, diffusion, and changing the content of the thoughts.

(continued)

Table 3.3 (continued)

Issue	Shared	REBT	ACT	CT	DBT
Behavioral strategies e.g., exposure, behavioral activation, assertiveness training	All models use interventions that encourage alternative, adaptive behaviors.	Behavioral strategies are utilized in the service of achieving one's goals. Uses exposure, assertiveness training and behavioral activation. Adaptive behavior is flexible and allows one to reach one's goals	Behavioral strategies utilized to promote psychological flexibility in the context of increased willingness to experience distressing private experiences.	Behavioral strategies utilized in the service of reducing negative affect and achieving one's goals. Uses exposure, assertiveness training, and behavioral activation. Adaptive behavior is flexible and allows one to reach one's goals	Behavioral strategies utilized to promote willingness to experience distressing negative affect and to avoid engaging in symptomatic behaviors.
Emphasis on affective expression	All models seek to facilitate emotional expression as a means to an end.	The depth, permanence, and effectiveness of cognitive restructuring is theorized to be enhanced when performed in the context of heightened affect.	Therapy encourages the expression of difficult affect as part of the goal of reduction of experiential avoidance, leading to greater psychological flexibility.	The depth, permanence, and effectiveness of cognitive restructuring is theorized to be enhanced when performed in the context of heightened affect.	Therapy encourages the expression of difficult affect as part of the goal of reduction of experiential avoidance, leading to greater psychological flexibility.

Therapeutic relationship	All models emphasize a collaborative relationship. However, they do not see the relationship as curative.	Therapeutic relationship is considered an important element that facilitates therapeutic change but is not curative in itself. Therapists display acceptance of the client and models self-acceptance and high discomfort tolerance.	Strong emphasis on principles applying to therapist & patient alike.	Therapist role is that of a benevolent coach, gently leading toward cognitive change through collaborative empiricism; solicits feedback from client at the conclusion of every session.	Therapeutic relationship is considered an important element that facilitates therapeutic change but is not curative in itself
Aspects of therapists' behavior that influence the therapeutic alliance	All models emphasize accurate empathy with collaboration in the context of acceptance of the client to facilitate change.	Specifically teaches patients about the proposed mechanism of changing and seeks agreement on the tasks of therapy.	Less likely to seek agreement on the task of therapy, as suggesting that certain activities are preferred could lead to rule being rigid adhered to and lead to inflexibility.	Specifically teaches patients about the proposed mechanism of changing and seeks agreement on the tasks of therapy.	Given the invalidating life experience of patients with BPD, emphasis is placed on the validation of the patients' suffering and adverse life experience as crucial and ongoing over the course of treatment.

Ellis worked as a private practitioner over his 60 year clinical career, personally delivered an estimated 180,000 hour-long psychotherapy sessions working with patients most of whom experienced multiple clinical problems and diagnoses (Ellis, 2002). Thus, REBT was cultivated in a real world clinical setting and developed a trans-diagnostic perspective from the outset. As a result, Ellis developed a flexible approach rooted in philosophy, semantics, and scientific thinking. His extensive clinical experience showed him that faulty cognitive processing of empirical reality was insufficient for producing emotional disturbance. Instead, he believed that rigid, absolutistic beliefs, a process he referred to as absolutizing, was at the core of emotional disturbance, which gave rise to extreme evaluative beliefs (awfulizing, LFT, global evaluations). In his view, extreme evaluative beliefs derived from these primary absolutistic beliefs and were secondary to them. Ellis urged patients to adopt scientific, flexible, and non-extreme beliefs after challenging the empirical validity and logical consistency of their absolutistic and extreme beliefs as well as helping them to see the functional impairment resulting from these irrational beliefs. This disputing or reflective process aimed to help patients experience healthy and functional reactions to their adverse realities and facilitate adaptation to them. Ellis found that if distorted automatic thoughts (i.e. cognitive distortions) of reality were present, they were likely the consequence of absolutistic beliefs and extreme evaluations tacitly held and brought to the adversity by the patient. Furthermore, Ellis appreciated how his patients frequently qualified for multiple diagnoses and often faced a grim reality and their thoughts about their difficult circumstances were not necessarily distorted. Consequently, Ellis focused on teaching deeper level, rational beliefs that would foster adaptation, accommodation, and acceptance of reality in response to the harsh situations faced by his patients.

Beck was a clinical scientist and academic who developed CT in the controlled confines of a university laboratory setting. As a result, CT was created with carefully selected patients who fit strict diagnostic criteria. Beck scientifically tested and refined his theory from the application of tightly controlled protocols with closely monitored psychotherapists following treatment manuals. The structured style of CT reflects this discipline to a manualized protocol. Beck's thesis from the outset was that faulty information processing was a foundational variable of all psychopathology. After testing this thesis with depressed patients, Beck focused on anxiety disorders (Beck, Emery, & Greenberg, 1985), substance abuse disorder (Beck, Wright, Newman, & Liese, 1993), personality disorders (Beck, Davis & Freemna et al., 2015), and now schizophrenia (Beck, Rector, Stolar, & Grant, 2008). Additionally, the CT model encompasses deeper level, dysfunctional core beliefs, also known as schema. These dysfunctional core beliefs are more central or fundamental types of cognitions that usually are developed in childhood as a result of ongoing aversive conditions. According to CT theory these core beliefs largely become activated when the person experiences stress and the schema contribute to the creation of distorted automatic thoughts. Over his career, he never abandoned the thesis that faulty information processing leads to psychopathology and a structured style of conducting psychotherapy, which was necessary for conducting clinical trials.

REBT and Cognitive Therapy

REBT and Cognitive Therapy are the oldest and most widely practiced forms of CBT. They have many similarities. Both rely on the A-B-C model of emotional disturbance. They both attempt to change automatic thoughts and beliefs that theoretically lead to emotional disturbance. In challenging dysfunctional cognitions, both encourage patients to adopt a more rigorous scientific outlook. They both foster behavior change between sessions and both rely on developing alternative adaptive cognitions.

Which Cognitions Are Targeted First in Therapy? Perhaps, the most important difference between these two therapies are the cognitions that they target for change at the outset of therapy. Because of its adaptation from an information processing model of psychopathology, CT emphasizes and, therefore, initially targets the negative automatic thoughts and cognitive distortions that are associated with the patients' experience of disturbed emotions. It is only after eight to ten sessions that the targeting of deeper level, dysfunctional cognitions occurs. Although these schema are important, fundamental and deeply held by the patient, they are not initially addressed in CT. It is hypothesized that the therapist does not have sufficient credibility, as well as, sufficient clinical data to accurately identify and then effectively treat such longstanding, fundamental beliefs until eight to ten sessions have been held. Therefore, the patient's attention is guided to the identification of automatic thoughts pertaining to the self, others, the future, and the world and encouraged to learn how to test these thoughts empirically against reality. Thus, CT sees the patients' disturbance as resulting from the inaccurate processing of data pertaining to the self, others, the future, and the world. CT identifies 11 different types of cognitive distortions, the majority of which are variations on logic errors of overgeneralizations formed by invalid inductive reasoning.

It should be noted that when the underlying core schema are eventually identified in CT, the therapist's review of automatic thoughts and discussion with the patient the therapeutic process differs from REBT practice in a couple of important ways. The core beliefs that are addressed often concern themes of helplessness, unloveability, and worthlessness. The CT therapist attempts to help the patient evaluate these beliefs by placing the targeted dysfunctional core belief on a continuum and has the patient compare his or herself to others in regards to the core belief (Padesky, 1994). Patients are encouraged to put into perspective the degree to which they differ on characteristics like incompetence, attractiveness, or their subjective assessment of worth as compared to others. Patients are taught to make finer distinctions when evaluating themselves and reduce bias and to take into account information they may have discounted. Effort is made to help the patient develop more adaptive core beliefs that structure processing from dichotomous categories, like helpless, unlovable, or worthless categories to more moderate beliefs along a continuum that more closely align with reality, improve mood, and promote behavioral functioning. A REBT therapist, at least initially, would not attempt to help the patient adopt a more moderate assessment of a negative characteristic, but question the imperative demand that the person absolutely must possess the desired characteristic at all. The discussion would take a philosophical turn focusing on the value and validity of unconditional acceptance of the self with or without the desired characteristic. Furthermore, the REBT therapist aims to do this from the outset of therapy instead of waiting for eight to ten sessions before attempting to intervene at the level of core beliefs.

A distinctive feature of REBT is that it initially assumes that cognitions like automatic thoughts to be true and goes on to targets for change two types of underlying beliefs. The first, considered to be primary, is the imperative, absolutistic beliefs that the self, others, and life conditions must be a certain way. It also targets three derivative or secondary evaluative beliefs which are theorized to stem from the absolutistic beliefs at the core of disturbance. The first derivative belief being that the situation is extremely negative, beyond 100% bad, and the second derivative belief being that the situation is so bad that the person cannot stand it (referred to as frustration or discomfort intolerance). The third derivative belief targeted is the evaluative beliefs that reflect that the self or another person is worthless or lesser as a person because of how they behave or the characteristics they possess. Beck's work does acknowledge that extreme evaluations are thoughts that can lead to disturbance, and even refers to some distortions using words similar to those found in REBT such as catastrophizing, and should statements. But these types of beliefs are examples of his 11 types of distorted thinking and hold no special place in the theory or therapy.

REBT sees at least five advantages of selectively focusing on the one primary and three derivative beliefs. First, sometimes a patient's automatic thoughts and core beliefs are true and not distortions of reality; therefore, targeting for change the underlying philosophical beliefs associated with negative realities is the better strategy. Second, even if the patients' automatic thoughts and beliefs are a distortion of reality, challenging these thoughts provides a coping mechanism only when the experienced thoughts are false; it fails to teach patients how to cope when reality is exceptionally bad. When the thoughts are consistent with the grim facts of reality the CT therapist resorts to problem solving, but this strategy can be quite limited in very difficult circumstances when the negative reality cannot be readily or ideally changed especially when problem solving largely comes down to choosing between two highly undesirable choices. Third, the disturbed negative extreme beliefs targeted early on in therapy by REBT are likely to produce subsequent distorted negative automatic thoughts and changing these imperative and extreme beliefs is a more fundamental cognitive change achieved earlier in therapy that will help the patient to avoid generating negative distorted thinking in the future. Fourth, the resulting flexible and non-extreme beliefs encouraged by REBT serve to inoculate patients from disturbance when adversity strikes in the future due to the profound "philosophical" change achieved. Fifth, given that these four beliefs are hypothesized to lie at the core of disturbance and quickly reveals where to focus interventions, the REBT therapist can achieve therapeutic efficiency by identifying and targeting core beliefs for therapeutic change from the outset of therapy.

The Nature of Emotions Over the years, Beck theorized that dysfunctional emotions represented exaggerated adaptive responses (Beck & Haigh, 2014). By viewing disturbance this way, Beck placed dysfunctional negative emotions on a continuum at the opposite end of adaptive responding. This view was similar to that of Wolpe's (1958) model that disturbed emotions were represented by a point along a continuum. This view is similar to the basic universal, evolutionary, and essentialist model of emotions postulated in psychology and has its roots in the work of Aristotle, and Darwin, and presently promoted by Ekman (see Feldman Barrett, Lewis, & Haviland-Jones, 2018). This stands in contrast to REBT's conceptualization of emotion. REBT posits that negative emotions fall on two continua: one healthy and associated with adaptive, functional behaviors, and one unhealthy associated with dysfunctional, maladaptive behaviors. Recent research has supported REBT's hypothesis that negative emotions probably fall on two continua, one healthy and adaptive and one unhealthy and maladaptive (Hyland & Boduszek, 2012). Recently, Feldman-Barret (2017) has challenged the traditional theory of emotions and has promoted a more constructivist model consistent with REBT. Her model recognizes that within any category of basic emotions such as fear, sadness, and anger, there are multiple emotions that people can experience and that the more emotions that people can conceptualize, the more adaptive they become.

It should be noted that both CT and REBT theories are interactional whereby they both see thinking, feeling, and behaving as mutually interactional. In both theories conceptualization, assessment, and treatment are influenced by this interactional premise. Although both models agree on the interactional relationships between thinking, feeling, and behaving only REBT argues for two separate continuums of thoughts, feelings, and behaviors whereby one continuum is self-helping and one self-defeating.

Position on Construction and Responsibility for Human Emotion Ellis believed that humans construct their thoughts and beliefs, and therefore have choice and a large degree of control over their beliefs and the subsequent emotions they experience in the face of adversity (Ellis, 1958, 1976) despite individual's differing biological tendencies toward irrationality. This choice makes them largely responsible for their subsequent emotional and behavioral disturbances. Ellis (1958) opposed the idea that humans have virtually no choice in determining their emotional reactions, and he suggested just the opposite by stating, *"The idea that one has virtually no control over one's emotions and that one cannot help feeling certain things – instead of the idea that one has enormous control over one's emotions if one chooses to work at controlling them and to practice saying the right kinds of sentences to oneself."* This REBT theoretical position on choice in emotion is called the Principle of Emotional Responsibility. Ellis's constructivist philosophical position importantly shapes the message given to the patient. A distinctive feature of REBT is the notion that patients disturb themselves about adversity.

CT does not take an explicit position on cognitive-behavioral-emotive choice and instead emphasizes the role of stimuli that trigger latent schema linked to ongoing adverse conditions of childhood, that determine the content of current automatic thoughts (Beck & Haigh, 2014). CT more heavily emphasizes the role of environmental events in the development of psychopathology. REBT chooses to emphasize the biological predisposition humans have towards irrationality while also emphasizing human choice in resisting this predisposition. This is an important difference. An REBT therapist would likely ask a patient and also emphasize how they are *constructing* their emotional disturbance or *making themselves upset and angry* about the adversity they were facing despite that upset having roots in one's biological nature. Instead, the cognitive therapist would encourage the patient to notice the temporal correlation between external events and their internal reactions (i.e. automatic thoughts, feelings, memories, or physical symptoms) and as well as how this way of responding has a basis in one's personal history of environmental adversity. Although both models teach the patients to help themselves, and both emphasize cognitive change as a path to adjustment, REBT clearly sends the message that acceptance of self-responsibility for one's own emotional disturbance despite its biological underpinnings, is a major therapeutic goal. Whereas a cognitive therapist sets out to teach skills aimed at changing automatic thoughts for responding to dysfunctional emotions and changing behavior, and only later in therapy with more chronic psychiatric conditions tend to address latent schema associated with early childhood trauma, an REBT psychotherapist goes beyond this and from the outset attempts to foster a more profound philosophical change. REBT posits that patients achieve greater emotional health when they appreciate the degree of responsibility they have for their own emotional disturbance in response to any adversity. This insight serves to inoculate the patient from future self-created and self-sustained emotional disturbance by showing them that their emotional destiny is largely determined by their self-created and self-maintained beliefs about adversity and not the adversity itself. Far from holding a position of blaming the patient for their disturbance, patients are shown that their adoption of responsibility for their emotional reactions represents a very self-liberating stance.

Positions on Self-Esteem Another major difference between these two therapies is their positions on self-esteem. CT's assumption of faulty or biased information processing of reality leads therapists to focus their efforts on helping patients to correct idiosyncratic distorted thoughts and core beliefs as these relate to the patient's self-concept and corresponding self-esteem. Patients are encouraged to examine the evidence for and against conclusions that lead to reduced self-esteem and an inaccurate self-concept. The CT therapist works to help the patients reframe cognitions and esteem or value themselves even when the data in a particular domain of life suggests failure. This can be accomplished in different ways one of which includes a broadening of and more precisely defining the criteria whereby the self is conditionally measured. Patients are encouraged to reduce biased processing of data and to take into account overlooked and undervalued strengths, roles, and accomplishments in order to put the patient's failures and weaknesses into a more balanced perspective in the service of more accurately measuring the self. In short the CT therapist teaches a patient how to more accurately rate himself or herself to improve mood and behavior.

In contrast to the efforts to improve patients' self-esteem through more accurate consideration of the available data, REBT rejects the construct of self-esteem and self-rating (Ellis, 1962, 2005). Ellis argued that it was both unproductive and philosophically invalid to attempt to summate human worth and compare people's ratings of worth according to any set of criteria. REBT posits that humans are properly viewed as living organisms in a constant state of evolution that possess almost an infinite number of traits, behaviors, and cognitions – some of which may be defined as good while others may be defined as bad. Because there is no universally agreed upon set of characteristics for determining human worth and that future behaviors and characteristics of the self are presently unknown, human self-rating and self-valuing at any point prior to death makes no sense and sets the stage for neurotic disturbance.

Ellis pointed out that a considerable amount of emotional disturbance resulted from the patient myopically, prematurely, and arbitrarily rating the self and then devaluing the self for its inadequacies. REBT recognizes that patients could function far more effectively and be motivated by healthy negative emotions if they limited their ratings to various components of the self, such as skills, traits, behaviors, and cognitions in the context of their personal goals. Traits, feelings, behaviors, and the beliefs that facilitate goal attainment can be evaluated as good and defined as rational while the self is not rated and is unconditionally accepted. Ruggiero, Spada, Caselli, and Sassaroli (2018) suggests that CT explores self-knowledge that would present a more accurate and corrective view of the self while REBT strives for self-acceptance regardless of one's flaws.

Discomfort Disturbance and Biology in Human Disturbance Ellis revolutionized the psychotherapeutic understanding of maladaptive motivation and behavior when he introduced the construct of discomfort disturbance leading to discomfort anxiety, depression, self-pity, and anger (Ellis, 1979a). His extensive clinical experience revealed that many patients experienced emotional disturbance and held themselves back from goal achievement due to inertia and their unwillingness to tolerate the discomfort inherent in working towards desired goals (Ellis, 1958, 1976). REBT shows patients how to rehabilitate their emotional and behavioral disturbance by learning to tolerate the discomfort of their negative emotions and doing behavioral assignments (Ellis, 1979a, 1979b). This discomfort disturbance and associated emotional and behavioral avoidance led to what Ellis also referred to as secondary emotional disturbance (Ellis & Dryden, 1987, 1997). The initial or primary emotional disturbance a patient experiences becomes an activating event about which the patient then has irrational beliefs that they cannot stand the discomfort of the initial disturbance, which then leads to the secondary emotional disturbance. This concept of becoming emotionally upset about one's emotional experience is now a common aspect of both ACT and DBT as we discuss below. CT's early protocols did not emphasize secondary emotional disturbance. More recently CT has begun to integrate mindfulness techniques thereby moving more closely towards the position taken by ACT and DBT on secondary disturbance.

What is important to note is that Ellis saw disturbance and associated irrationality as being largely biologically based and innate and to a far lesser extent environmentally taught (Ellis, 1976). Beck takes a considerably more balanced interactional view of the relative importance of adverse environmental life events interacting with genetic factors along with selective allocation of attentional resources in the development of negatively biased, dysfunctional core beliefs (Beck & Haigh, 2014). Ellis defined irrationality as thinking, emoting, and behaving that leads to self-defeating consequences that then undermine the goals of survival and happiness. He cited as evidence for the biological origins of irrationality (1) the ubiquity of human irrationality, (2) the ease with which humans hold rigid beliefs and extreme evaluations towards their desires and values, (3) the observation that the irrationality displayed by humans often goes against the environmental teaching of parents, teachers, and culture, and (4) that humans seem prone to lapse, relapse and replace particular irrationalities with other irrationalities. He also highlighted the biological predisposition of humans to learn and acquire both rational and irrational beliefs and behaviors. Ellis argued that although humans can modify their self-defeating ways, they will never eliminate their propensity for irrational thinking, emoting, and behaving.

The concept of discomfort disturbance and Ellis's emphasis on innate leanings towards irrationality found across all individuals is absent from Beck's writings and theorizing. Beck will acknowledge that negative cognitive biases underpinning depression could result from an individual variation of relatively greater influence of subcortical emotion processing brain regions in conjunction with weakened higher cortex cognitive control (Disner, Beevers, Haigh, & Beck, 2011). However, the concept of an innate discomfort disturbance is not a focus of the theory and practice of CT as it clearly is in Ellis's writings. Although Beck does discuss the identification and targeting of a patient's dysfunctional avoidance strategies, formal recognition of discomfort disturbance as a fundamental aspect of the human condition is absent in CT.

Theoretical Specificity and Parsimony REBT is quite specific and parsimonious in its theoretical position of the four rigid and extreme beliefs that underpin emotional disturbance across disorders. Absolutistic beliefs, expressed as absolute "shoulds" and "musts", are theorized to be at the core of emotional disturbance. The primacy of absolutistic, inflexible thinking leading to disturbance is a hallmark of REBT theory and determines the key cognitive target of the therapeutic process (Ellis & Dryden, 1987, 1997). From this hypothesized core, three extreme evaluative beliefs are derived known as awfulizing, discomfort intolerance, and global rating leading to the devaluation of self, others, and life. The parsimony of REBT is unique and contrasts to the intricate generic cognitive model advanced by Beck & Haigh, 2014. Whereas Beck organizes disorders into modes (a depressive mode, an anxiety mode, etc.) which represent a complex organization of automatic thoughts, beliefs, distortions, and schemas, he also ambitiously attempts to theoretically account for normal adaptations as well as mechanisms of activation and deactivation of schemas. This intricate generic cognitive model serves as a guide for clinicians in conceptualizing and tailoring treatment to the unique features of particular disorders.

Acceptance as a Therapeutic Process Over the course of his long clinical career Ellis refined his theory from roughly twelve irrational beliefs underpinning emotional disturbance and came to see the importance of a central absolutizing belief process and how a dogmatic insistence of how reality absolutely should and must be was at the core of emotional disturbance. Consequently, this insight led him to appreciate and emphasize the emotional leverage offered by the development of philosophical acceptance (Ellis, 1957). REBT teaches patients to cultivate three types of unconditional acceptance, namely acceptance of oneself, others, and life. By contrast, CT fails to have any corresponding rational, therapeutic process similar to acceptance, opting instead only for the empirical testing of inferences and core beliefs that might not be supported by empirical data or adaptive, along with teaching problem-solving skills for changing adversity when cognitions are not distorted. Acceptance, first mentioned by REBT in 1957, has become exceptionally popular and is one of the key concepts in many forms of CBT such as ACT and DBT discussed here, as well as in psychotherapy in general.

Philosophical Foundations The philosophical underpinnings of both REBT and CT concerning epistemology are important to note. CT's information processing model rests heavily on logical empiricism and logical positivism. The philosopher of science, Popper (1959), appreciated the limitations of strict empirical verification and argued that science derives more knowledge by establishing theories and then attempting to falsify them. Popper (1972) said, *"Philosophers are as free as others to use any method in searching for truth. There is no method peculiar to philosophy"* (cited in Ellis, 1958, preface p. xix). Ellis appreciated Popper's idea that the human mind, both the clinician's and the patient's, naturally made hypotheses; and therefore he took a nomothetic theoretical approach. REBT theory and practice encourages clinicians to take a hypothetico-deductive stance in assessment and treatment resting on the four theorized rigid and extreme beliefs underpinning emotional disturbance. REBT's interventions stem from hypotheses that are confirmed or rejected with empirical data.

CT follows the philosophy of Hume and other British Empiricists (Morris & Brown, 2017) that is disinclined to engage in normative, hypothetico-deductive clinical reasoning. Beck has remained a strict empiricist in theory and practice. The model relies on inductive clinical reasoning and devised clinical protocols taking an inductive and idiographic approach in assessment and treatment. An individual patient's automatic thoughts and cognitive distortions are systematically collected over the first 8–10 sessions to complete an individualized case conceptualization. This conceptualization includes relevant early life traumas, the patient's conditional rules, intermediary beliefs, and deeper level schemas. REBT in contrast starts to help patients see, from the outset of therapy, that one or more of his four rigid and extreme beliefs about adversity are likely to underpin his self-defeating feelings and behaviors.

The philosophical roots of REBT and CT exert influence over how clinicians assesses for the presence of dysfunctional cognitions and then intervene to help patients evaluate and modify their dysfunctional cognitions. Ellis subscribes to Popper's critical realism and hypothetically-deductively attempts to identify dysfunctional cognitions using REBT theory instead of exclusively relying on inductively identifying dysfunctional cognitions as is advocated in CT (Ellis, 1962). REBT, again following Popper, encourages multiple methods to challenge and falsify rigid and extreme beliefs (Popper, 1959). REBT will use a functional analysis of the impact the targeted belief has on emotional and behavioral functioning, an empirical evaluation to determine if the belief is supported by observable data, and a logical evaluation to determine if the belief is in accord with the principles of logic. The cognitive psychotherapist, by contrast, remains true to empiricism and largely prefers clinical interventions aimed at empirical analysis of the dysfunctional cognitions.

Disorder Specific Treatment As previously noted, REBT and CT were nurtured in radically different environments. REBT has its roots in philosophy and clinical practice, while CT has its roots in medicine and academic clinical research. Both are routinely applied to clinical disorders. CT starts with a generic cognitive model and developed disorder specific models that are tailored to the individual patient (Hofmann, Asmundson, & Beck, 2013). These disorder specific models presume that biased processing of reality leads to psychopathology, but they attempt to outline the specific thoughts and beliefs that occur in each disorder that will then give rise to biased information processing. This more case specific treatment plan is developed from the integration of the patient's history, past traumatic incidents, and other experiences, along with compensatory strategies that might have contributed to the development and maintenance of the patient's core beliefs. REBT does not hypothesize that one of the four irrational belief processes are largely responsible for the presence of any given formally recognized disorder. Instead, REBT hypothesizes that the core of all disturbance lies in primary absolutistizing regarding a patient's specific goals and values which then gives rise to derivative extreme beliefs that might be more disorder specific. For example, a rigid belief about uncertainty followed by a derivative belief of being unable to bear uncertainty and uncomfortable feelings are hypothesized and assessed when working with anxiety disorders. Absolute beliefs towards the self, others, and\or life, followed by a secondary beliefs of depreciation of the whole self and of life are hypothesized to occur in depressive disorders.

Applicability to Problems of Everyday Living and Happiness A major difference between these two therapies is their applicability to the broader issue of life satisfaction, meaning, and happiness. REBT's philosophical roots allow it to readily assist people who seek psychotherapy with sub-clinical problems of daily living and request help finding greater life satisfaction and meaning. REBT is interested in problems of everyday living and better able to assist with these than CT because Ellis was more interested in problems of modern-day living. Because REBT is rooted in ancient and modern philosophy (Ellis et al., 1982, 1987) it addressed the problems of non-clinical people and can guide people towards happiness and personal fulfillment. Because CT is rooted in a symptom and disorder-focused perspective it has had less focus on problems of everyday living. REBT states that two explicit fundamental values are held by most people-namely survival and enjoyment. However, unique to REBT are twelve subgoals (Ellis et al., 1987) that are consistent with these two fundamental values and constitute a REBT theory of an emotionally healthy human.

Bernard (2011) created a survey on Rationality and Happiness that enables the measurement of this construct in non-clinical samples. Bernard (2011) argued that many people wrongly believe REBT is primarily about emotional misery reduction. Ellis and Becker (1982) emphasized that the secondary goal of REBT is to assist people to self-actualize and grow in ways unique to their personal goals and values. Consistent with this view Martin Seligman has acknowledged that Ellis is the unsung hero of the now popular positive psychology movement in his testimonial for the book "Rationality and the Pursuit of Happiness" (Bernard, 2011). CT focuses on psychopathology and does not readily join in the zeitgeist of facilitating positive psychology.

REBT and ACT

Unlike REBT, but like CT, ACT largely developed within an academic research setting. Hayes was involved in the Functional Analysis of Behavior in the Skinnerian tradition and wanted to apply radical behavioral principles to all aspects of human behavior including psychotherapy (Hayes, Stroshal & Wilson, 1999).

Because language represents such a central aspect of human existence, Hayes first explored the relationship between language and other human behavior. He started where Skinner failed in his analysis of verbal behavior. Hayes spent many years researching language form a behavioral perspective and discovered that human language has some unique characteristics. Humans have the capacity to have shared associations between stimuli to form networks of meaning (Hayes, Barnes-Holmes, & Roche, 2001). Thus, a learned fear to a specific stimulus can have a cascading number of associations of that fear to many of the stimuli to which the first stimuli were connected. Hayes did not work primarily in delivering psychotherapy. Rather he built a conceptual foundation from the science of the functional, contextual analysis of behavior, and the study of language in relational frame theory before developing applications to clinical problems. Because Hayes did not work primarily delivering psychotherapy, in our opinion, the ACT model pays less attention to the common factors (Wampold & Imel, 2015) of psychotherapy than other forms of CBT.

Hayes rarely references Ellis or REBT in his writings, but he coauthored a paper critically reviewing the conceptual and empirical status of REBT (Zettle & Hayes, 1980), and he did report that one of his first clinical supervisors was trained by Ellis in REBT (Hayes S, 2015, Personal communication). Therefore, it is logical to assume that Hayes had some awareness of REBT theory and practice and this could have influenced the development of ACT.

Basic Theoretical Differences

In some ways ACT is closer to REBT than any other form of CBT and in some ways it is more different. Below we will review some of these theoretical differences.

The Role of Language Both models rely heavily on the study of language, the meaning of words, and their effect on our emotional and behavioral reactions. ACT relies on a revised version of Skinner's (1957) *Verbal Behavior* in relational frame theory (Hayes et al., 2001), while REBT builds on Korzybski's (1933, 1958) General Semantics theory. Both theories stress that the meaning associated with our use of language can be disturbing. Both theories agree that although language is a marvelous tool, humans generate many dysfunctional and invalid ideas from their use of language. A favorite quote by Hayes states, "You do not have to believe everything you think." Although REBT and General Semantics theory stresses examining the possible errors in one's thinking, language, and semantic imprecision before creating new adaptive meaning patterns, ACT believes that therapy helps clients form new more adaptive relations between what they think and feel with how they behave without challenging the validity of the content of one's thoughts.

Inflexibility as the Core of Disturbance ACT postulates that rigidity and lack of flexibility as the nature and cause of psychological disturbance. Disturbance is responding consistently and dysfunctionally to one's internal experience, whether they are thoughts or feelings. Adaption involves being able to respond differently to those internal stimuli based on what is one's long term interests. The therapy states that humans are prone to generate much dysfunctional thought content that moves us towards dysfunctional behavior. REBT shares several aspects with this notion that inflexibility is the core of disturbance. First, REBT has always seen rigidity and inflexibility in thinking, feeling, or acting as disturbance. REBT has long advocated that the process of therapy teaches people behave in their long term best interests. Also, REBT postulates that humans can take preferences and escalate them to rigid demands. REBT also states that humans have the biological capacity to create dysfunctional thoughts and emotions.

Hayes' research found that humans easily take guidelines and suggestions for adaptive behavior literally and make them into rigid rules that they perniciously follow thereby becoming rigid. Hayes' (1989) book, *Rule Governed Behavior*, represents an affirmation of Ellis' idea that humans can take preferences and because of the nature of language and the way humans can form relational connections, escalate them into inflexible demands.

Given the focus on language as a central human skill, both REBT and ACT would advocate the use metaphors as a process to teach patients how an idea can be dysfunctional and how to act adaptively.

The Role of Secondary Disturbance or Discomfort Anxiety ACT postulates that most human disturbance results from what it calls "experiential avoidance." That is, patients engage in avoidance or escape behaviors that are negatively reinforced (the avoidance makes the discomfort go away) to avoid the discomfort of their emotions or any private experiences. This is similar to the REBT concept of secondary emotional problems and discomfort anxiety (Ellis & Dryden, 1987, 1997). ACT thus targets experiential avoidance by teaching people to evaluate whether it is best to face their fears and teaches them to behave in their long term best interests despite feeling badly. REBT postulates that much human disturbance results from negatively evaluating one's emotions as unbearable. REBT would teach patients to tolerate their dysfunctional emotions, think of them as just uncomfortable, and behave in one's long term best interests. The difference is that ACT sees almost all disturbance as resulting from this process, while REBT sees it as one possible mechanism leading to disturbance or worsening an already existing disturbance. As a result, most ACT sessions and interventions focus on targeting experiential avoidance, while in REBT it would be a possible target.

The Role of Cognitions in Disturbance ACT clearly fits in the radical behaviorist camp and does not see cognitions, thoughts, or beliefs as central to disturbance, but as covert behaviors in need of an explanation. Cognitions are not an independent variable that causes emotions or behavior but independent variable to be studied. In ACT, cognitions, emotions, or any private experiences are stimuli that people have learned to differently associate with overt behaviors. The therapy focuses on changing the overt behaviors and their relationship with cognitions and emotions, rather than changing the cognitions or emotions themselves. In fact, ACT teaches patients to stop trying to change their specific cognitions and emotions, to accept these negative internal experiences and at the same time to learn to perform behaviors that will achieve their goals and values (and will be reinforcing) despite the desire to escape these uncomfortable experiences. Thus, therapeutic activities are designed to break the connections between one's dysfunctional thoughts and emotions with dysfunctional behaviors by teaching patients they can have those thoughts and emotions and still behave effectively, i.e. in accordance with their chosen values. Therapeutic activities break the connections or change the relations between patients' dysfunctional thoughts and emotions with their dysfunctional behaviors and teaches patients to perform new behaviors instead. To do this, therapists help patients see that their thoughts are not practically helpful. This is similar to what REBT would consider functional disputing. However, in ACT there would be no attempt to employ philosophical, logical, or empirical challenges to the thoughts. This strategy is similar to what Ellis called behavioral disputation, that is getting patients to act against their irrational beliefs.

Disputing Versus Defusion Although ACT does not see cognitive change as necessary for therapeutic change, it goes so far as to suggest that challenging of beliefs can be iatrogenic. It recommends that patients do not try to dispute or challenge the beliefs and that doing so might strengthen the thoughts. The rationale for this idea is epitomized in the "White Bear Effect" (Wegner & Schneider, 2003). This represents the notion that attempts at not experiencing a thought or thought suppression will lead to an increase in the frequency and intensity of the thought one is trying to suppress. If a person tries not to think of a polar bear, he or she will think about it more and more. Empirical or logical challenging of ideas requires that one hold the thought in working memory and examine it. This process keeps the thought or emotion in one's consciousness, and is proposed to be equivalent of thought suppression. This idea runs counter to the overwhelming research that suggests that interventions designed to challenge thoughts and beliefs in CT (Hofmann, Asnaani, Vonk, Sawyer, & Fang, 2012) and REBT (Vîslă, Flückiger, Grosse Holtforth, & David, 2016) have a great deal of efficacy. We think that the analogy of challenging thoughts to thought suppression is false. Thought suppression represents attempt to strike the thoughts from one's mind, which cannot be done if one is truly examining the validity of the thought.

ACT attempts to weaken the connection between thoughts and emotions with adaptive behavior and to avoid strengthening cognitions by using diffusion. In diffusion a person attempts to have a nonjudgmental acceptance attitude towards their thoughts and emotions, recognizing them as nothing more or nothing less than thoughts and emotions, and to avoid any attempt to change or fix them. By being present in the moment and noticing thoughts as "just a thought," patients can focus on the overt behaviors that the patient can do that are consistent with their goals. Producing such behaviors becomes more probable when people defuse or distance themselves from the experience of the thought rather than struggle to change it. Notice however, that this commonly used phrase in ACT, "Your experiences are JUST thoughts." conveys that the thoughts in question are unlikely to be true. One might therefore ask if this type of response is in fact a subtle disputation of the thought. We think so.

We question whether the analogy of challenging thoughts as being similar to the White Bear effect and whether labeling challenging beliefs as thought suppression is accurate. As referenced above, much research supports the efficacy of challenging negative automatic thoughts and irrational beliefs and has helped many patients because it gets them to stop believing these thoughts and beliefs. We think diffusion represents an alternative means of changing the believability of thoughts and helps people behave more flexibly and in line with their goals not a replacement for challenging thoughts. Much of the criticism of traditional CBT by ACT-affiliated therapists has been aimed at the challenging of the negative automatic thoughts, and we are not aware of this criticism being aimed at changing the evaluative or demanding beliefs targeted in REBT. REBT challenges and disputes irrational beliefs and teaches patients to replace them with rational ones. It is therefore important to note that the targets of REBT challenges are the evaluative and imperative beliefs not the veracity of reality statements. ACT has been less specific if its criticism of cognitive challenges apply equally to REBT.

Acceptance as a Therapeutic Processes ACT shares with REBT the importance of acceptance. However, our reading of the ACT literature and attending conference presentations indicates that, as with DBT that we will discuss below, acceptance in ACT primarily focuses on accepting internal stimuli of thoughts and emotions. Not much mention is made in the ACT literature on accepting the external reality of the world or the behavior of others. This does not mean that accepting the world and others would be antithetical to ACT; it just does not appear to be as important or explicit as it is in REBT.

Philosophical Foundations ACT takes a definitive stand on epistemology and the nature of arguments to determine truth. ACT is based on the pragmatic philosophy of functional contextualism proposed by philosopher Stephen Pepper (1942). This position stresses that the only evidence needed to determine a meaningful conclusion is practicality, or whether an idea works to help one achieve one's goals. REBT uses a three pronged approach to challenge beliefs that includes (1) an idea is logically consistent, (2) is consistent with empirical reality, and (3) it is functional and helps one achieve one's goals. Only the last of these is considered important in functional contextualism. One is left with the thought that truth is totally relative and if something works for the individual, it is true for that person. Thus, a world view that advocated slavery, genocide, or coercion would be considered true if it worked for the individual. We think that functional contextualism is wanting in promoting a moral philosophy.

This focus on practicality is consistent with ACT's pragmatic truth criterion and in contrast to CBT's correspondence truth criterion, which would place more emphasis on challenging the empirical reality of negative automatic thoughts, or to use empirical disputes against demands and musts. It is not important within ACT if an idea corresponds to something called "reality – whatever that means" – but whether it works. Thus, viability, not veracity as understood in a correspondence theory of truth, is the touchstone of evidence.

Position on Construction and Responsibility in Human Emotion ACT's foundation in behaviorism would lead it to conclude that people are not responsible for their disturbance. People's history of exposure to stimuli and reinforcers create who we are. Thus, ACT would be opposed to the constructivist philosophy that is present in many aspects of cognitive psychotherapies.

Specificity and Parsimony of Theory and Disorder-Specific Treatment Like REBT, ACT is a transdiagnostic therapy that focuses on processes and functional relationships rather than disorders. Hayes argued that significant strides in clinical treatments can only occur when we understand the underlying mechanisms involved in clinical problems. Hayes' research has aimed at understanding basic mechanisms of human disturbance. ACT is a transdiagnostic treatment because the same functional relationships are thought to apply across the problems that are defined as mental disorders. The processes of acceptance and diffusion are always the same because ACT views being disturbed about anything occurs in the same way, namely emotional avoidance and cognitive fusion. The differences in an ACT treatment of different patients would be in the new behaviors that they patient would work to increase. These behaviors are based on the patient's values and goals and thus it is appropriate that they would differ by patient.

Applicability to Problems of Everyday Living and Happiness Like REBT and differing from CT, ACT concerns itself with problems of everyday living, personal meaning, and satisfaction. Although less concerned about the pursuit of happiness than the pursuit of personal meaning, ACT argues for embracing the discomfort involved when one tries to live in a way that is consistent with their valued life. The procedures used in ACT to treat disturbance would be the same in pursuing a more meaningful satisfactory life.

Hayes promotes the pursuit of one's values in order to achieve a meaningful life. Unlike Ellis who showed that individuals have a good degree of choice in the beliefs they held, the feelings and behaviors that went along with these beliefs, as well as the paths they took to find happiness and meaning Hayes focused his attention mainly on the behaviors consistent with living a meaningful life. REBT also stresses a fulfilling and meaningful life. ACT does this as well. We think that these theories both distinguish between short term pleasurable goals, being happy in a more enduring way, and long term goals, seeking meaning and fulfillment; and they consider the long term goals of meaning and fulfillment as being more important. They both seem to recognize that achieving fulfillment and meaning in the long-run requires one to do things that are painful or uncomfortable in the short-run.

REBT and DBT

Linehan's (1993) DBT emerged from her work with patients with serious histories of suicidal ideation and attempts, and acts of non-suicidal self-injurious behavior, who often met criteria for Borderline Personality Disorder (BPD). Linehan observed that traditional CBT that targeted negative automatic thoughts and cognitive distortions was often ineffective with these patients and resulted in unacceptably high dropout rates. Linehan noted that these patients found the targeting of negative thoughts invalidating due to the constant focus on change and lack of empathy and failure to acknowledge their degree of pain or the occurrence of negative life events. They often responded to treatment with anger and/or withdrawal. In addition to the problem of attendance, the severity and quantity of the problems experienced by these patients made it impossible for therapists to adequately address each problem *and* teach the necessary adaptive skills to the patients. Thus, Linehan's goal was to modify the traditional CBT approach. It should be noted that many of these changes had already been incorporated into REBT and represented elements of Eastern and Western philosophy. These included promoting unconditional acceptance and validation of patients (Ellis, 1957). In addition, she developed a system of treatment that includes individual psychotherapy, structured skills training, and strategies that reduced any behaviors that interfered with therapy.

Philosophical Foundations DBT developed from the roots of traditional CBT. Linehan hoped to better adapt and enhance CBT for multi-disordered, chronically suicidal patients. Thus, DBT, like REBT, and CT share many characteristics. These include a collaborative approach to therapy, teaching and practicing skills, and assigning homework for patients to complete between sessions. DBT is similar to CT in terms of adherence to a manualized treatment for a specific disorder. Unlike CT however, DBT is designed to treat individuals who have multiple comorbid disorders and places a great emphasis on the teaching and practicing of behavioral skills as a mechanism for change.

At the foundation of DBT is the dialectic philosophy that acknowledges that people can hold two contradictory ideas simultaneously. The central dialectic in DBT is the validation and acceptance of patients and their suffering while simultaneously encouraging them to change (Linehan & Schmidt, 1995). Failure to validate and acknowledge patients' suffering leads to their not believing they are understood, the development of a rupture in the therapeutic alliance, and anger at not being understood. Failure to encourage change results in continued suffering. DBT emphasizes that the synthesis of these opposites lead to replacement of rigid beliefs about the world. This is similar to REBT's view on rigid beliefs being at the core of disturbance – DBT and REBT aim to change rigid patterns of thinking.

Linehan (1993) stated that DBT focuses on dialectics and validation because many patients with BPD felt that the CT strategy of challenging negative automatic thoughts invalided and denied the difficulty that patients faced and the strong negative emotions they experienced. Validation of their experiences accepts that very negative things have happened to them, that they feel very strong negative emotions, and that these facts are accepted by their therapists and not challenged. The dialectic represents the possibility that one can acknowledge and cope with the very negative events and strong negative feelings. This core strategy of DBT is similar to the REBT strategy of not challenging negative automatic thoughts, but assuming that they are true, acknowledging them, and learning to cope with the negative reality by changing the evaluation and reaction to the harsh reality (Robins & Rosenthal, 2011).

Acceptance in DBT appears to focus more on the acceptance and tolerance of internal experiences such as dysregulated emotions, which is indistinguishable from the REBT concept of secondary disturbance (Ellis & Dryden, 1987, 1997) and tolerance of discomfort (Ellis, 2004). Some differences in acceptance do exist between REBT and DBT. REBT stresses that clients accept both the external world and the internal world, whereas DBT focuses more on accepting ones' internal experiences. However, the therapeutic stance of validating clients' reality is a form of acceptance of the external world.

As in both REBT and ACT, Linehan's DBT combines elements of Eastern philosophy (Ellis & Dryden, 1987, 1997) with more traditional elements of Western psychotherapy. In DBT, acceptance is achieved largely using mindfulness exercises, in addition to therapeutic strategies that promote validation and acceptance (Dimeff & Linehan, 2001). These philosophies focus on accepting what is and developing coping strategies with the world as we find it, and not attempting to change one's image of the world.

Position on Constructivism and Responsibility in Human Emotion Like Ellis, Linehan believed that individuals have the ability to change, grow, and learn to reduce their distress and to improve their quality of life. Like REBT's principle of emotional responsibility, DBT places the onus of change on the patient, but provides patients with a framework, support, and set of skills with which to make these changes. Within the context of a supportive, accepting, though often irreverent, therapist and consultation team, patients are encouraged to participate in skills training and strengthening, and psychotherapy to make changes that are more conducive to leading a meaningful life. Similar to REBT, DBT emphasizes the clients' capacity to change, and by helping them to understand this capacity and instill hope and optimism in their ability to improve their lives.

The means by which DBT accomplishes this, however, are substantially more directive and related to the higher dose than REBT. Whereas Ellis's approach focused on replacing absolute beliefs with rational beliefs, and acceptance of self, others, and life through psychotherapy and practice, DBT works to enhance dialectical thinking as a replacement for absolutistic thinking through a manualized, multi-stage, multi-component approach. DBT postulates that for patients to change and improve their quality of life, they must first learn (through structured skills-training groups and psychotherapy) the strategies with which to regulate their emotions, tolerate distress, and foster functional relationships.

An integral aspect of DBT is an increase in the dose of therapy. The treatment usually involves weekly therapy groups that teach emotional regulation skills, individual psychotherapy sessions, the opportunity for patients to have phone consultations with their therapists concerning how to use the skills, and meetings for the therapists to support each other and discuss their cases. This increase in dose recognizes that DBT was designed for those with serious disorders; inpatient therapy is costly, and usually is not available long enough to achieve noticeable results and the outpatient tradition of once a week sessions is not sufficient. DBT has recognized that the need to a gradation of treatment does and challenges traditional service delivery models.

Discomfort Disturbance and Biology Linehan adopted a biosocial theory of psychopathology for BPD. Specifically, DBT is based on the idea that at the core of disturbance is a continuous interplay between biological factors (which manifest in emotion dysregulation) and an invalidating social environment. This interplay results in each of these factors exacerbating the other and resulting in a patient's extreme emotion dysregulation and self-invalidation (two hallmark aspects of BPD). DBT proposes that patients need to be taught skills in a supportive environment to address and reduce the distressing symptoms that have occurred because of these biosocial interactions. In many ways, this is similar to Ellis's understanding of emotional and behavioral disturbance as stemming from both biological and environmental origins. In both REBT and DBT, the patient learns that experiencing and acknowledging the discomfort associated with both experiencing adversity and learning to cope with it are necessary for change and growth to occur.

DBT does not rely on cognitive interventions to help clients regulate their emotions. It proposes that emotional arousal can remain high and dysregulated without any cognitive distortions due to biological predispositions. DBT teaches clients to use self-soothing techniques. These are behaviors that provide a comforting, nurturing, kind, and gentle way to sooth their strong disturbed negative emotions. Although this use of self-soothing activities is not unique to DBT, it uses these techniques more frequently than other forms of CBT.

Specificity and Parsimony of Theory Much like REBT, DBT is specific and parsimonious in its view of the origins and mechanisms of disturbance. Both Ellis and Linehan believe that disturbance stems from the rigid beliefs and thought patterns that one has, and that this is at the core of disorders. REBT is guided by the idea of flexible and non-extreme beliefs replacing absolute and extreme ones. DBT is guided with the idea of flexible, dialectical thinking replacing dichotomous thought patterns. However, whereas REBT was designed for and has been effective in treating a broad range of disorders and severity levels in patients, DBT was designed for and has been implemented in the treatment of a much narrower and more specific scope of disorders. DBT is most applicable to severe and chronic disorders like BPD. Despite the many stages and components that comprise the DBT manualized treatments, both DBT and REBT are parsimonious in their theoretical framework and treatment goals. Both treatments aim to reduce symptoms that are causing an individual distress and interfering with their functioning, in order for them to live a more meaningful and fulfilling life.

Acceptance as a Therapeutic Process Similar to REBT and ACT, DBT relies heavily on the concept of acceptance. However, DBT also emphasizes that acceptance of the patient by the therapist is of vital importance in establishing an effective therapeutic alliance, and through this, therapists teach acceptance to the patient. In DBT, as in REBT, the concept of unconditional other-acceptance, the therapist's validation and acceptance of a patient's feelings and experiences is a core element of treatment. A fundamental tenet of DBT is that therapists simultaneously accept and validate patients as they are, while also encouraging their change and progress. DBT uses the term "radical acceptance" for encouraging global acceptance of self, life, and others, much like REBT. Patients are also encouraged to practice acceptance through mindfulness and attending to the present in a non-judgmental way, similar to Hayes's ACT. Rather than viewing thoughts as just thoughts to be examined as ACT suggests, DBT, and REBT, help patients learn to replace rigid and maladaptive thoughts with more adaptive ones, thereby actively working to change while simultaneously accepting themselves and their situations as they are.

Disorder Specific Treatment DBT was initially developed for treatment of individuals with chronic suicidality and extensive trauma histories, which was prominent in patients with a diagnosis of BPD. In this respect, DBT is a disorder-specific therapy. Although much of the research literature on DBT has focused on its effectiveness for treating BPD, DBT has also been shown to be effective in treating eating disorders and substance use disorders. Due largely to its conceptual origins, DBT is more a disorder-specific approach to treatment than REBT is. REBT is a more transdiagnostic approach that is applicable to a wide range of disorders and psychopathology. However, elements of DBT, such as dialectical thinking, assertiveness training, and validation seem to be transdiagnostic constructs that would be helpful in treating a variety of clinical problems and can be readily applied as a transdiagnostic treatment to other serious disorders beyond BPD.

Dosage of Therapy DBT differs from all other forms of psychotherapy in proscribing more and intensive interventions over the course of a week. DBT usually includes three aspects of treatment: (1) individual psychotherapy sessions, (2) skills training groups, (3) therapist consultation to help each of them deal with the difficulty in treating such a difficult population. It would be interesting to see the degree to which the dose effect accounts for the success of DBT with difficult to treat patients. Perhaps any form of CBT would be more effective with these patients if they were given in the same dosages. REBT and CT have long advocated skills building activities such as bibliotherapy, the use of homework forms to teach the challenging of beliefs, assertiveness training, problem-solving skills and in vivo activities. They just do not do it in such a systematized way as DBT does.

Applicability to Problems of Everyday Living and Happiness REBT and DBT both have the goal of improving a patient's quality of life and improving well-being through symptom reduction. Compared to DBT, REBT is far more readily applicable and able to address the more frequent, common, everyday problems that patients experience. In this way, REBT is perhaps the more versatile of the two therapies, being able to treat patients with severe psychopathology as well as those with sub-clinical symptoms that interfere with life functioning and satisfaction.

Conclusions

This chapter examined the similarities and differences of the four major CBT therapies popularly practiced today, namely Ellis's REBT, Beck's CT, Hayes's ACT, and Linehan's DBT. With the exception of Ellis's REBT all the subsequent CBT therapies were cultivated in academic environments and were developed subsequent to REBT. All share many similarities such as having a problem focused therapeutic agenda, emphasis on the role cognition plays in emotional and behavioral disturbance, the development of alternative ways of thinking or behaving to either reduce symptomatology or cope with external reality. Despite the many similarities one should take note of the very important differences, which were discussed throughout this chapter and in our view, gives REBT a distinct advantage over the other CBT approaches that followed in its footsteps. Given the similarities of the other therapies that we identified and discussed in this chapter, as well as the prominence of Ellis and his revolutionary views, these subsequent CBT therapies have inadequately acknowledged the influence of Ellis and the role his pioneering theoretical and clinical work has had. With this said it is also true to add that each has been strongly shaped by the individual who was the leading force in the development of their particular brand of CBT therapy. REBT stands alone in being the product of a master clinician who spent approximately 180,000 hours in face-to-face clinical contact treating patients. The other CBT therapies are somewhat more popular today because of their broader research base, which would be expected from therapies developed by theorists who had academic affiliations and were clinical scientists conducting randomized clinical trials on the therapy they were developing. REBT is the CBT approach that is the most versatile therapy when it comes to addressing both a wide range of emotional and behavioral disorders and problems of daily living. This is to be expected when one takes into consideration that Ellis, more than any of the other theorists, practiced the psychotherapy he carefully refined over the 60 years of a long clinical career.

References

Beck, A. T. (1976). *Cognitive therapy and the emotional disorders*. New York, NY: International University Press.

Beck, A. T., Emery, G., & Greenberg, R. L. (1985). *Anxiety disorders and phobias: A cognitive perspective*. New York, NY: Basic Books.

Beck, A. T., & Haigh, E. A. P. (2014). Advances in cognitive theory and therapy: The generic cognitive model. *Annual Review of Clinical Psychology, 10*, 1–24.

Beck, A. T., Rector, N. A., Stolar, N., & Grant, P. (2008). *Schizophrenia: Cognitive theory. Research, and therapy*. New York, NY: Guilford.

Beck, A. T., Wright, F., Newman, C., & Liese, B. (1993). *Cognitive therapy of substance abuse*. New York, NY: Guilford.

Bernard, M. E. (2011). *Rationality and the pursuit of happiness: The legacy of Albert Ellis*. Chichester, UK: Wiley-Blackwell.

Dimeff, L., & Linehan, M. M. (2001). Dialectical behavior therapy in a nutshell. *The California Psychologist, 34*(3), 10–13.

Disner, S. G., Beevers, C. G., Haigh, E. A. P., & Beck, A. T. (2011). Neural mechanisms of the cognitive model of depression. *Nature Reviews Neuroscience, 12*, 467–477.

Dryden, W. (2016). *Attitudes in rational emotive behaviour therapy: Components, characteristics and adversity related consequences*. London, UK: Rationality Publications.

Ellis, A. (1957). *How to live with a neurotic*. New York, NY: Crown Publishers.

Ellis, A. (1958). Rational psychotherapy. *Journal of General Psychology, 59*, 35–49.
Ellis, A. (1962). *Reason and emotion in psychotherapy*. New York, NY: Lyle Stuart.
Ellis, A. (1976). The biological basis of human irrationality. *Journal of Individual Psychology, 32*, 145–168.
Ellis, A. (1979a). Discomfort anxiety: A new cognitive-behavioral construct (Part 1). *Rational Living, 14*, 3–8.
Ellis, A. (1979b). The issue of force and energy in behavioral change. *Journal of Contemporary Psychotherapy, 10*(2), 83–97.
Ellis, A. (1993). Changing rational-emotive therapy (RET) to rational emotive behavior therapy (REBT). *Behavior Therapist, 16*, 257–258.
Ellis, A. (1994). *Reason and emotion in psychotherapy, revised and updated*. Secaucus, NJ: Carol Publishing Group.
Ellis, A. (2002). *Overcoming resistance – A rational emotive behavior therapy integrated approach* (2nd ed.). New York: Springer.
Ellis, A. (2004). *The road to tolerance*. Amherst, NY: Prometheus Books.
Ellis, A. (2005). *The myth of self-esteem: How REBT can change your life forever*. Amherst, NY: Prometheus Books.
Ellis, A., & Becker, I. (1982). *A guide to personal happiness*. North Hollywood, CA: Wilshire.
Ellis, A., & Dryden, W. (1987). *The practice of rational-emotive behavior therapy*. New York, NY: Springer.
Ellis, A., Young, J., & Lockwood, G. (1987). Cognitive therapy and rational-emotive therapy: A dialogue. *Journal of Cognitive Psychotherapy, 1*(4), 137–187.
Ellis, A., & Dryden, W. (1997). *The practice of rational emotive behavior therapy* (2nd ed.). New York, NY: Springer.
Feldman-Barret, L. (2017). *How emotions are made*. New York: Houghton Mifflin Harcourt.
Feldman Barrett, L., Lewis, M., & Haviland-Jones, J. M. (2018). *Handbook of emotions* (4th ed.). New York, NY: Guilford.
Flaxman, P. E., Blackledge, J. T., & Bond, F. W. (2011). *Acceptance and commitment therapy: The CBT distinctive features series*. Oxon, UK: Routledge.
Follette, V. M., & Hazlett-Stevens, H. (2016). Mindfulness and acceptance therapies (pp. 273–302). In J. C. Norcross, G. R. VandenBos, & D. F. Freedheim (Eds.), *The handbook of clinical psychology. II of V: Theory and research*. Washington, DC: American Psychological Association. The Associate Editor for this volume II is Bunmi O. Olatunji.
Hayes, S. (Ed.). (1989). *Rule governed behavior*. New York, NY: Plenum.
Hayes, S.C., Strosahl, K. D., Wilson, K. G. (1999). *Acceptance and commitment therapy: An experiential approach to behavior change*. New York, NY: Guilford Press.
Hayes, S. C., Barnes-Holmes, D., & Roche, B. (Eds.). (2001). *Relational frame theory: A post-Skinnerian account of language and cognition*. New York, NY: Plenum.
Hofmann, S., Asnaani, A., Vonk, I., Sawyer, A., & Fang, A. (2012). The efficacy of cognitive behavioral therapy: A review of meta-analyses. *Cognitive Therapy & Research, 36*(5), 427–440. https://doi.org/10.1007/s10608-012-9476-1
Hofmann, S. G., Asmundson, G. J., & Beck, A. T. (2013). The science of cognitive therapy. *Behavior Therapy, 44*(2), 199–212. https://doi.org/10.1016/j.beth.2009.01.007
Hyland, P., & Boduszek, D. (2012). Resolving a difference between cognitive therapy and rational emotive behaviour therapy: Towards the development of an integrated CBT model of psychopathology. *Mental Health Review Journal, 17*(2), 104–116.
Korzybski, A. (1958). *Science and sanity: An introduction to non-Aristotelian systems and general semantics* (4th ed.). Lakeville, CT: The International Non-Aristotelian Library Publishing Co. (now part of the I. G. S., Englewood, NJ).
Korzybski, A. (1933). *Science and sanity*. San Francisco, CA: the International Society of General Semantics.

Linehan, M. M. (1993). *Cognitive–behavioral therapy of borderline personality disorders*. New York, NY: Guilford Press.
Linehan, M. M., & Schmidt, H. (1995). The dialectics of effective treatment of borderline personality disorder. In W. T. O'Donohue & L. Krasner (Eds.), *Theories of behavior therapy: Exploring behavior change* (pp. 553–584). Washington, DC: American Psychological Association.
Morris, W. E., & Brown, C. R. (2017, Spring). David Hume, In E. N. Zalta (Ed.), *The Stanford encyclopedia of philosophy* (Spring 2017 Edition). https://plato.stanford.edu/cgi-bin/encyclopedia/archinfo.cgi?entry=hume
Padesky, C. (1994). Schema change processes in cognitive therapy. *Clinical Psychology and Psychotherapy, 1*(5), 267–278.
Pepper, S. C. (1942). *World hypotheses: A study in evidence*. Berkeley, CA: University of California Press.
Popper, K. (1959). *The logic of scientific discovery*. New York, NY: Harper & Bros.
Popper, K. (1972). *Objective knowledge; an evolutionary approach*. Oxford, UK. Clarendon Press.
Ruggiero, G. M., Spada, M. M., Caselli, G., & Sassaroli, S. (2018). A historical and theoretical review of cognitive behavioral therapies: From structural self-knowledge to functional processes. *Journal of rational Emotive and Cognitive Behavior Therapies, 36*, 378–403.
Skinner, B. F. (1957). *Verbal behavior*. New York, NY: Prentice Hall.
Swales, M. A., & Heard, H. L. (2017). *Dialectical behavior therapy* (The CBT distinctive features series) (2nd ed.). Oxon, UK: Routledge.
Vîslă, A., Flückiger, C., Grosse Holtforth, M., & David, D. (2016). Irrational beliefs and psychological distress: A meta-analysis. *Psychotherapy and Psychosomatics, 85*(1), 8–15. https://doi.org/10.1159/000441231
Wampold, B. E., & Imel, Z. E. (2015). *The great psychotherapy debate*: The evidence for what makes psychotherapy work, 2nd ed. New York, NY: Routledge/Taylor & Francis Group.
Wegner, D. M., & Schneider, D. J. (2003). The white bear story. *Psychological Inquiry, 14*, 326–329. https://doi.org/10.1207/s15327965pli1403&4_24
Wolpe, J. (1958). *Psychotherapy by reciprocal inhibition*. Palo Alto, CA: Stanford University.
Zettle, R., & Hayes, S. (1980). Conceptual and empirical status of rational emotive therapy. *Progress in Behavior Modification, 9*, 125–166.

Chapter 4
The Measurement of Irrationality and Rationality

Daniel O. David, Raymond DiGiuseppe, Anca Dobrean, Costina Ruxandra Păsărelu, and Robert Balazsi

Introduction

Rational Emotive Behavior Therapy (REBT) assumes that when people are faced with adverse, activating events, their irrational beliefs generate dysfunctional feelings and maladaptive behaviors, while their rational beliefs generate functional feelings and adaptive behaviors (Ellis, 1994).

Generally speaking, irrational beliefs are beliefs, which have no logical, empirical, and/or functional support, while rational beliefs are beliefs, which have logical, empirical, and/or functional support. Rational and irrational beliefs can be defined generally as cognitive errors/distortions and beliefs or they can be defined more narrowly (Ellis, 1977). In the general view of beliefs, rational and

D. O. David (✉)
Department of Clinical Psychology and Psychotherapy, The International Institute for the Advanced Studies of Psychotherapy and Applied Mental Health, Babeş-Bolyai University, Cluj-Napoca, Romania

Icahn School of Medicine at Mount Sinai, New York, NY, USA
e-mail: danieldavid@psychology.ro

R. DiGiuseppe
Department of Psychology, St. John's University, Jamaica, NY, USA
e-mail: digiuser@stjohns.edu

A. Dobrean · C. R. Păsărelu
Department of Clinical Psychology and Psychotherapy, The International Institute for the Advanced Studies of Psychotherapy and Applied Mental Health, Babeş-Bolyai University, Cluj-Napoca, Romania
e-mail: anca.dobrean@ubbcluj.ro; costinapasarelu@psychology.ro

R. Balazsi
Department of Psychology, Babeş-Bolyai University, Cluj-Napoca, Romania
e-mail: robertbalazsi@psychology.ro

© Springer Nature Switzerland AG 2019

M. E. Bernard, W. Dryden (eds.), *Advances in REBT*,
https://doi.org/10.1007/978-3-319-93118-0_4

irrational beliefs include descriptions/inferences (i.e., cold cognitions) and their evaluations (i.e., hot cognitions) (see David, 2003; Wessler, 1982). By way of contrast, REBT (Ellis, 1977) proposed four irrational beliefs processes – which do not have logical, empirical, and functional support – and their counterpart rational beliefs processes, which have logical, empirical, and functional support. In this REBT view, rational and irrational beliefs refer only to evaluations/appraisal. The REBT irrational beliefs processes are demandingness (i.e., inflexible/rigid/absolutistic thinking), catastrophizing/awfulizing, frustration intolerance/low frustration tolerance, and global evaluation of self, other, and/or life. The alternative REBT rational beliefs processes are preferences (i.e., flexible/accepting thinking), badness, frustration tolerance/high frustration tolerance, and unconditional self, other, and/or life acceptance. While demandingness and preferences are primary beliefs, the other rational and irrational beliefs mentioned above are according to Ellis derivatives, more proximally related to various emotional and behavioral consequences.

Irrational beliefs (IBs) and rational beliefs (RBs) represent the core conceptual elements of Rational Emotive Behavioral Therapy (Ellis, 1994) that contribute to emotional and behavioral disturbance. Therefore, investigations into the mechanisms involved in the etiology of emotional disturbance, requires that irrational and rational beliefs are assessed rigorously, accurately, using instruments with sound psychometric properties.

A brief history of irrational beliefs assessment begins with the development of self-report instruments in accordance to Ellis' (1962) original list of 11 irrational beliefs. Initially, almost all the assessment instruments (Bessai, 1977; Jones, 1968; Malouff & Schutte, 1986; Newmark, Ann Frerking, Cook, & Newmark, 1973; Shorkey & Whiteman, 1977) were developed in accordance with these beliefs, most of them containing only one item for each belief (Macavei & McMahon, 2010). A major limitation of these instruments resides in the fact that the items did not reflect pure cognitive content (e.g., irrational beliefs), as many questions in these instruments were confounded by reference to emotional states (Smith, 1989). The mixture of cognitive and emotional items from those instruments was extremely problematic in terms of discriminant validity (Smith & Zurawski, 1983). Furthermore, another problem of the incipient measures of irrationality was the fact that they did not contain items formulated differently for rational and irrational beliefs, but almost exclusively assessed only irrational beliefs. Rationality scores were computed as the reverse of the irrationality scores. This is a major shortcoming of these instruments given the fact that (a) REBT theory assigns different roles for rational (e.g. support functional feelings and adaptive behaviors) and irrational beliefs (e.g., support dysfunctional feelings and maladaptive behaviors), (b) empirical evidence shows that higher scores on rational beliefs do not imply lower scores on irrational beliefs (Bernard, 1998) and (c) The distinction between cognitive processes and content areas is another limitation of the previously developed instruments for the assessment (David, Szentagotai, Kallay, & Macavei, 2005).

In an attempt to overcome these limitations in the assessment of irrational beliefs, several instruments have been developed (DiGiuseppe, Leaf, Gorman, & Robin, 2017; Hyland, Shevlin, Adamson, & Boduszek, 2014; Lindner, Kirkby, Wertheim, & Birch, 1999; Mogoase, Stefan, & David, 2013), that take into consideration: (a) the contamination problems (e.g., the newly developed instruments contained only cognitive items), (b) the separate assessment of rational and irrational beliefs (e.g., providing items that tackled either rational or irrational beliefs, offering separate subscales for rational and irrational beliefs) and (c) distinguish between cognitive processes and areas of content.

The assessment of irrational and rational beliefs is essential for evaluating the efficacy of REBT interventions, and to estimate accurately the relationship between irrational and rational beliefs and other constructs (e.g., distress). For instance, Vîslă, Flückiger, Holtforth, and David (2016) conducted a meta-analysis on the relationship between irrational beliefs and distress and demonstrated that the specific irrational beliefs assessment instruments used in the studies were a significant moderator of the relationship between IBs and emotional outcomes (e.g., anxiety and depression). The contamination of some items that overestimate the relationship between irrational beliefs and distress and the high reliabilities of several scales appeared to account for this moderation effect. Another important moderator that Vîslă et al. (2016) found was the developer/validator status of an author of the assessment instrument, which leads to smaller effect sizes. Namely, smaller effect sizes resulted for the association between irrational beliefs and anger or depression when the author of an article was also the developer/validator of an irrational beliefs scale.

Considerable debate exists in the literature concerning which is the best instrument to assess irrational beliefs (Hyland et al., 2017). An important aspect that has not been investigated in previous reviews of irrational beliefs assessment is the existence of self-reported instruments developed for specific populations or persons with specific disorders or clinical problems in addition to assessing general irrational beliefs and their psychometric properties.

This chapter presents available instruments designed for the assessment of IBs and rational beliefs as defined in REBT, as well as the existent research concerning their psychometric properties. First of all, concepts such as reliability, validity, diagnostic accuracy, responsiveness, and the close relationship between these psychometric concepts and clinical practice will be discussed. Then, self-report instruments that assess general irrational beliefs or specific cognitive irrational processes, as well as instruments designed for specific populations (e.g., women, parents, children, teachers), or specific content irrational beliefs scales (e.g., heath-related, academic performance-related), together with the empirical support will be presented in the corresponding section. Other means of assessing irrational beliefs, such as content analysis, or behavioral analog tasks will be discussed. One sub-section focuses on the individualized assessment of irrational beliefs (e.g., personalizing assessment according to patient's unique characteristics, such as religion, or culture). Finally, future directions of research in the evidence-based assessment of irrationality are presented in the last section of this chapter.

Psychometric Characteristics of Clinical Measurement Instruments

Clinical measures must have strong psychometric evidence (Hunsley & Mash, 2008), the most important of which are high, or at least acceptable reliability, validity, and responsiveness. When choosing a measurement instrument, clinical researchers most often focus only on reliability and validity, while responsiveness is frequently an ignored psychometric attribute (Bagozzi, 1981). Reliability as a psychometric characteristic of a scale quantifies the degree of non-systematic error contained in a clinical score and usually is expressed by indicators such as internal consistency, test-retest reliability, and inter-rater agreement. Higher reliability means more consistent scores over time or across different raters. According to the existing standards, instruments used clinically should have internal consistency coefficient (estimated by Cronbach's Coefficient) of 0.80 or above, test-retest coefficient at least between 0.75 and 0.85 and inter-rater agreement (estimated by intra-class correlation coefficient or Kappa coefficient, depending on the measurement scale, interval or categorical) above 0.70 (Baer & Blais, 2010). Reliability is a necessary, but not a sufficient, psychometric property of useful clinical scale. Validity refers to the degree of correspondence between what a scale actually measure and what it was intended to measure. According to this standard, scales of irrationality will be considered to have high validity only if they truly measure irrational beliefs and no other marginally or unrelated constructs to these. The types of validity are content validity, criterion validity, and construct validity (Foster & Cone, 1995). Content validity of a scale represents the extent to which the items of the scale express all relevant aspects of the measured construct. Distinct from criterion and construct-related validity, content validity is not directly estimated. Usually, it involves agreement among expert raters regarding how important a particular item is from the perspective of the measured theoretical concept (Haynes, Richard, & Kubany, 1995). Criterion (concurrent and predictive) and construct (convergent and discriminant) related validity are all expressed as a correlation coefficient between scale/subscale score and: (a) other scales that measure the same construct (concurrent validity), (b) future behavior (predictive validity), (c) other scales that measure related constructs (convergent validity) and, (d) other scales that measure different constructs (discriminant validity) (Borsboom, Mellenbergh, & van Heerden, 2004).

Self-report Instruments that Assess Irrational Beliefs

Table 4.1 describes the instruments included in this chapter and their psychometric properties.

Table 4.1 Characteristics of irrationality instruments included

Name of the instrument, acronym and authors	No. of items	Scales/subscales	Population	Reliability	Validity
Jones Irrational Beliefs Test (IBT; Jones, 1968)	100	10 subscales (Demand for approval, High self-expectations, Blame-proneness, Frustration Reactivity. Emotional irresponsibility, Anxious overconcern, Problem avoidance, Dependency, Helplessness, and Perfectionism)	Adults	α between 0.45 and 0.72 Test-retest (1 day) = 0.92[a]	No support the divergent validity relative to anxiety and depression; Convergent validity with RBI (Smith & Zurawski, 1983)
The Rational Behavior Inventory (RBI; Shorkey & Whiteman, 1977)	38	11 subscales (Catastrophizing, Guilt, Perfectionism, Need for approval, Caring and helping, Blame and punishment, Inertia and avoidance, Independence, Self-downing, Projected misfortune, and Control of emotions)	Adults Youth	$\alpha = .86$[a]; α between −0.01 and 0.43[b]; test-retest 3 days = 0.82[a]; test-retest at 10 days = 0.71[a]	Limited divergent validity (when separating emotional and non-emotional items, there were very small correlations with distress; Kienhorst, van den Bout, & de Wilde, 1993); Mixed support for convergent validity (small correlations with IBT)
The Irrational Belief Questionnaire (IBQ; Newmark et al., 1973)	11	Irrational beliefs (corresponding to Ellis originally identified beliefs)	Adults	$\alpha = 0.85$[a]	Not investigated
The Common Beliefs Survey III (CBS; Bessai, 1977)	54	6 subscales (Perfectionism, Self-downing, Need for approval, Blame proneness, Importance of the past, Control of emotions)	Adults	$\alpha = 0.85$[a] (Thorpe, Parker, & Barnes, 1992)	Convergent - Correlated with other measures of cognitions (SSASI) (Thorpe et al., 1992); Divergent validity (with scales that assess emotions)
The Idea Inventory (II; Kassinove, Crisci, & Tiegerman, 1977)	33	11 subscales corresponding to Ellis originally identified beliefs	Youths	$\alpha = 0.59$[a] Test-retest (4–6 weeks) between 0.81 and 0.87	Moderate divergent validity with neuroticism

(continued)

Table 4.1 (continued)

Name of the instrument, acronym and authors	No. of items	Scales/subscales	Population	Reliability	Validity
The Belief Scale (BS; Malouff & Schutte, 1986)	20	Irrational beliefs	Adults	$\alpha = 0.80$[a] Test-retest at 2 weeks = 0.89	Convergent validity (correlated with IBT); Divergent validity - negative correlations with measures of social desirability (Malouff & Schutte, 1986), positive correlations with depression scores and with neuroticism; Warren and Zgourides (1989); Treatment sensibility
The Common Belief Inventory for Students (CBIS; Hooper & Layne, 1983)	45	Irrationality 11 subscales corresponding to Ellis originally identified beliefs	Youths	$\alpha = 0.85$[a] Test-retest reliability over 6 weeks ($r = 0.84$)	Treatment sensibility (changes in irrational beliefs after an RBT education program)
The Attitudes and Belief Inventory (ABI: Burgess, 1986, 1990)	48	13 subscales (Demandingncss, Awfulizing, Low frustration tolerance,Global worth, Approval, Success, Comfort, Rational, Irrational, Self-referential, Non-self-referential, Focused, Unfocused)	Adults	α between 0.84 and 0.95[b] (DiGiuseppe & Leaf, 1990)	Discriminant validity (participants from the clinical sample endorsed more irrational beliefs than non-clinical participants)
The Attitudes and Belief Scale 2 (ABS-2; DiGiuseppe et al., 2017)	72 items	Global Irrationality Score Irrationality, Rationality 4 Cognitive Processes domains (Demandingness, Awfulizing, Frustration Intolerance, Global evaluations of human worth, either of the self or others) 3 Content domains (Affiliation, Achievement, Comfort)	Adults	$\alpha = 0.97$[a], α between 0.83 and 0.97[b]	Convergent validity (correlated with other measures of dysfunctional thinking); Divergent validity (Correlated with measures of anxiety, affective disorders, alcohol dependence, and thought disorders); Discriminates between clinical and non-clinical samples

The Abbreviated Version of the Attitudes and Belief Scale 2 (AV-ABS2; Hyland et al., 2014)	24	4 irrational belief processes (Demandingness, Catastrophizing, Frustration Intolerance, Self-downing), 4 rational belief processes (Preferences, Realistic evaluation of badness, Frustration tolerance, and Self-acceptance)	Adults	Composite reliability = 0.32–0.78[b]	Not investigated
The General Attitude and Belief Scale (GABS; Bernard, 1998)	55	7 subscales (Need for Approval, Need for Achievement, Need for Comfort, Self-Downing, Other-Downing, Demands for Fairness, and Rationality)	Adults	$\alpha > 0.80$[a,b]	Divergent validity (correlated with measures of emotional distress and with measures of life satisfaction)
The Shortened General Attitude and Belief Scale (SGABS; Lindner et al., 1999)	26	8 subscales (Irrationality, Rationality, Need for achievement, Need for comfort, Self-downing, Other-downing, Need for approval, Demand for fairness)	Adults	Test-retest (3 days) = 0.91[a], between 0.65 and 0.87[b] α between 0.77 and 0.85[b]	Convergent & divergent validity (Stronger correlations with others measures of irrationality than with measures of psychological distress)
The Survey of Personal Beliefs (SPB; Demaria, Kassinove, & Dill, 1989)	50	5 subscales (Self-directed shoulds, Other-directed shoulds, Awfulizing beliefs, Low frustration tolerance, and Self-worth)	Adults	$\alpha = 0.89$[a], between 0.57 and 0.72[b] Test-retest at 21 days = 0.87[a], between 0.65 and 0.87[b]	Convergent & divergent validity - higher correlations with a measure of irrationality than with measures of depression, hopelessness, and anxiety (Nottingham, 1992)
The Ellis Emotional Efficiency Inventory (EEEI; Ellis, 1992)	60	3 factors (Anti-awfulizing, Anti-self-downing and Anti-low frustration tolerance)	Adults	$\alpha = 0.72$	Divergent validity (correlated with measures of the domains of the five-factor personality model; Blau, Fuller, & Vaccaro, 2006)
The Evaluative Beliefs Scale (EBS; Chadwick, Trower, & Dagnan, 1999)	18	3 subscales (Self-self statements, Other-self statements, Self-other statements)	Adults	α between 0.86 and 0.92[b]	Divergent validity (Other-self and self-self negative evaluations, but not self-other, correlated with measures depression and anxiety)

(continued)

Table 4.1 (continued)

Name of the instrument, acronym and authors	No. of items	Scales/subscales	Population	Reliability	Validity
The Unconditional Self-Acceptance Questionnaire (USAQ; Chamberlain & Haaga, 2001)	20	Unconditional self-acceptance	Adults	$\alpha = 0.72$[a]	Poor discriminant validity – highly positively correlated with a measure of self-esteem; negatively correlated with measures of anxiety and depression (Chamberlain & Haaga, 2001)
Unconditional Acceptance Questionnaire (UAQ; D. David, Cotet, Szentagotai, McMahon, & DiGiuseppe, 2013)	34	Unconditional acceptance	Adults	$\alpha = 0.95$[a]	Convergent validity (positively correlated with other measures of unconditional acceptance and negatively correlated with a measure of self-esteem; David et al., 2013); Divergent validity (UAQ negatively associated with distress, automatic thoughts, and irrational beliefs)
The Rational and Irrational Beliefs Scale (RAIBS; Mogoase et al., 2013)	44	2 subscales (Rational, Irrational)	Adults	α between 0.87 and 0.94[b]	Convergent (correlated with ABS2) & divergent validity (correlated with general distress, with functional/dysfunctional emotions)
The O'Kelly Women's Belief Scales (O'Kelly, 2011)	92	5 subscales (Demandingness, Awfulizing, Low Frustration Tolerance, Self-Downing, and General Traditional Belief)	Adults	Test-retest between 0.79 and 0.91 $\alpha = 0.95$[a], α between 0.75 and 0.84[b]	Convergent (correlated with other instruments measuring attitudes and schemas); Divergent validity (not associations with extroversion)
The Child and Adolescent Scale of Irrationality (CASI; Bernard & Cronan, 1999)	49	Self-downing, Intolerance of frustrating rules, Intolerance of work frustration and Demands for fairness	Youths	$\alpha = 0.92$[a]; α between 0.62 and 0.86[b]	Divergent validity (correlations with measures of emotions and behavioral problems)

The Parent Irrational Beliefs – Revised (PIB; Joyce, 1995)	24	3 subscales (Low Frustration Tolerance, Demandingness, and Self Worth)	Adults	$\alpha = 0.75$[a]	Discriminant validity (correlated with emotional measures); Treatment sensibility (changes in several subscales correlated with changes in measures of emotions); no significant correlation between the Demandingness subscale and measures of emotions
Parent rational and irrational scale (P-RIBS; Gavița, David, DiGiuseppe, & DelVecchio, 2011)	24	3 subscales (Rational beliefs, Irrational beliefs, Global evaluation)	Adults	α between 0.71 and 0.83[b]; α 0.73[a] Test-retest = 0.78	Convergent (correlated with GABS, USAQ) & divergent validity (correlated with parent distress)
The Teacher Irrational Belief Scale (TIBS; Bernard, 1988, 2016)	25	4 subscales (Self-downing, Authoritarianism, Demands for Justice, and Low Frustration Tolerance)	Adults	$\alpha = 0.85$[a], α between 0.70 and 0.78[b] (Bernard, 2016) Test-retest = 0.80[a] between 0.64 and 0.79 (Bora, Bernard, Trip, Decsei-Radu, & Chereji, 2009)	Moderate convergent validity with ABS2 (Bora et al., 2009) Divergent validity (with stress) (Bernard, 2016); Treatment sensitivity (Ugwoke et al., 2017)
The Employee Rational and Irrational Beliefs Scale (E-RIBS; Gavița & Duță, 2013)	30	3 subscales (Rational beliefs, Irrational beliefs, Global evaluation)	Adults	$\alpha = 0.74$[a], α between 0.70 and 0.83[b]	Convergent validity (correlated with GABS-SF subscales); Divergent validity (Correlated with measures of total emotional distress, dysfunctional negative emotions, anxious and depressed mood)
The Manager Rational and Irrational Beliefs Scale (M-RIBS; O. A. David, 2013)	30	3 subscales (Rational beliefs, Irrational beliefs, Global evaluation)	Adults	$\alpha = 0.76$[a]	Convergent validity (correlated with GABS subscales)

(continued)

Table 4.1 (continued)

Name of the instrument, acronym and authors	No. of items	Scales/subscales	Population	Reliability	Validity
The Work-Related Irrational Beliefs Questionnaire (WIB-Q; van Wijhe, Peeters, & Schaufeli, 2013)	20	4 subscales (Performance demands, Co-workers' approval, Failure, and Control)	Adults	α between 0.77 and 0.83[b]	Divergent validity (correlated with measures of negative emotions and workaholism)
The irrational food beliefs scale (IFB; Osberg, Poland, Aguayo, & MacDougall, 2008)	57	2 subscales (Irrational food beliefs, Rational food beliefs)	Adults	α between 0.74 and 0.89[b]	Divergent validity (scores were only weakly to moderately related to various dimensions of psychopathology)
Irrational performance beliefs inventory (iPBI; Turner et al., 2016)	28	4 subscales (Primary irrational beliefs, Low-frustration tolerance, Awfulizing, and Depreciation subscale)	Adults	α between 0.90 and 0.96[b]	Convergent (correlated with SGABS subscales) and divergent validity (correlated with measures of anger, anxiety, and depression)
The Exam-Related Beliefs Scale (EBS; Montgomery, David, Dilorenzo, & Schnur, 2007)	8	2 subscales (Rational beliefs, Irrational beliefs)	Adults	$\alpha = 0.74$[a]	Divergent validity (correlated with distress and response expectancies)

Note. [a]alpha Cronbach computed for the total scale, [b]alpha Cronbach for subscales, *GABS-SF* General Attitudes and Beliefs Scale–Short Form, *RET* rational emotive therapy

General Irrational Beliefs Assessment Instruments

Scales Assessing' Original Model of Irrational Beliefs

Many of the earlier instruments attempted to assess these 11 irrational beliefs and had subscales that corresponded to these categories. The beliefs included factual errors, demands, catastrophizing statements, condemnations of the self and others, and a lack of endurance and/or perseverance. Ellis (1977) changed his theory and proposed that absolutistic thinking and rigidity thinking, called demandingness, represented the core or central cognitive processes underlying psychopathology. *Demandingness* as expressed in words such as "*Must,*" "*Should,*" "*Demand,*" or "*Ought*" to do something, think something, or feel something. Ellis' revised theory proposed that three other irrational beliefs *Awfulizing* (AWF), *Low Frustration Tolerance* (now called *Frustration Intolerance*), and *Global Evaluations of Human Worth* concerning the self or others were derivatives of demandingness. Measures of irrational and rational beliefs differ in the types of beliefs they measure -either the original 11 irrational beliefs or the more recent conceptualization of the four cognitive processes.

Scales included in this category are: *Jones Irrational Beliefs Test* (IBT; Jones, 1968), *The Rational Behavior Inventory* (RBI; Shorkey & Whiteman, 1977), *The Irrational Belief Questionnaire* (IBQ; (Newmark et al., 1973), *The Common Beliefs Survey III* (CBS; Bessai, 1977), *The Idea Inventory* (II; Kassinove et al., 1977), *The Belief Scale* (Malouff & Schutte, 1986) and *The Common Belief Inventory for Students* (CBIS; Hooper & Layne, 1983).

Scales Assessing Ellis' Revised Theory of Four Cognitive Processes

Below, we consider scales that reflect Ellis's (1977) revised theory and categorized irrational beliefs into the four cognitive processes of demandingness, awfulizing, frustration intolerance and global evaluations of human worth.

The scales included in this category are:

- *The Attitudes and Belief Inventory* (ABI: Burgess, 1986, 1990)
- *The Attitudes and Belief Scale 2* (ABS-2; DiGiuseppe et al., 2017)
- *The Abbreviated Version of the Attitudes and Belief Scale 2* (AV-ABS2; Hyland et al., 2014)
- *The General Attitude and Belief Scale* (GABS; Bernard, 1998)
- *The Shortened General Attitude and Belief Scale* (SGABS; Lindner et al., 1999)
- *The Survey of Personal Beliefs* (SPB; Demaria et al., 1989), with two abbreviated forms, namely a 30-items SPB (Flett, Hewitt, & Cheng, 2008) and a 12-item SPB (Watson, Simmons, Weathington, O'Leary, & Culhane, 2009)
- *The Irrational Beliefs Inventory* (IBI; Koopmans, Sanderman, Timmerman, & Emmelkamp, 1994)
- *The Ellis Emotional Efficiency Inventory* (EEEI; Ellis, 1992)
- *The Evaluative Beliefs Scale* (EBS; Chadwick et al., 1999)

Scales Assessing Specific Cognitive Irrational Processes Scales included in this category are: *the Unconditional Self-Acceptance Questionnaire* (USAQ; Chamberlain & Haaga, 2001), the *Unconditional Acceptance Questionnaire* (UAQ; (D. David et al., 2013), and *the Rational and Irrational Beliefs Scale* (RAIBS; Mogoase et al., 2013).

Scales for Specific Populations

In this category, we included scales developed specifically for:

- *Women. The O'Kelly Women's Belief Scales* (O'Kelly, 2011);
- *Youths. The Child and Adolescent Scale of Irrationality* (CASI; Bernard & Cronan, 1999) which is an adaptation and expansion of *the Child and Adolescent Scale of Irrationality* (CASI; Bernard & Laws, 1988)
- *Parents. The Parent Irrational Beliefs – Revised* (PIB; Joyce, 1995) which is, in fact, a revision of the *Belief Scale for Parents* (Berger, 1983); *Parent rational and irrational scale* (P-RIBS; Gavița et al., 2011);
- *Teachers. The Teacher Irrational Belief Scale* (TIBS; Bernard, 1988, 2016);
- *Managers and employees. The Employee Rational and Irrational Beliefs Scale; The Manager Rational and Irrational Beliefs Scale* (M-RIBS; O. A. David, 2013); *The Work-Related Irrational Beliefs Questionnaire* (WIB-Q; van Wijhe et al., 2013).

Specific Content Irrational Beliefs

In this category we included scales developed specifically to assess:

- *Health-related irrational beliefs. The irrational food beliefs scale* (IFB; Osberg et al., 2008);
- *Academic performance-related irrational beliefs. Irrational performance beliefs inventory* (iPBI; Turner et al., 2016); *The Exam-Related Beliefs Scale* (EBS; Montgomery et al., 2007).

Strengths and weaknesses of the existent instruments One main limitation of the existing instruments that assess rational and irrational beliefs is the contamination of items with terms of distress and behavior problems. This could have resulted in spuriously higher correlations between the instruments that assess irrational beliefs (e.g., IBT) and measures of disturbance. This limitation is a characteristic of those instruments developed to assess the original model of irrational beliefs (e.g., IBT, RBI, IBQ, CBS III, II, BS). Another limitation is related to the fact that several scales do not have reverse items (e.g., BS). The factorial structure of the scales was investigated in several papers, however, in different replication studies conducted, the initial proposed factorial structure did not fit the data well.

For instance, the factorial structure of ABS-2 was investigated in a sample of participants recruited from the Republic of Ireland and the Republic of Kosovo; however, the model fit indicators indicated poor model fit (Hyland et al., 2014). Despite the fact that more recently developed scales were developed so as to overcome major limitations regarding the contamination problems, still, several problems exist that affected the validity of such instruments. For instance, Hyland et al. (2017) examined several of the problems in the manner in which the items of one of the most frequently used instruments (ABS-II) are formulated, which could have affected the validity of the scale. Namely, the proposed reasons were: (a) items are formulated so that they refer to the cognitive process and the context in which they appear; (b) there is a high similarity between items, as for instance items that measure frustration intolerance correlated highly with items measuring demandingness; (c) rational beliefs items have very low item loadings, they have a poor discrimination among factors, therefore the rational scale of this instrument could be highly problematic.

Another limitation is related to their psychometric properties, namely to internal consistency, where for instance we found instruments with unacceptable Alpha Cronbach coefficients. Test-retest reliability is investigated in very few studies. Very few of the instruments have been used with clinical participants in addition to community samples. Other limitations previously documented in Macavei and McMahon review (2010) is the fact that several scales have only a total irrationality score, stating that a rationality score could be computed by summing the items reverse coded.

Also, by using the item response theory, strong evidence exists for several items of frequently used instruments that have a higher discriminative power. For instance, using item-response-theory, Thorpe et al. (2007) investigated how well the items discriminate between participants with low and high trait level of irrational beliefs. Their results indicated that almost half of the items discriminated moderately, while four items discriminated highly and ten items had a very high discrimination value. Their results showed that CBS was an adequate instrument only when participants had an irrationality level situated with half of a deviation unit above the sample's mean. Given the fact that the item response theory framework used showed that the instrument failed to measure irrationality adequately, Thorpe et al. (2007) proposed the development of a new instrument, namely an irrationality screening instrument, comprised of four items of the CBS, namely those items that had satisfactory discrimination among male and female participants, covered a large interval of difficulty, and met the goodness-of-fit criteria of the proposed model.

The item response theory was also used for another instrument, namely for GABS (Bernard, 1998). Owings et al. (2013) selected the best six items from each subscale with the most informative value in order to develop a briefer scale that could be used in clinical settings. Furthermore, the authors investigated the most informative items representing the four irrational themes (e.g., Needs for Achievement, Approval, Comfort, and Demands for Fairness) and processes (e.g., Demandingness, Awfulizing, Low frustration tolerance, and Self-downing). Furthermore, it seemed that for all four processes, the item reflecting global rating was the most informative for irrationality, while low frustration was the lowest. This means participants with high levels of irrationality agree with global evaluation items, while those who have low irrationality tend to choose low frustration tolerance items (Owings et al., 2013).

Another important aspect is that instruments have been refined across time, and where limitations have been found, revised versions with fewer items were developed, or with items that assess important irrational beliefs that were not accounted. This is the case of the USAQ scale (Chamberlain & Haaga, 2001). Two important limitations of this instrument were: a) the scale assesses only self-acceptance, with no information regarding other and life-acceptance, relevant to the REBT theory and b) it also contains items related to self-esteem, which leads to a contamination effect. Therefore, UAQ scale (D. David et al., 2013) was developed in order to overcome existent limitations in the assessment of unconditional acceptance.

Towards a gold standard in the assessment of irrationality/rationality Cohen et al. (2008) propose a framework for the evidence-based assessment that is very similar to that used in the assessment for evidence-based treatment. Namely, instruments could be included in one of the three categories: well-established assessment, approaching well-established assessment and promising assessment, according to the existent evidence for their psychometric properties (good validity and reliability), number of teams that has published in a peer-review journal, and the amount of information regarding the instrument (instrument and manual) that allows replication.

Therefore, given this framework, in order to include in the category of *well-established assessment,* instruments that assess rational and irrational beliefs should fulfill three criteria: (a) at least two-peer reviewed articles published by different teams of investigators; (b) the instrument and a manual should be provided upon request, and (c) adequate psychometric properties (reliability and validity) published in at least one peer-reviewed article.

Other Types of Assessment

Content Analysis

Given the fact that self-reported instruments can present biases in capturing irrational beliefs (e.g., social desirability), other means of assessment need to be considered in the measurement of irrational beliefs. Solomon, Haaga, Brody, Kirk, and Friedman (1998) used the Articulated Thoughts in Simulated Situations (ATSS; Davison, Robins, & Johnson, 1983) to assess irrational beliefs along with the Beliefs Scale (Malouff & Schutte, 1986). Namely, participants were required to imagine themselves in four negative scenarios, which were presented on an audiotape, and they were instructed to think aloud, their thoughts were audio-taped and transcribed for the content analysis. The two relevant scenarios referred to rejection from boyfriend or rejection at a book club, while the two autonomy related scenarios referred to being demoted at work or owing a large sum of money for taxes, therefore, having an increased risk for prosecution. Five raters, trained in this procedure as well as in REBT, used a 7 point scale, ranging from 1 (*Not at all irrational*) to 7 (*Very irrational*) in order to code participants' answers and to provide an overall irrationality score.

Eckhardt, Barbour, and Davison (1998) used the ATSS in an anger arousal situation with martially violence men nonviolent men who were satisfied with their marital relationship. The total irrational beliefs score had very high intercoder reliability ($r = .92$); while the interrater reliability for the four irrational belief score ranged from 0.67 (Awfulizing) to 0.94 (Low frustration tolerance), with a mean of 0.85. Using discriminant function analyses they found that the ATSS irrational belief scores differentiated between maritally violent men and their nonviolent peers, and between severely aggressive and mildly aggressive husbands.

Behavior Analogue Tasks for Frustration Intolerance

Rodman, Daughters, and Lejuez (2009) summarized the existent behavioral analogue laboratory tasks that can be used in the assessment of frustration intolerance. Behavioral analog tasks have been used to assess parenting-related frustration intolerance. For instance, a study showed that parental irrational beliefs, namely parental frustration intolerance, can be assessed effectively using analog tasks assessment (Rodriguez, Russa, & Kircher, 2015). In this study, to assess parenting-related frustration intolerance, participating parents completed an unsolvable task while listening to a child's crying or tantrums. Another analog task that has been investigated is called the Frustration Intolerance Task (McElroy & Rodriguez, 2008). During this task, participants perform a task on computers where they have to find the exit to a grocery store while listening to a crying baby. In both tasks, frustration intolerance is measured as the amount of time, in seconds, in which participants quit the sessions. Lower time to quitting is associated with low frustration tolerance.

Tailoring Assessment According to Clients' Unique Characteristics

As previously stated, the REBT assessment is a dynamic process (DiGiuseppe, Doyle, Dryden, & Backx, 2013); therefore, it can be adapted to clients' development (e.g., children's age, clients with mental disability), religion (see Johnson & Nielsen, 1998), and culture (see Agiurgioaei, 2014). There are significant differences in how clients with depression versus non-clinical participants respond to a self-reported questionnaire on irrationality (DiGiuseppe et al., 2013). Taking this into consideration, the existing differences between participants, some authors proposed that clinicians and researchers individualize the assessment of irrationality (see for example of such a task in Solomon, Arnow, Gotlib, & Wind, 2003).

Discussion

Despite the fact that many instruments exist to assess rational and irrational beliefs, both generally, for specific populations (children and adolescents, parents, teachers) and in specific organizations (e.g., organizational, academic etc.) much research needs to be conducted to ascertain their psychometric properties. For most of the instruments reviewed, only data pertaining internal consistency was reported, with no further investigation of other psychometric properties such as measurement invariance and validity for instance.

Also, considering reliability, even though for most of the instruments the internal consistency for the overall scale was adequate, for the instruments' subscales the reliability (e.g., Cronbach alpha) coefficients were much lower. This raises some questions regarding their usefulness in capturing several types of irrational beliefs (e.g., demandingness, low frustration tolerance, awfulizing or global evaluation), or for rational beliefs assessment. There could be differences in how men and women, community and clinical samples, or participants from different cultures understand and interpret the items related to rational and irrational beliefs. Before conducting group comparisons, it is highly important to establish the measurement invariance. Only by conducting such investigations might we conclude that indeed there are significant differences in the latent irrationality variable, rather than measurement artifacts.

Despite the fact that there is an important movement in the literature towards evidence-based assessment concerning emotional outcomes both in adult and child populations (e.g., depression, anxiety, obsessive compulsive disorder, post-traumatic stress disorder), research is scarce regarding the evidence-based assessment of cognitive processes involved in various forms of CBT, particularly of interest here, irrational and rational beliefs. Therefore, the ongoing cross-cultural research program started at the Albert Ellis Institute, focused on the measurements of rational and irrational beliefs in various cultures, is fundamental for the REBT field (http://albertellis.org/international-research-program-cognitive-behavioral-theorytherapy-cbt-at-a-countryculturenationsociety-level-the-cognitive-behavioral-national-profile/). The development of sound instruments for the assessment of rational and irrational beliefs can have important relevance for research, but also for clinical practice. Having adequate instruments could inform treatment, could help in monitoring treatment effects and could help investigate their evolution over time.

The vast majority of the existing studies on psychometric qualities of rationality and irrationality ratings scales (excepting a few, see for example Owings et al., 2013; Thorpe et al., 2007) have been run within the framework of classical theory of measurement, which is based on relatively „weak assumptions" (Kean & Reilly, 2014). As a consequence, the estimated psychometric indices (item discrimination, item difficulty, Cronbach's Alpha, etc.) do not reflect any particularities of the clinical assessment instrument, as they are specific to the sample on the basis of which they were estimated (Graham, 2006; Miller, 1995). These psychometric indicators might provide information about the target population only to the extent that the sample is representative of a given population (Reise & Waller, 2009). The use of Item Response Theory (IRT) as a methodological framework of psychometric analysis of assessment instruments is not a common practice in clinical research (Reise & Waller, 2009). IRT is a measurement theory based on strong assumptions. Its main aim is to establish a mathematical relationship between the used items, the response to these items, and how these responses are linked to the measured trait (Hambleton & Jones, 1993). In the context of clinical research, two of the most commonly cited IRT procedures are exploring the relationship between the trait level variations and the measurement standard error variations and determining the individual differences in the assessed trait independently of the sample of items used (Embretson & Reise, 2000). Even if the IRT approach can increase the construct validity of a measure, only a few studies have used this method to investigate the relationship between items and construct (Owings et al., 2013). We recommend that further psychometric studies should take into account this perspective.

A major limitation of many cognitive measures in the field of cognitive-behavior therapies is that they are highly contaminated with distress items. However, in this regard, REBT is somehow more advanced, as the more recent scales of rational and irrational beliefs (e.g., ABS II; GABS), controlled for such a contamination. Moreover, many cognitive measures in the CBT field combined different cognitive constructs under the same measure, thus contaminating the measures and complicating the test of the specific CBT theories. For example, Automatic Thoughts Questionnaire/ATQ, Young Schema Questionnaire, or Dysfunctional Attitudes Scale combine items referring to descriptions/inferences with those referring to evaluations/appraisal. Vîslă, Holtforth, and David (2015) found that in the ATQ the relationship between descriptive/inferential cognitions and distress was mediated by evaluative beliefs (i.e., IBs). These is in line with the REBT's claim that cold cognitions lead to psychological disturbance only if evaluated.

Future research conducted on the assessment of rational and irrational beliefs should take into consideration the existent limitations and develop sound instruments that are sensitive to differentiate between rational and irrational beliefs involved in functional and dysfunctional emotions. Furthermore, as irrational beliefs are considered mechanisms of change in REBT, we need to have assessment instruments sensitive to changes during treatment (e.g., weekly assessments).

Given the different modalities in which clinical assessment can be conducted, we should take into consideration the existence of remotely-delivered assessments (e.g., delivered via online platforms, computerized, or smartphone apps) that have the potential to overcome several problems associated with traditional assessment of irrational beliefs (e.g., social desirability). The investigation of the accuracy of such technology drive administration in capturing rational and irrational beliefs, as well as their sensitivity to changes in rational and irrational beliefs over time or as a function of treatment is a desiderate that needs to be considered by future investigations related to REBT assessment.

References

Agiurgioaei, B. (2014). *Measuring irrational beliefs across culture new directions in the rational emotive behavior therapy* (Psy.D.). St. John's University, New York, NY, USA. Retrieved from https://search.proquest.com/docview/1543358272/abstract/1CC8CCCF60904B56PQ/1

Baer, L., & Blais, M. A. (2010). *Handbook of clinical rating scales and assessment in psychiatry and mental health*. New York: Humana Press.

Bagozzi, R. P. (1981). An examination of the validity of two models of attitude. *Multivariate Behavioral Research, 16*, 323–359.

Berger, A. (1983). *The role of irrational cognitions in the phenomenology of anger and guilt in parents of disturbed children* (Unpublished Ph.D. Dissertation). Hofstra University, July, 1983.

Bernard, M. E. (1988). *Teacher irrationality and teacher stress*. Paper presented at the 24th International Congress of Psychology, Sydney, Australia.

Bernard, M. E. (1998). Validation of the general attitude and beliefs scale. *Journal of Rational-Emotive and Cognitive-Behavior Therapy, 16*(3), 183–196.

Bernard, M. E. (2016). Teacher beliefs and stress. *Journal of Rational-Emotive & Cognitive-Behavior Therapy, 34*(3), 209–224. https://doi.org/10.1007/s10942-016-0238-y

Bernard, M. E., & Cronan, F. (1999). The child and adolescent scale of irrationality: Validation data and mental health correlates. *Journal of Cognitive Psychotherapy, 13*(2), 121–132.

Bernard, M. E., & Laws, W. (1988). *Childhood irrationality and mental health*. Paper presented at the 24th International Congress of Psychology, Sydney, Australia.

Bessai, J. L. (1977, June). *A factored measure of irrational beliefs*. Paper presented at the Second National Conference on Rational-Emotive Therapy, Chicago.

Blau, S., Fuller, J. R., & Vaccaro, T. P. (2006). Rational-emotive disputing and the five-factor model: Personality dimensions of the Ellis Emotional Efficiency Inventory. *Journal of Rational-Emotive and Cognitive-Behavior Therapy, 24*(2), 87–100. https://doi.org/10.1007/s10942-005-0020-z

Bora, C., Bernard, M. E., Trip, S., Decsei-Radu, A., & Chereji, S. (2009). Teacher irrational belief scale - preliminary norms for Romanian population. *Journal of Evidence-Based Psychotherapies, 9*(2), 211.

Borsboom, D., Mellenbergh, G. J., & van Heerden, J. (2004). The concept of validity. *Psychological Review, 111*, 1061–1071.

Burgess, P. (1986). *Belief systems and emotional disturbance: Evaluation of the rational emotive model* (Unpublished doctoral dissertation). University of Melbourne, Parkville, Melbourne, Australia.

Burgess, P. M. (1990). Toward resolution of conceptual issues in the assessment of belief systems in rational-emotive therapy. *Journal of Cognitive Psychotherapy, 4*(2), 171–184.

Chadwick, P., Trower, P., & Dagnan, D. (1999). Measuring negative person evaluations: The evaluative beliefs scale. *Cognitive Therapy and Research, 23*(5), 549–559. https://doi.org/10.1023/A:1018776522497

Chamberlain, J. M., & Haaga, D. A. F. (2001). Unconditional self-acceptance and psychological health. *Journal of Rational-Emotive and Cognitive-Behavior Therapy, 19*(3), 163–176. https://doi.org/10.1023/A:1011189416600

Cohen, L. L., La Greca, A. M., Blount, R. L., Kazak, A. E., Holmbeck, G. N., & Lemanek, K. L. (2008). Introduction to special issue: Evidence-based assessment in pediatric psychology. *Journal of Pediatric Psychology, 33*(9), 911–915. https://doi.org/10.1093/jpepsy/jsj115

David, D. (2003). Rational Emotive Behavior Therapy (REBT): The view of a cognitive psychologist. In W. Dryden (Ed.), *Rational emotive behaviour therapy: Theoretical developments* (pp. 130–159). New York: Brunner-Routledge.

David, D., Cotet, C. D., Szentagotai, A., McMahon, J., & DiGiuseppe, R. (2013). Philosophical versus psychological unconditional acceptance: Implications for constructing the unconditional acceptance questionnaire. *Journal of Evidence-Based Psychotherapies, 13*(2A), 445.

David, D., Szentagotai, A., Kallay, E., & Macavei, B. (2005). A synopsis of Rational-Emotive Behavior Therapy (REBT); fundamental and applied research. *Journal of Rational-Emotive and Cognitive-Behavior Therapy, 23*(3), 175–221. https://doi.org/10.1007/s10942-005-0011-0

David, O. A. (2013). The online Prescriptive Index platform for the assessment of managerial competencies and coaching needs: Development and initial validation of the experience sampling Mood Wheel and the Manager-Rational and Irrational Beliefs Scale. *Romanian Journal of Applied Psychology, 15*(2), 41–50.

Davison, G. C., Robins, C., & Johnson, M. K. (1983). Articulated thoughts during simulated situations: A paradigm for studying cognition in emotion and behavior. *Cognitive Therapy and Research, 7*(1), 17–39. https://doi.org/10.1007/BF01173421

Demaria, T. P., Kassinove, H., & Dill, C. A. (1989). Psychometric properties of the survey of personal beliefs: A rational-emotive measure of irrational thinking. *Journal of Personality Assessment, 53*(2), 329–341. https://doi.org/10.1207/s15327752jpa5302_10

DiGiuseppe, R., & Leaf, R. C. (1990). The endorsement of irrational beliefs in a general clinical population. *Journal of Rational-Emotive and Cognitive-Behavior Therapy, 8*(4), 235–247. https://doi.org/10.1007/BF01065807

DiGiuseppe, R., Leaf, R., Gorman, B., & Robin, M. W. (2017). The development of a measure of irrational/rational beliefs. *Journal of Rational-Emotive & Cognitive-Behavior Therapy*, 1–33. https://doi.org/10.1007/s10942-017-0273-3

DiGiuseppe, R. A., Doyle, K. A., Dryden, W., & Backx, W. (2013). *A practitioner's guide to rational-emotive behavior therapy*. London: Oxford University Press.

Eckhardt, C. I., Barbour, K. A., & Davison, G. C. (1998). Articulated thoughts of maritally violent and nonviolent men during anger arousal. *Journal of Consulting and Clinical Psychology, 66*(2), 259–269. https://doi.org/10.1037//0022-006X.66.2.259

Ellis, A. (1962). *Reason and emotion in psychotherapy*. Secaucus, NJ: Lyle Stuart.

Ellis, A. (1977). Basic clinical theory of rational-emotive therapy. In A. Ellis & R. Grieger (Eds.), *Handbook of rational-emotive therapy* (pp. 3–34). New York: Springer Publishing Company.

Ellis, A. (1992). *Questionnaire: The elegant solution to emotional and behavioral problems*. New York: Albert Ellis Institute.

Ellis, A. (1994). *Reason and emotional in psychotherapy: A comprehensive method of treating human disturbance. Revised and updated*. New York: Birch Lane Press.

Embretson, S. E., & Reise, S. P. (2000). *Item response theory for psychologists*. Mahwah: Lawrence Erlbaum Associates, Inc..

Flett, G. L., Hewitt, P. L., & Cheng, W. M. W. (2008). Perfectionism, distress, and irrational beliefs in high school students: Analyses with an abbreviated survey of personal beliefs for adolescents. *Journal of Rational-Emotive & Cognitive-Behavior Therapy, 26*(3), 194–205. https://doi.org/10.1007/s10942-007-0066-1

Foster, S. L., & Cone, J. D. (1995). Validity issues in clinical assessment. *Psychological Assessment, 7*, 248–260.

Gavița, O. A., David, D., DiGiuseppe, R., & DelVecchio, T. (2011). The development and validation of the parent rational and irrational beliefs scale. *Procedia - Social and Behavioral Sciences, 30*(Supplement C), 2305–2311. https://doi.org/10.1016/j.sbspro.2011.10.449

Gavița, O. A., & Duță, T. (2013). The employee rational and irrational beliefs scale: Preliminary validation. *Transylvanian Journal of Psychology, 14*(1), 19–39.

Graham, J. M. (2006). Congeneric and (essentially) tau-equivalent estimates of score reliability: What they are and how to use them. *Educational and Psychological Measurement, 66*(6), 930–944. https://doi.org/10.1177/0013164406288165

Hambleton, R. K., & Jones, R. W. (1993). Comparison of classical test theory and item response theory and their applications to test development. *Educational Measurement: Issues and Practice, 12*(3), 38–47.

Haynes, S. N., Richard, D. C. S., & Kubany, E. S. (1995). Content validity in psychological assessment: A functional approach to concepts and methods. *Psychological Assessment, 7*(3), 238–247.

Hooper, S. R., & Layne, C. C. (1983). The common belief inventory for students: A measure of rationality in children. *Journal of Personality Assessment, 47*(1), 85–90. https://doi.org/10.1207/s15327752jpa4701_10

Hunsley, J., & Mash, E. J. (2008). Developing criteria for evidencebased assessment: An introduction to assessments that work. In J. Hunsley & E. J. Mash (Eds.), *A guide to assessments that work* (Oxford series in clinical psychology) (pp. 3–14). New York, NY: Oxford University Press.

Hyland, P., Fox, R., Treacy, G., Maguire, P., Boduszek, D., & Vallières, F. (2017). Assessing the factorial validity of the attitudes and belief scale 2 – Abbreviated version: A call for the development a gold standard method of measuring rational and Irrational beliefs. *Journal of Rational-Emotive & Cognitive-Behavior Therapy, 35*(2), 111–124. https://doi.org/10.1007/s10942-016-0243-1

Hyland, P., Shevlin, M., Adamson, G., & Boduszek, D. (2014). Modeling the structure of the Attitudes and Belief Scale 2 using CFA and bifactor approaches: Toward the development of an abbreviated version. *Cognitive Behaviour Therapy, 43*(1), 60–71. https://doi.org/10.1080/16506073.2013.777467

Johnson, W. B., & Nielsen, S. L. (1998). Rational-emotive assessment with religious clients. *Journal of Rational-Emotive and Cognitive-Behavior Therapy, 16*(2), 101–123. https://doi.org/10.1023/A:1024934311040

Jones, R. G. (1968). *A factored measure of Ellis' irrational beliefs systems with personality and maladjustment correlates* (Unpublished doctoral dissertation). Texas Tech College, Lubbock.

Joyce, M. R. (1995). Emotional relief for parents: Is rational-emotive parent education effective? *Journal of Rational-Emotive and Cognitive-Behavior Therapy, 13*(1), 55–75. https://doi.org/10.1007/BF02354557

Kassinove, H., Crisci, R., & Tiegerman, S. (1977). Developmental trends in rational thinking: Implications for rational-emotive, school mental health programs. *Journal of Community Psychology, 5*(3), 266–274. https://doi.org/10.1002/1520-6629(197707)5:3<266::AID-JCOP2290050312>3.0.CO;2-3

Kean, J., & Reilly, J. (2014). Classical test theory). In F. M. Hammond, J. F. Malec, T. Nick, & R. Buschbacher (Eds.), *Handbook for clinical research: Design, statistics and implementation* (pp. 192–194). New York, NY: Demos Medical Publishing.

Kienhorst, C. W. M., van den Bout, J., & de Wilde, E. J. (1993). Does the Rational Behavior Inventory (RBI) assess irrationality or emotional distress? *Personality and Individual Differences, 14*(2), 375–379. https://doi.org/10.1016/0191-8869(93)90137-R

Koopmans, P. C., Sanderman, R., Timmerman, I., & Emmelkamp, P. M. (1994). The Irrational Beliefs Inventory (IBI): Development and psychometric evaluation. *European Journal of Psychological Assessment, 10*, 15–27.

Lindner, H., Kirkby, R., Wertheim, E., & Birch, P. (1999). A brief assessment of irrational thinking: The shortened general attitude and belief scale. *Cognitive Therapy and Research, 23*(6), 651–663. https://doi.org/10.1023/A:1018741009293

Macavei, B., & McMahon, J. (2010). The assessment of rational and irrational beliefs. In D. David, S. J. Lynn, & A. Ellis (Eds.), *Rational and irrational beliefs: Research, theory, and clinical practice* (pp. 115–147). New York: Oxford University Press.

Malouff, J. M., & Schutte, N. S. (1986). Development and validation of a measure of irrational belief. *Journal of Consulting and Clinical Psychology, 54*(6), 860–862.

McElroy, E. M., & Rodriguez, C. M. (2008). Mothers of children with externalizing behavior problems: Cognitive risk factors for abuse potential and discipline style and practices. *Child Abuse & Neglect, 32*(8), 774–784. https://doi.org/10.1016/j.chiabu.2008.01.002

Miller, M. B. (1995). Coefficient alpha: A basic introduction from the perspectives of classical test theory and structural equation modeling. *Structural Equation Modeling: A Multidisciplinary Journal, 2*(3), 255–273. https://doi.org/10.1080/10705519509540013

Mogoase, C., Stefan, S., & David, D. (2013). How do we measure rational and irrational beliefs? The development of Rational and Irrational Beliefs Scale (Raibs) – A new theory-driven measure. *Journal of Evidence-Based Psychotherapies, 13*(2A), 529.

Montgomery, G. H., David, D., Dilorenzo, T. A., & Schnur, J. B. (2007). Response expectancies and irrational beliefs predict exam-related distress. *Journal of Rational-Emotive and Cognitive-Behavior Therapy: RET, 25*(1), 17–34. https://doi.org/10.1007/s10942-006-0029-y

Newmark, C. S., Ann Frerking, R., Cook, L., & Newmark, L. (1973). Endorsement of Ellis' irrational beliefs as a function of psychopathology. *Journal of Clinical Psychology, 29*(3), 300–302. https://doi.org/10.1002/1097-4679(197307)29:3<300::AID-JCLP2270290306>3.0.CO;2-R

Nottingham, E. J. (1992). Use of the Survey of Personal Beliefs Scale: Further validation of a measure of irrational beliefs with psychiatric inpatients. *Journal of Rational-Emotive and Cognitive-Behavior Therapy, 10*(4), 207–217. https://doi.org/10.1007/BF01062375

O'Kelly, M. (2011). Psychometric properties of the O'Kelly women's belief scales. *Journal of Rational-Emotive & Cognitive-Behavior Therapy, 29*(3), 145–157. https://doi.org/10.1007/s10942-010-0120-2

Osberg, T. M., Poland, D., Aguayo, G., & MacDougall, S. (2008). The Irrational Food Beliefs Scale: Development and validation. *Eating Behaviors, 9*(1), 25–40. https://doi.org/10.1016/j.eatbeh.2007.02.001

Owings, L. R., Thorpe, G. L., McMillan, E. S., Burrows, R. D., Sigmon, S. T., & Alley, D. C. (2013). Scaling irrational beliefs in the general attitude and belief scale: An analysis using item response theory methodology. *SAGE Open, 3*(2), 2158244013484156. https://doi.org/10.1177/2158244013484156

Reise, S. P., & Waller, N. G. (2009). Item response theory and clinical measurement. *Annual Review of Clinical Psychology, 5*(1), 27–48. https://doi.org/10.1146/annurev.clinpsy.032408.153553

Rodman, S. A., Daughters, S. B., & Lejuez, C. W. (2009). Distress tolerance and rational-emotive behavior therapy: A new role for behavioral analogue tasks. *Journal of Rational-Emotive & Cognitive-Behavior Therapy, 27*(2), 97–120. https://doi.org/10.1007/s10942-009-0090-4

Rodriguez, C. M., Russa, M. B., & Kircher, J. C. (2015). Analog assessment of frustration tolerance: Association with self-reported child abuse risk and physiological reactivity. *Child Abuse & Neglect, 46*, 121–131. https://doi.org/10.1016/j.chiabu.2015.02.017

Shorkey, C. T., & Whiteman, V. L. (1977). Development of the rational behavior inventory: Initial validity and reliability. *Educational and Psychological Measurement, 37*(2), 527–534. https://doi.org/10.1177/001316447703700232

Smith, T. W. (1989). Assessment in rational-emotive therapy: Empirical access to the ABCD model. In M. E. Bernard & R. DiGiuseppe (Eds.), *Personality, psychopathology, and psychotherapy* (Inside rational-emotive therapy: A critical appraisal of the theory and therapy of Albert Ellis) (Vol. 38, pp. 135–153). San Diego, CA: Academic Press.

Smith, T. W., & Zurawski, R. M. (1983). Assessment of irrational beliefs: The question of discriminant validity. *Journal of Clinical Psychology, 39*(6), 976–979.. https://doi.org/10.1002/1097-4679(198311)39:6<976::AID-JCLP2270390627>3.0.CO;2-X

Solomon, A., Haaga, D. A., Brody, C., Kirk, L., & Friedman, D. G. (1998). Priming irrational beliefs in recovered-depressed people. *Journal of Abnormal Psychology, 107*(3), 440–449. https://doi.org/10.1037//0021-843X.107.3.440

Solomon, A., Arnow, B. A., Gotlib, I. H., & Wind, B. (2003). Individualized measurement of irrational beliefs in remitted depressives. *Journal of Clinical Psychology, 59*(4), 439–455. https://doi.org/10.1002/jclp.10081

Thorpe, G. L., McMillan, E., Sigmon, S. T., Owings, L. R., Dawson, R., & Bouman, P. (2007). Latent trait modeling with the common beliefs survey III: Using item response theory to evaluate an irrational beliefs inventory. *Journal of Rational-Emotive & Cognitive-Behavior Therapy, 25*(3), 175–189. https://doi.org/10.1007/s10942-006-0039-9

Thorpe, G. L., Parker, J. D., & Barnes, G. S. (1992). The common beliefs survey III and its subscales: Discriminant validity in clinical and nonclinical subjects. *Journal of Rational-Emotive and Cognitive-Behavior Therapy, 10*(2), 95–104. https://doi.org/10.1007/BF01061385

Turner, M. J., Allen, M. S., Slater, M. J., Barker, J. B., Woodcock, C., Harwood, C. G., & McFayden, K. (2016). The development and initial validation of the Irrational Performance Beliefs Inventory (iPBI). *European Journal of Psychological Assessment, 34*, 1–7. https://doi.org/10.1027/1015-5759/a000314

Ugwoke, S. C., Eseadi, C., Igbokwe, C. C., Chiaha, G. T. U., Nwaubani, O. O., Orji, C. T., … Abugu, L. I. (2017). Effects of a rational-emotive health education intervention on stress management and irrational beliefs among technical college teachers in Southeast Nigeria. *Medicine, 96*(31), e7658. https://doi.org/10.1097/MD.0000000000007658

van Wijhe, C., Peeters, M., & Schaufeli, W. (2013). Irrational beliefs at work and their implications for workaholism. *Journal of Occupational Rehabilitation, 23*(3), 336–346. https://doi.org/10.1007/s10926-012-9416-7

Vîslă, A., Holtforth, M. g., & David, D. (2015). Descriptive/inferential cognitive processes and evaluative cognitive processes: Relationships among each other and with emotional distress. *Journal of Rational-Emotive & Cognitive-Behavior Therapy, 33*(2), 148–159. https://doi.org/10.1007/s10942-015-0207-x

Vîslă, A., Flückiger, C., Holtforth, M. g., & David, D. (2016). Irrational beliefs and psychological distress: A meta-analysis. *Psychotherapy and Psychosomatics, 85*(1), 8–15. https://doi.org/10.1159/000441231

Warren, R., & Zgourides, G. (1989). Further validity and normative data for the Malouff and Schutte belief scale. *Journal of Rational-Emotive and Cognitive-Behavior Therapy, 7*(3), 167–172. https://doi.org/10.1007/BF01076188

Watson, P. J., Simmons, N. M., Weathington, B. L., O'Leary, B. J., & Culhane, S. E. (2009). Psychometric analysis and tentative shortening of survey of personal beliefs. *Journal of Rational-Emotive & Cognitive-Behavior Therapy, 27*(4), 201–212. https://doi.org/10.1007/s10942-007-0077-y

Wessler, R. L. (1982). Varieties of cognitions in the cognitively-oriented psychotherapies. *Rational Living, 17*, 3–10.

Chapter 5
Empirical Research in REBT Theory and Practice

Daniel O. David, Mădălina Sucală, Carmen Coteț, Radu Șoflău, and Sergiu Vălenaș

Introduction

The theory of REBT was developed by Ellis (1962, 1994), being seen by many in the field as the first form of CBT (e.g., Hollon & DiGiuseppe, 2010) and as a major contributor to the cognitive revolution in psychology and psychotherapy (David, 2015). First labeled Rational Therapy, it was renamed Rational Emotive Therapy before receiving the current name: Rational Emotive Behavior Therapy (David, 2015). In a personal communication to one of the chapter's authors (Dr. David), Albert Ellis in 2005 would have liked to finally name it Cognitive Affective Behavior Therapy.

The original REBT theory was systematically adjusted, as it continuously incorporated different empirical findings. Although some authors criticized REBT by claiming that it needs more empirical research (see for details Terjesen, Salhany, & Sciutto, 2009), since the first appearance of the REBT theory, hundreds of papers have been published aiming to investigate REBT's theory and practice. As the

D. O. David (✉)
Department of Clinical Psychology and Psychotherapy, "Babeș-Bolyai" University of Cluj-Napoca, Cluj-Napoca, Romania

Ichan School of Medicine at Mount Sinai, New York, NY, USA
e-mail: danieldavid@psychology.ro

M. Sucală
Department of Clinical Psychology and Psychotherapy, "Babeș-Bolyai" University of Cluj-Napoca, Cluj-Napoca, Romania
e-mail: madalinasucala@psychology.ro

C. Coteț · R. Șoflău · S. Vălenaș
International Institute for the Advanced Studies of Psychotherapy and Applied Mental Health, "Babeș-Bolyai" University of Cluj-Napoca, Cluj-Napoca, Romania
e-mail: carmen.cotet@ubbcluj.ro; radu.soflau@ubbcluj.ro

© Springer Nature Switzerland AG 2019
M. E. Bernard, W. Dryden (eds.), *Advances in REBT*,
https://doi.org/10.1007/978-3-319-93118-0_5

REBT theory evolved, so did the research testing both its theory and practice. Although the first REBT studies had methodological limitations (e.g., questionable psychometric properties of the scales employed for assessing irrationality of beliefs, lack of randomization in studies investigating REBT efficacy on mental health outcomes), most of the recent research conducted within the REBT framework is of high quality (see David, Coteț, Matu, Mogoașe, & Ștefan, 2017; David, Szentagotai, Eva, & Macavei, 2005). Moreover, in recent years, there has been renewed interest in REBT research concerning both theory and practice, and recent studies generally employ state of the art methodological approaches.

There are a number of available systematic reviews and meta-analyses that summarize this literature, some of these focus on specific aspects of the REBT theory (e.g., Vîslă, Flückiger, Grosse Holtforth, & David, 2016) and/or practice (David et al., 2017). Thus, this chapter will briefly review the available empirical data concerning the theory and practice of REBT.

Current Status of REBT Theory

In this section we will briefly overview the main theoretical claims of the REBT theory (based on Ellis, 1994) as well as the empirical status of published research.

In the REBT approach the concept of irrational beliefs refers only to evaluations/appraisal (i.e., hot cognitions), which have no logical, empirical, and functional support while REBT rational beliefs refers to evaluations/appraisal (i.e., hot cognitions), which have logical, empirical, and functional support (see for details David, 2003; Wessler, 1982).

According to REBT's ABC(DE) model, beliefs' irrationality is the main determinant of psychological disturbance, while rationality is a sanogenetic mechanimsm. REBT claims that in the presence of an activating event irrational beliefs (IBs) lead to dysfunctional/maladaptive consequences at the behavioral, emotional, and cognitive levels, while rational beliefs (RBs) result in functional/adaptive consequences on the same outcomes. Thus, changes in the irrationality of beliefs should lead to changes in the functionality of the displayed emotions and behaviors, as well as in the functionality of other cognitive factors (e.g., descriptions/inferences (attributions).

REBT makes an important distinction between primary IBs (absolutes)/RBs (i.e., demandingness – DEM/preference – PRE) and derivative (secondary) IBs (evaluations)/RBs (i.e., (a) awfulising – AWF/badness – BAD; (b) low frustration tolerance – LFT/ frustration tolerance – FT; and (c) global evaluation – GE/non-global evaluation – non-GE). People holding irrational primary beliefs (DEM; e.g., "I must be respected by all people") would also have irrational derivative beliefs, such as AWF (e.g., It is awful to be disrespected"), LFT (e.g., "I cannot stand to be disrespected"), and/or GE (e.g., "I am worthless/bad, others are bad, and/or life is unfair if I am not respected"). In contrast, people holding rational primary beliefs (PRE; e.g., "I would prefer to be respected and I do what is in my powers for this to happen, but I accept that it might not happen") would further endorse rational derivative beliefs derived from these primary beliefs, such as FT (e.g., "I can accept/tolerate that other people do not respect me"), BAD (e.g., "It would be difficult/bad if other people did not respect me, but it would not be the worst thing that could happened"), and non-GE (e.g., "Although it may not be reasonable/just for others to behave disrespectfully towards me, this does not mean that I am, others are, and/or life is worthless/totally bad").

Primary beliefs are central/core beliefs (i.e., are interposed between activating events and derivative beliefs), while derivative beliefs/appraisals are proximal to psychological disturbance/psychological health (David, 2003). Thus, the impact of DEM on dysfunctional outcomes would be mediated by derivative appraisals (AWF, LFT, and/or SD) according to recent developments of REBT. Of importance, REBT claims that these beliefs can be represented at the conscious or the subconscious level (e.g., they function automatically).

Even if the REBT theory is focused mainly on evaluation/appraisal (i.e., hot cognitions) in the form of RBs/IBs, it does not ignore other cognitions (i.e., cold cognitions: descriptions and inferences/attributions). The REBT model assumes that the "B" component includes both hot and cold cognitions and claims a bidirectional dynamic between the two types of cognitions. Thus, cold cognitions can be both triggers for IBs/RBs and consequences of IBs/RBs. As REBT assumes that cold cognitions do not lead to dysfunctional outcomes unless appraised, it is hypothesized that the relationships between negative descriptions and inferences/attributions and psychological disturbance would be mediated by IBs. Of importance for this issue is the nuanced view of REBT concerning the nature of IBs/RBs. According to REBT, IBs/RBs can be represented at multiple levels in the cognitive system. Thus, IBs/RBs are primary coded as schemas (i.e., general core IBs/RBs; complex propositional networks). Subsequently, in the presence of activating events the schemas bias the perception and representation of reality, thus generating context-specific IBs/RBs (i.e., with contents/themes that are specific to a particular context/activating event) that appear in the form of automatic thoughts. The automatic IBs/RBs further reinforce the general core IBs/RBs (see David, 2003).

Moreover, in the expanded ABC model (David, 2003) it is claimed that information (B) is partially processed implicitly in the cognitive system (see Fig. 5.1). Here, a distinction between (a) structural (both consciously unavailable and functions unconsciously) and (b) functional subconscious information processing (can be consciously available, but functions rather subconsciously) is proposed. The expanded model maintains that classic (i.e., explicit) IBs/RBs amplify the "C" that are generated by these implicit processes, through further appraisal. Therefore, the empirical investigations concerning links between hot, cold cognitions, and distress should also take into consideration the REBT assumptions that IBs/RBs can be represented as both general and specific/automatic beliefs and can be processed both explicitly and implicitly.

The distinction between functional (healthy) and dysfunctional (unhealthy) negative emotions is another central aspect of the REBT theory. The first type is assumed to be associated with functional/adaptive behaviors, while the latter to dysfunctional/maladaptive behaviors. Within the REBT framework, two competing models have been developed for this distinction. The first model (i.e., the

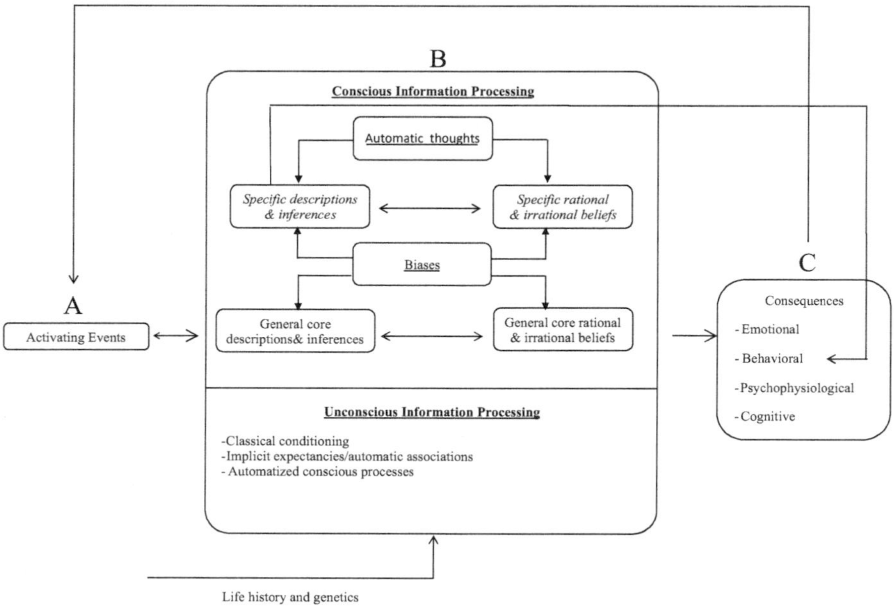

Fig. 5.1 The expanded ABC model

quantitative model) assumes that the difference between functional and dysfunctional negative emotions is quantitative in nature. The second model (i.e., the binary model) claims that there is not just a quantitative, but mainly a qualitative distinction between functional (e.g., sadness) and dysfunctional (depression) negative emotions (see David, 2003).

Now, once that we have presented the REBT theory in details, let us analyze its empirical support.

Links Between IBs/RBs and Dysfunctional Outcomes

REBT claims that the irrationality of beliefs is the core determinant of psychological disturbance. Thus, testing whether IBs/RBs are linked to changes concerning psychological disturbance is a necessary first step towards validating the REBT theory. It needs to be noted that the comprehensive systematic reviews described below comprised both high-quality REBT studies, as well as some early studies with certain methodological limitations. The first empirical studies conducted within the REBT framework generally failed to assess/manipulate IBs/RBs in the presence of a specific activating event, despite the fact that the stress-vulnerability ABC model claims that IBs (i.e., a vulnerability factor) lead to dysfunctional outcomes only when triggered by relevant activating events (i.e., a stressor).

Overall, the recent meta-analysis of David and colleagues (2017) systematically analyzed all the available literature concerning the links between IBs/RBs and outcomes of the REBT interventions, indicating significant associations between effect sizes on IBs/RBs (i.e., mechanisms of change) and effect sizes on study outcomes (i.e., emotional, behavioral, cognitive, psychophysiological, and other psychological outcomes) at both post-test ($B = .38$, $p < .001$ - between groups; $B = .42$, $p < .001$ - within group) and follow-up ($B = .43$, $p = .008$ - between groups; $B = .74$, $p = .42$ - within group). In other words, the findings of this meta-analysis suggest that changes in RBs/IBs correspond to changes in the functionality of psychological consequences. Additional empirical data concerning the relationships between IBs/RBs and emotional, behavioral, cognitive, and psychophysiological factors is briefly described below.

A strong test of this relationship must always involve an activating event. Indeed, Vîslă et al. (2016) found that the association between irrational beliefs and depression is much higher during the presence on an activating event ($d = .30$ vs. d .67) or if the activating event is more relevant ($d = .43$ vs. $d = .26$).

A. *Emotional disturbance*

There are a number of studies that aimed to investigate associations or causal links between IBs/RBs and emotional disturbance. Still, the meta-analysis of David and colleagues (2017) assessed only data from trial-based studies, given that its focus was mainly concerned with the efficacy of REBT. Thus, there are some other studies providing relevant data concerning the links between IBs/RBs and dysfunctional outcomes, including emotional disturbance. For example, a recent meta-analysis based on 83 primary studies providing primary data concerning the relationship between IBs and psychological distress (Vîslă et al., 2016) found a medium effect size for the association ($r = .38$). Moreover, the associations between IBs and distress were significant for each type of negative emotion that has been investigated (i.e., general distress, $r = .36$; depression, $r = .33$; anxiety, $r = .41$; anger, $r = .25$; and guilt, $r = .29$), IBs being most closely related to anxiety.

B. *Behavioral outcomes*

There are several studies that aimed to investigate relationships/causal links between IBs/RBs and behavioral outcomes. In line with REBT theory, the review of Szentagotai and Jones (2010) showed that most studies confirm the claim that IBs/RBs also impact on the behavioral level. An additional indirect support for this claim comes from the meta-analysis of David et al. (2017) that found a medium effect size for the impact of REBT on behavioral outcomes ($d = .56$, $p < 0.01$), based on 13 comparisons. These results suggest that REBT interventions that are designed to change IBs/RBs lead to changes in behavior. Still, the associations between changes in IBs/RBs and changes in behavioral outcomes (i.e., IBs/RBs as mechanisms of change) were not directly assessed in the studies included in this meta-analysis. Although David et al. (2017) computed a meta-regression and found positive associations between effect sizes for changes on IBs/RBs and effect sizes for changes on psychological outcomes (i.e., including behavioral outcomes), the association was not specifically investigated for behavioral outcomes (due to reduced number of studies). Thus, more empirical data are needed.

C. *Cognitive outcomes*

As a test of REBT theory, a number of studies aimed to evaluate links between IBs/RBs and other cognitive factors (e.g., Bond & Dryden, 1996, 1997, 2000; Dryden, Ferguson, & Clark, 1989; Dryden, Ferguson, & McTeague, 1989; McDuff & Dryden, 1998; Szentagotai & Freeman, 2007). Most of these correlational and experimental studies are focused on dysfunctional inferences and automatic thoughts and have been recently systematically reviewed (Şoflău & David, 2017). As it was the case for the associations between IBs/RBs and psychological disturbance, the meta-analysis indicated a medium effects size ($r = .43$) for the relationships between IBs and negative/dysfunctional automatic thoughts (Şoflău & David, 2017). Similarly, the meta-analysis of David et al. (2017) provided some indirect support for this relationship, indicating a significant impact of REBT (i.e., designed to change IBs/RBs) on cognitive outcomes ($d = .32$, $p < 0.01$). It should be noted that the indirect support from this meta-analysis share the shortcomings that have been detailed above for the behavioral outcomes.

Some of the studies investigating the impact of IBs/RBs on dysfunctional inferences aimed to ascertain which of the primary and derivative IBs is the active component. The findings indicated that derivative IBs lead to more dysfunctional inferences than DEM. Still, the meta-analysis of Şoflău and David (2017), which also included some correlational data, found no statistical differences in the magnitude of the associations between IBs and inferences based on the type of beliefs (i.e., primary, derivative or primary & derivative IBs combined).

D. *Psychophysiological outcomes*

It was claimed (e.g., Goldfried & Sobocinski, 1975) that IBs might also be associated with intense physiological arousal and other psychophysiological indicators. The incipient studies generally failed to support this claim (see David et al., 2005 for a review). However, other studies with improved methodological apparatus added some empirical support for this hypothesis with IBs being correlated with physiological arousal (e.g., Eckhardt, Barbour, & Davidson, 1998), with plasma inflammatory markers (Papageorgiou et al., 2006), as well as with various biological indicators of pathology (Lyons & Woods, 1991; Woods & Lyons, 1990). However, results are generally rather mixed (see David, 2014).

The Impact of REBT on IBs and RBs

A second central assumption is that REBT works through targeting IBs (i.e., identifying, disputing and changing IBs to RBs). Thus, testing whether REBT interventions are successful in changing IBs/RBs is an essential next step towards confirming the evidence based status of the REBT theory.

A recent meta-analysis (David et al., 2017) summarized the empirical research concerning the impact of REBT on RBs and IBs by analyzing data from trial-based studies. The study reported a significant medium effect size for the impact of REBT on combined RBs and IBs, both relative to different comparison groups (i.e., between groups effect size; $d = 0.70$ - post-intervention; $d = 0.57$ - maintained at follow-up) and relative to the baseline level (i.e., within group effect size; $d = 0.61$). When taking into account the type of REBT intervention (i.e., educational – REE, psychotherapy, counseling), results for between groups analysis revealed a significant large effect size for REE ($d = 0.82$), a significant medium effect size for psychotherapy ($d = 0.74$), and a non-significant effect for counseling interventions ($d = -0.31$) concerning the impact on IBs/RBs. In addition, it appears that the magnitude of the impact of REBT on IBs/RBs depends on the type of comparison. Thus, the effect size was significant and large relative to waitlist/no treatment ($d = 1.35$), but small/medium when compared to treatment as usual ($d = 0.33$), different psychological interventions ($d = 0.37$) and minimal/supportive interventions ($d = 0.47$), while relative to placebo it was medium, but non-significant ($d = 0.58$, $p > .05$ – however, in this case only a small number of studies were available, supporting only three comparisons).

A similar result was reported in another meta-analysis that aimed to investigate the effectiveness of REE (Trip, Vernon, & McMahon, 2007), an intervention derived from the REBT theoretical corpus. The authors found a medium effect size for the impact of REE on IBs ($d = .73$) and inferential beliefs ($d = .50$).

The Interplay Between Primary and Derivative RBs/IBs

REBT claims that DEM/PRE are central beliefs (i.e., primary appraisals), while GE/non-GE, AWF/BAD and LFT/FT are derivative beliefs (appraisals) derived from these beliefs. The hypothesized mediational role of derivative appraisals for the relationships between primary appraisals and dysfunctional outcomes (David, Schnur, & Belloiu, 2002) has gained some empirical support. For example, Buschmann, Horn, Blankenship, Garcia, and Bohan (2017) tested multiple structural models integrating both appraisals and automatic thoughts as predictors of anxiety and depression, using a cross-sectional design. They found that DEM leads to LFT and SD, which subsequently lead to distress both directly and indirectly (through negative automatic thoughts). Similarly, another study (DiLorenzo, David, & Montgomery, 2007) found that the predictive value of DEM for distress appears to be mediated by AWF, LFT, and GE. Hyland and colleagues reported a similar pattern, showing indirect links between DEM and posttraumatic stress disorder (Hyland, Shevlin, Adamson, & Boduszek, 2014a) and anxiety/depression (Oltean, Hyland, Vallières, & David, 2017), with derivative IBs as mediators. Thus, it appears that the available empirical findings support the hypothesis of the primacy of DEM among IBs.

Although RBs are assumed to play a protective role against psychopathology, the hypothesis was more closely investigated only more recently. The existing empirical investigations are generally in line with this claim, thus supporting the REBT model of mental health. For example, Hyland, Maguire, Shevlin, and Boduszek (2014) uncovered significant negative associations between RBs and PTSD symptoms. In another study, Hyland and colleagues (2014b) found additional support for the hypothesis. They showed that RBs (i.e., PRE and non-GE) are linked to lower levels of posttraumatic stress symptomatology. Moreover, their findings suggest that RBs might moderate the links between IBs and posttraumatic stress symptomatology. However, only non-GE (acceptance), but not other RBs, significantly moderated the impact of IBs. These data have been summarized in a recent meta-analysis that aimed to systematically review all the articles reporting empirical data concerning links between RBs and psychological distress (Oltean & David, 2018). Based on 26 studies, the meta-analysis revealed a medium negative relationship between RBs and distress. Overall, these findings confirm that RBs might be a factor of resilience. Still, the protective effect of RBs has not yet been compared to the detrimental effect of IBs, so these results need to be taken with caution.

Links Between RBs/IBs, Cold Cognitions and Psychological Disturbance

A few researchers investigated the interplay between IBs and automatic thoughts in generating distress (e.g., anxiety, depression, exam-related distress) and generally found that automatic thoughts mediated the effects of IBs on distress (Buschmann et al., 2017; Montgomery, David, DiLorenzo, & Schnur, 2007; Oltean et al., 2017; Szentagotai & Freeman, 2007; Vîslă, Cristea, Tătar, & David, 2013). A limit of these studies is that "automatic thoughts" contained both "hot" and "cold" cognitions (i.e., combined automatic IBs and inferences/attributions). Therefore, although of importance, these studies do not provide a direct test of the REBT hypothesis that IBs/RBs mediate the links between "cold" cognitions and dysfunctional emotions.

A more recent study (Vîslă, Grosse Holtforth, & David, 2015) separated automatic thoughts into appraisals/evaluative and non-evaluative cognitions (i.e., descriptive/inferential cognitions). They found that although both types of cognitions were related to distress, the association between descriptive/inferential cognitions and distress was mediated by evaluative beliefs (i.e., IBs). These results support REBT's claim that "cold" cognitions could lead to psychological disturbance only by triggering subsequent IBs. Future studies are needed to examine the stability of these results, as well as to explore the causal sequence between IBs, cold cognitions and emotions/behaviors.

To date, there are few studies that investigated the role of general core (schema like) and specific (automatic thoughts like) IBs/RBs within the same design. For example, Montgomery and colleagues (2007) found that both general and specific (i.e., exam-related) IBs were linked with exam-related distress. Interestingly, specific IBs predicted distress only when assessed before the exam (i.e., in the presence of the activating event), but not when assessed at the beginning of the semester. The authors of the paper suggest that specific IBs are more relevant to distress in an "acute" context. Similarly, another study (Gavița, David, DiGiuseppe, & DelVecchio, 2011) indicated that general and specific (i.e., parenting-related) IBs/RBs are positively associated and that specific IBs/RBs are linked with parental distress, but the mediation relationships between general an specific IBs/RBs were not investigated in this study (as it was a validation study for the scale assessing IBs/RBs). Given that these studies did not assess the interplay between general and specific IBs/RBs and distress, it is yet unclear whether the two types of IBs/RBs play different roles in generating psychological disturbance. Upcoming empirical studies employing longitudinal studies with multiple assessment points/experimental designs and focusing on different outcomes (e.g., emotional, behavioral, cognitive) are necessary in order to clarify this issue.

The Nature of Functional and Dysfunctional Emotions

A number of studies attempted to test the claims of the quantitative and binary models concerning the distinction between functional and dysfunctional emotions. First, in a series of studies Cramer and colleagues (see for a review David & Cramer, 2010) found that IBs were associated with both functional and dysfunctional negative emotions in imagined scenarios. Although somewhat in line with the quantitative model, these results do not invalidate the binary model as the former also assumes a quantitative difference. Unfortunately, most of these studies did not use an activating events context, as REBT theory requires.

In contrast, a couple of subsequent studies provided empirical support for the binary model by showing that high levels of IBs are linked to both functional and dysfunctional distress, while low levels of IBs (i.e., interpreted by authors as higher rationality) are associated only with functional distress (see David & Cramer, 2010 for a review). Moreover, it was found that the level of arousal alone does not discriminate between functional and dysfunctional negative emotions (David, Schnur, & Birk, 2004). Although these findings are somewhat debatable due to certain methodological limitations (e.g., rationality operationalized as low levels of IBs), overall, the data appear to favor the binary model. Thus, in accordance to Ellis and Harper's (1975) reconceptualization, functional and dysfunctional negative emotions seem to differ both qualitatively and quantitatively. However, most of these studies did not use an activating events context, as REBT theory requires.

In the case of positive emotions, the distinction between functional and dysfunctional positive emotions has been somewhat more recently proposed (Bernard, Froh, DiGiuseppe, Joyce, & Dryden, 2010; Szentagotai & David, 2013; Tiba & Szentagotai, 2005). Thus, there is little empirical research on the topic, the study conducted by Tiba and Szentagotai (2005) being the only empirical investigation, to the best of our knowledge.

Empirical Status of REBT Practice

Further, we will summarize the most relevant pillars of REBT practice, by presenting the state of the art in REBT intervention efficacy for different types of outcomes and populations.

REBT has been applied in several areas targeting different recipients, such as psychotherapy for mental health patients, education for children and adolescents (e.g., REE), industrial and organizational psychology for employees (e.g., Rational Assertiveness Training), and self-development and optimization (i.e. in nonclinical populations) (David et al., 2005). Empirical research data presented below demonstrate that REBT may be efficient for a large spectrum of psychological conditions and disorders.

REBT Practice Over the Years

In its early stage, REBT practice has not been rigorously tested (David et al., 2005). Prior to the 1970s, most articles were case studies or contained quasi-experimental designs. After the 1970s, a few controlled clinical studies emerged, albeit containing trans-diagnostic interventions mostly set in a clinical environment. At the time, REBT did not stand out by conducting these types of investigations, although in the present trans-diagnostic approaches are returning into the funding agencies' spotlight. Still, several early qualitative reviews did offer support for the idea that REBT practice could be efficacious, offering suggestions for the future (e.g., DiGiuseppe, Miller, & Trexler, 1977; Haaga & Davidson, 1989a, 1989b; Zettle & Hayes, 1980).

In the past three decades, however, a series of randomized clinical trials investigated REBT efficacy across numerous psychological disorders and encompassing all age groups. REBT became more visible and its results were disseminated through several good practice guides. Thus, REBT seems to be equally effective for children, adults or elders in both clinical and nonclinical populations (David et al., 2005).

As Barlow (2004) noted, there is a fine distinction between the general framework of a type of psychotherapy (i.e., REBT) and specific psychological treatments (e.g., REBT psychological treatments) for various mental health issues derived from the aforementioned framework. In this line of thought, numerous REBT psychological treatments (derived from the general REBT framework but catered for specific mental health issues) have been tested for efficacy both under the name of REBT and under the CBT umbrella.

Thus, REBT has been evaluated for efficacy/effectiveness as CBT in the treatment of various disorders or symptoms in children (e.g. disruptive behavior – Gavița, David, Bujoreanu, Tiba, & Ionuțiu, 2012) and adult populations (e.g. obsessive-compulsive disorder – Emmelkamp & Beens, 1991; psychotic symptoms – Meaden, Keen, Aston, Barton, & Bucci, 2013; side effects of breast cancer treatment – Montgomery et al., 2014; Schnur et al., 2009; social phobia – Mersch, Emmelkamp, Bogels, & van der Sleen, 1989).

Further, REBT has been investigated under the specific name of REBT and proven to be efficacious/effective in targeting several different outcomes such as depression (David, Szentagotai, Lupu, & Cosman, 2008; Macaskill & Macaskill, 1996; Sava, Yates, Lupu, Szentagotai, & David, 2009; Szentagotai, David, Lupu, & Cosman, 2008), providing support for including REBT as a "probably efficacious" treatment in the National Institute for Health and Clinical Excellence (NICE) Guidelines and in the Research Supported Psychological Treatments List of the 12th Division of the American Psychological Association (APA). Similarly, due to its efficacy in reducing parental distress (Greaves, 1997; Joyce, 1995), REBT was included in Barlow, Coren, and Stewart-Brown's (2003) Cochrane Review on parent training programs.

REBT efficacy/effectiveness has also been examined in several meta-analyses focused on children and adolescents (Gonzalez et al., 2004; Trip et al., 2007), or adult populations (David et al., 2017; Engels, Garnefsky, & Diekstra, 1993; Lyons & Woods, 1991).

REBT Efficacy in the 1990s

REBT was investigated under the name of RET in a couple of early meta-analyses. Engels and colleagues (1993) used a meta-analytic approach on 28 studies on adult populations comparing RET with passive controls (wait-list, no treatment), placebo, systematic desensitization and combination treatments (where RET was combined with behavioral components). Results showed a large effect size for RET at posttest as compared to passive controls (wait-list or no treatment) ($d = 1.62$). Although a trend was found which might indicate the superiority of REBT in comparison with placebo at posttest, the differences did not reach significance ($t(14.67) = 1.94$, $p = .07$). Additionally, the authors found that RET had the same effects as other active forms of treatments (e.g., systematic desensitization and combination treatments, $p > .05$). The study also found no significant differences between the results of RET studies employing only cognitive methods, those using primarily cognitive techniques, and those of studies using primarily behavioral methods. At follow-up, overall efficacy of RET was large ($d = 1.46$), but few studies reported follow-up measures.

Another meta-analysis on adult populations investigating the efficacy of RET (Lyons & Woods, 1991), comprising 70 articles, showed medium effect sizes for non-clinical adult samples ($d = 0.52$), and large effect sizes for clinical samples (Cohen's d effect size estimates ranging from 0.82–1.92), with a large overall effect size of $d = 0.95$. Analyses for all types of outcome measures provided medium and large effect sizes, with the highest effect sizes for physiological measures ($d = 3.88$). Further, moderation analysis showed that high internal validity ratings yielded higher effect size estimates than ratings with medium internal validity. However, the overall effect size in this meta-analysis was comprised of both effect sizes from posttest comparisons between controls, as well as effect sizes from baseline to posttest comparisons within RET groups.

When assessing the differential effects of RET as compared to control groups at posttest, the authors found large effect sizes for the comparison with no treatment ($d = 0.98$) and wait-list controls ($d = 1.02$), as well as placebo controls ($d = 0.80$), but small effect sizes when compared to active interventions such as Behavior Therapy or Cognitive Behavior Modification ($d = 0.30$ and $d = 0.14$, respectively; Lyons & Woods, 1991). This last finding is probably due to the behavioral component of RET (that was present even before it changed its name to REBT) and, thus, the similarities between RET and the aforementioned controls.

Current Status of REBT Practice

Two meta-analyses that investigated the efficacy of REBT in children and adolescents showed positive and significant effect sizes (Gonzalez et al., 2004; Trip et al., 2007). In the meta-analysis conducted by Gonzales and colleagues (2004), five outcome categories (i.e., anxiety, disruptive behaviors, irrationality, self-concept, and grade point average) were investigated in addition to the overall effect, in a total of 19 studies. Results revealed that the overall effect size of REBT as compared to no treatment and active controls at posttest was large (weighted mean $Z_r = 0.5$), while the largest effect size of REBT on the studied outcomes was on disruptive behavior ($Z_r = 1.15$; Gonzalez et al., 2004). Furthermore, they found that overall children benefited from REBT more than adolescents, but that REBT has the same effects for both clinical and subclinical problems (Gonzalez et al., 2004). Another significant moderator of effect size was the length of treatment, with REBT interventions of medium and high duration yielding larger effect sizes than shorter REBT programs.

Similarly, Trip and colleagues (2007) investigated the effect of REE on dysfunctional behaviors and emotions in children, adolescents and youth. Results showed a medium effect size for reducing dysfunctional emotions ($d = 0.60$), and a large effect size for reducing dysfunctional behaviors ($d = 0.85$) in 26 published articles. When compared to passive or placebo controls, REE provided medium effect sizes at posttest ($d = 0.64$ and $d = 0.60$, respectively), while in comparison with active controls, effect sizes were large ($d = 0.85$). Gains were maintained at follow-up ($d = 2.69$).

A recent REBT meta-analysis (David et al., 2017), which took into consideration all REBT published literature up to 2015, provided a medium effect size estimate for REBT compared to all types of controls at post-test ($d = 0.58$) for all types of interventions (psychotherapy, REE, counselling) and encompassing the whole range of populations (non-clinical, subclinical, clinical) and age groups. When looking at outcome categories, most remained significant, with effect sizes ranging from 0.32 to 0.94 (only the effects on psychophysiological outcomes were non-significant). Frequently studied outcomes in REBT trials included emotional (anger, anxiety, depression, and distress), behavioural, health, or psychophysiological variables, as well as quality of life, school performance or social skills.

The meta-analysis also identified a number of factors that could impact on the efficacy of REBT. Thus, it appears that the number of therapy sessions predicted better outcomes at the end of the REBT treatment. More recent studies also provided larger effect size estimates than older studies, while studies of higher quality (as assessed by risk of bias) yielded smaller effect sizes than studies of lower quality. Neither number of sessions, nor study year remained significant moderators at follow-up, but increased study quality still negatively predicted the outcome. Importantly, the medium effect size of REBT as compared to controls was maintained at follow-up ($d = 0.66$).

When assessing the effectiveness of REBT as compared to passive control groups (wait-list or no-treatment), effect sizes were larger than relative to any other types of control, at both posttest and follow-up. Still, REBT proved more effective than any other type of control condition (placebo, treatment as usual, pharmacotherapy, other psychotherapies or psychoeducation), with small effect sizes, both at posttest and follow-up. When taking into consideration only clinical samples, however, REBT was as effective as pharmacotherapy or other types of psychotherapy, and more effective than other forms of control conditions. This result is also supported by a more recent study investigating the effect of REBT on youth depression (Iftene, Predescu, Stefan, & David, 2015).

Recent investigations published since 2015 mainly in organizational and school settings on non-clinical populations also follow the trend of results described above. Thus, REBT-based interventions seem to reduce distress (measured as occupational stress, anxiety and depression, or psychological distress) in instructors (Ogbuanya et al., 2017), high school students (Sælid & Nordahl, 2017), or teachers (Ugwoke et al., 2017), in comparison with passive and placebo control groups. Similarly, in a sample of cancer patients and their family caregivers, REBT significantly reduced distress and death anxiety, as compared to treatment as usual, gains which were maintained at follow-up (Onyechi et al., 2016).

Discussion and Conclusions

Overall, the literature published on REBT theory and practice is positive. The overview of the literature suggests that there is good empirical support for the core assumptions of the REBT framework, as well as for the efficacy/effectiveness of the REBT therapeutic packages.

Concerning REBT theory, there is consistent evidence showing that REBT has the ability to change IBs/RBs (i.e., decrease IBs and increase RBs) and that IBs/RBs are linked to dysfunctional emotional, behavioral and cognitive outcomes. Still, less is known about the causal links between IBs and psychophysiological indicators. This might be due to the lack of a detailed theory concerning the types of psychophysiological indicators that should be impacted by IBs/RBs (David, 2014). More specific hypotheses/predictions concerning which psychophysiological indicators should be linked to IBs/RBs are needed in order to advance the current status.

Empirical findings are also in line with REBT's claim that RBs are a resilience factor (DiLorenzo, David, & Montgomery, 2011; Hyland, Maguire, et al., 2014), playing a protective role against psychopathology. Still, the results regarding the role of IBs/RBs in psychopathology need to be cautiously interpreted. The conclusions are based mainly on correlational data or on experimental studies with some methodological limitations. For example, although the research conducted within the REBT framework concerning links between IBs/RBs and other cognitions is promising, the field needs certain methodological refinements. The available experimental studies on this topic are mainly based on a role-play methodology. Although role play could be a useful tool, its internal validity is debatable due to demand characteristic issues. The correlational studies, on the other hand, seem to generally assess the cognitive factors in the absence of specific activating events. Since REBT assumes that IBs lead to dysfunctional outcomes only while activated by specific triggers (Dryden & David, 2008), the procedure employed in the correlational studies may not represent a valid investigation of the ABC model. Future studies need to employ different manipulation procedures (e.g., priming) and to adjust the methodological approach in order to assess IBs/RBs in the presence of an activating event (e.g., using virtual reality-based stressful scenarios).

In the recent developments of the REBT theory it has been claimed that IBs/RBs can manifest both at the conscious or subconscious level (David, 2003). However, most of the available assessment tools for irrational beliefs are self-report. Thus, it is highly desirable to develop additional assessment instruments that are not based on the awareness of subjects in order to test different aspects of the REBT theory. Implicit measures and priming tasks might be examples of useful tools for an indirect assessment of beliefs' irrationality, but their methodology still needs refinements.

The debate concerning the nature of the distinction between functional and dysfunctional emotions represents a good illustration for REBT as an empirically-based approach. The two concurent explanatory models (i.e., quantitative and binary) developed within the REBT framework generated a significant number of empirical studies that aimed to test the hypotheses derived from these theoretical models. Although the findings appear to favor the binary model, future studies are needed to establish the validity of the two models, as well as to clarify different implications (e.g., does the binary model also stand for the disticntion between functional/dysfuncitonal positive emotions?). Upcoming research on this topic should also incorporate the theoretical developments concerning the bidimensional nature of RBs-IBs (i.e., taking into account that lower levels of IBs do not necessary imply higher levels of RBs).

In which concerns REBT practice, early meta-analyses indicated large effect sizes overall, especially regarding clinical populations, in comparison with passive and placebo controls. Effects of REBT were found to be similar to or slightly better than other active interventions. This was perhaps due to the overlap between the behavioral components of REBT and of other types of psychotherapies studied at the time. The state-of-the-art in REBT practice now shows that it offers medium effects overall, which are preserved at follow-up. When compared to non-active controls, REBT is more effective with large effect sizes, while compared placebo and active controls, REBT fairs better, with small effect sizes overall. Clinical samples are, however, impacted equally by REBT and active controls such as pharmacotherapy or other forms of psychotherapy. This comes to show a certain maturation of the REBT practice, with effect sizes becoming more stable and reliable.

Duration of REBT treatment seems to positively impact its effectiveness, with longer treatments having better outcomes. Having in mind that REBT is usually classified as a short-term form of psychotherapy, this is not a surprising finding. Another important factor is the quality of the studies, with more rigorously controlled studies reporting a smaller (and probably more accurate) effect. As in the case of any scientific approach, the quality of future studies needs careful monitoring, in order to appropriately reflect the true impact of REBT.

Of importance, REBT has been proven to be efficacious for a somewhat wide range of psychopathologies and among different age segments (i.e., from children to adults). Although most of the research concerning clinical practice in REBT shows promising evidence, less is known about the effectiveness/efficacy of REBT for optimization and health promotion (David, 2015). Although recent studies have started to investigate the effectiveness of REBT on positive outcomes in non-clinical and subclinical samples, more research in these tiers is needed. Moreover, future research should take into account the cultural context of the individuals, as well as more diverse clinical samples (given that most clinical studies focus on depression and anxiety). Also, more effectiveness studies are needed to ensure that the delivery of REBT intervention packages is equally useful in ecological setting as it is in well controlled experimental settings.

In conclusion, REBT can be construed as an evidence-based oriented psychotherapy, securely moving from mixed results and tentative data towards well supported therapeutic packages and theory research (see David & Montgomery, 2011). Sharing the limitations of any scientific approach to mental health, REBT has not yet clarified the etiological factors involved in psychopathology and mental health. Moreover, REBT is less effective in tackling the etiological factors in some patients, even when the causal mechanisms are known. More research is needed in order to detect the etiopathogenetic factors and the mechanisms of change involved in REBT, as well as to develop more effective techniques for addressing these factors in different patients.

References

Barlow, D. H. (2004). Psychological treatments. *American Psychologist, 59*, 869–878. https://doi.org/10.1037/0003-066X.59.9.869

Barlow, J., Coren, E., & Stewart-Brown, S. (2003). Parent-training programmes for improving maternal psychosocial health. *Cochrane Database of Systematic Reviews, 4*, CD002020.

Bernard, M. E., Froh, J. J., DiGiuseppe, R., Joyce, M. R., & Dryden, W. (2010). Albert Ellis: Unsung hero of positive psychology. *The Journal of Positive Psychology, 5*, 302–310. https://doi.org/10.1080/17439760.2010.498622

Bond, F. W., & Dryden, W. (1996). Testing an REBT theory: The effects of rational beliefs, irrational beliefs, and their control or certainty contents on the functionality of interferences: II. In a personal context. *International Journal of Psychotherapy, 1*(1), 55–77.

Bond, F. W., & Dryden, W. (1997). Testing an REBT theory: The effects of rational beliefs, irrational beliefs, and their control or certainty contents on the functionality of inferences: I. In a social context. *Journal of Rational-Emotive & Cognitive-Behavior Therapy, 15*(2), 157–188. https://doi.org/10.1023/A:1025042522741

Bond, F. W., & Dryden, W. (2000). How rational beliefs and irrational beliefs affect people's inferences: An experimental investigation. *Behavioural and Cognitive Psychotherapy, 28*(1), 33–43.

Buschmann, T., Horn, R. A., Blankenship, V. R., Garcia, Y. E., & Bohan, K. B. (2017). The relationship between automatic thoughts and irrational beliefs predicting anxiety and depression. *Journal of Rational-Emotive & Cognitive-Behavior Therapy*, 1–26. https://doi.org/10.1007/s10942-017-0278-y

David, D. (2003). Rational Emotive Behavior Therapy (REBT): The view of a cognitive psychologist. In W. Dryden (Ed.), *Rational Emotive Behaviour Therapy: Theoretical developments* (pp. 130–159). New York, NY: Brunner-Routledge.

David, D. (2014). Rational Emotive Behavior Therapy. In D. S. Dunn (Ed.), *Oxford bibliographies in psychology*. New York, NY: Oxford University Press.

David, D. (2015). In R. L. Cautin & S. O. Lilienfeld (Eds.),. *The encyclopedia of clinical psychology Rational emotive behavior therapy (REBT)*. Hoboken, NJ: Wiley. https://doi.org/10.1002/9781118625392.wbecp077

David, D., Coteț, C., Matu, S., Mogoașe, C., & Ștefan, S. (2017). 50 years of Rational-Emotive And Cognitive-Behavioral Therapy: A systematic review and meta-analysis. *Journal of Clinical Psychology*, 1–15. https://doi.org/10.1002/jclp.22514

David, D., & Cramer, D. (2010). Rational and irrational beliefs in human feelings and psychophysiology. In D. David, S. J. Lynn, & A. Ellis (Eds.), *Rational and Irrational Beliefs in Human Functioning and Disturbances* (pp. 99–112). Oxford: Oxford University Press.

David, D., & Montgomery, G. H. (2011). The scientific status of psychotherapies: A new evaluative framework for evidence-based psychosocial interventions. *Clinical Psychology: Science and Practice, 18*(2), 89–99. https://doi.org/10.1111/j.1468-2850.2011.01239.x

David, D., Schnur, J., & Belloiu, A. (2002). Another search for the "hot" cognitions: Appraisal, irrational beliefs, attributions, and their relation to emotion. *Journal of Rational-Emotive and Cognitive-Behavior Therapy, 20*(2), 93–131.

David, D., Schnur, J., & Birk, J. (2004). Functional and dysfunctional emotions in Ellis' cognitive theory: An empirical analysis. *Cognition and Emotion, 18*, 869–880. https://doi.org/10.1080/02699930341000185

David, D., Szentagotai, A., Eva, K., & Macavei, B. (2005). A synopsis of Rational-Emotive Behavior Therapy (REBT): Fundamental and applied research. *Journal of Rational-Emotive and Cognitive-Behavior Therapy, 23*(3), 175–221. https://doi.org/10.1007/s10942-005-0011-0

David, D., Szentagotai, A., Lupu, V., & Cosman, D. (2008). Rational Emotive Behavior Therapy, Cognitive Therapy, and medication in the treatment of major depressive disorder: A randomized clinical trial, posttreatment outcomes, and six-month follow-up. *Journal of Clinical Psychology, 64*, 728–746. https://doi.org/10.1002/jclp.20487

DiGiuseppe, R., Miller, N. J., & Trexler, L. D. (1977). A review of Rational Emotive psychotherapy studies. *The Counseling Psychologist, 7*, 64–72. https://doi.org/10.1177/001100007700700109

DiLorenzo, T. A., David, D., & Montgomery, G. H. (2007). The interrelations between irrational cognitive processes and distress in stressful academic settings. *Personality and Individual Differences, 42*(4), 765–776. https://doi.org/10.1016/j.paid.2006.08.022

DiLorenzo, T. A., David, D., & Montgomery, G. H. (2011). The impact of general and specific rational and irrational beliefs on exam distress: A further investigation of the binary model of emotional distress as an emotional regulation model. *Journal of Cognitive and Behavioural Psychotherapies, 11*, 121–142.

Dryden, W., & David, D. (2008). Rational Emotive Behavior Therapy: Current status. *Journal of Cognitive Psychotherapy, 22*(3), 195–209. https://doi.org/10.1891/0889-8391.22.3.195

Dryden, W., Ferguson, J., & Clark, T. (1989). Beliefs and inferences: A test of a rational-emotive hypothesis: I. Performing in an academic seminar. *Journal of Rational-Emotive & Cognitive-Behavior Therapy, 7*(3), 119–129. https://doi.org/10.1007/BF01076184

Dryden, W., Ferguson, J., & McTeague, S. (1989). Beliefs and inferences: A test of a rational-emotive hypothesis: II. On the prospect of seeing a spider. *Psychological Reports, 64*(1), 115–123. https://doi.org/10.2466/pr0.1989.64.1.115

Eckhardt, C. I., Barbour, K. A., & Davidson, G. C. (1998). Articulated thoughts of maritally violent and non-violent men during anger arousal. *Journal of Consulting and Clinical Psychology, 66*, 259–269. https://doi.org/10.1037/0022-006X.66.2.259

Ellis, A. (1962). *Reason and emotion in psychotherapy*. Oxford, UK: Lyle Stuart.

Ellis, A. (1994). *Reason and emotion in psychotherapy* (Rev Sub ed.). Secaucus, NJ: Citadel.

Ellis, A., & Harper, R. A. (1975). *A new guide to rational living*. North Hollywood, CA: Wilshire.

Emmelkamp, P. M., & Beens, H. (1991). Cognitive Therapy with obsessive-compulsive disorder: A comparative evaluation. *Behavior Research and Therapy, 29*, 293–300. https://doi.org/10.1016/0005-7967(91)90120-R

Engels, G. I., Garnefsky, N., & Diekstra, R. F. (1993). Efficacy of Rational-Emotive Therapy: A quantitative analysis. *Journal of Consulting and Clinical Psychology, 61*, 1083–1090. https://doi.org/10.1037/0022-006X.61.6.1083

Gavița, O. A., David, D., Bujoreanu, S., Tiba, A., & Ionuțiu, D. (2012). The efficacy of a short cognitive-behavioral parent program in the treatment of externalizing behavior disorders in Romanian foster care children: Building parental emotion-regulation through unconditional self- and child-acceptance strategies. *Children and Youth Services Review, 34*(2), 1290–1297. https://doi.org/10.1016/j.childyouth.2012.03.001

Gavița, O. A., David, D., DiGiuseppe, R., & DelVecchio, T. (2011). The development and validation of the Parent Rational and Irrational Beliefs Scale. *Procedia-Social and Behavioral Sciences, 30*, 2305–2311. https://doi.org/10.1016/j.sbspro.2011.10.449

Goldfried, M. R., & Sobocinski, D. (1975). Effect of irrational beliefs on emotional arousal. *Journal of Consulting and Clinical Psychology, 43*(4), 504. https://doi.org/10.1037/h0076787

Gonzalez, J. E., Nelson, J. R., Gutkin, T. B., Saunders, A., Galloway, A., & Shwery, C. S. (2004). Rational Emotive Therapy with children and adolescents: A meta-analysis. *Journal of Emotional and Behavioral Disorders, 12*, 222–235.

Greaves, D. (1997). The Effect of Rational-Emotive Parent Education on the stress of mothers of children with Down syndrome. *Journal of Rational-Emotive and Cognitive-Behavior Therapy, 15*, 249–267. https://doi.org/10.1023/A:1025063425172

Haaga, D. A. F., & Davidson, G. C. (1989a). Slow progress in Rational-Emotive Therapy outcome research: Etiology and treatment. *Cognitive Therapy and Research, 13*, 493–508. https://doi.org/10.1007/BF01173908

Haaga, D. A. F., & Davidson, G. C. (1989b). Outcome studies of rational emotive therapy. In M. E. Bernard & R. DiGiuseppe (Eds.), *Inside Rational-Emotive Therapy: A critical appraisal of the theory and therapy of Albert Ellis* (pp. 155–260). New York, NY: Academic.

Hollon, S. D., & Digiuseppe, R. (2010). *Cognitive psychotherapies. History of psychotherapy: Continuity and change* (2nd ed.). Washington, DC: American Psychological Association.

Hyland, P., Maguire, R., Shevlin, M., & Boduszek, D. (2014). Rational beliefs as cognitive protective factors against posttraumatic stress symptoms. *Journal of Rational-Emotive & Cognitive-Behavior Therapy, 32*(4), 297–312. https://doi.org/10.1007/s10942-014-0195-2

Hyland, P., Shevlin, M., Adamson, G., & Boduszek, D. (2014a). The organization of irrational beliefs in posttraumatic stress symptomology: Testing the predictions of REBT theory using structural equation modelling. *Journal of Clinical Psychology, 70*(1), 48–59. https://doi.org/10.1002/jclp.22009

Hyland, P., Shevlin, M., Adamson, G., & Boduszek, D. (2014b). The moderating role of rational beliefs in the relationship between irrational beliefs and posttraumatic stress symptomology. *Behavioural and Cognitive Psychotherapy, 42*(3), 312–326. https://doi.org/10.1017/S1352465813000064

Iftene, F., Predescu, E., Stefan, S., & David, D. (2015). Rational-Emotive and Cognitive-Behavior Therapy (REBT/CBT) versus pharmacotherapy versus REBT/CBT plus pharmacotherapy in the treatment of major depressive disorder in youth: A randomized clinical trial. *Psychiatry Research, 225*(3), 687–694. https://doi.org/10.1016/j.psychres.2014.11.021

Joyce, M. R. (1995). Emotional relief for parents: Is Rational-Emotive Parent Education effective? *Journal of Rational-Emotive and Cognitive-Behavior Therapy, 13*, 55–75. https://doi.org/10.1007/BF02354557

Lyons, L. C., & Woods, P. J. (1991). The Efficacy of Rational Emotive Therapy: A quantitative review of the outcome research. *Clinical Psychology Review, 11*, 357–369. https://doi.org/10.1016/0272-7358(91)90113-9

Macaskill, N. D., & Macaskill, A. (1996). Rational-Emotive Therapy plus pharmacotherapy versus pharmacotherapy alone in the treatment of high cognitive dysfunction depression. *Cognitive Therapy and Research, 20*(6), 575–592. https://doi.org/10.1007/BF02227962

McDuff, A. C., & Dryden, W. (1998). REBT and emotion: I. A role-play experiment using a shame/disappointment scenario to investigate the effects of rational, irrational and indifference beliefs on inferences and action tendencies. *Journal of Rational-Emotive & Cognitive-Behavior Therapy, 16*(4), 235–254. https://doi.org/10.1023/A:1024912518928

Meaden, A., Keen, N., Aston, R., Barton, K., & Bucci, S. (2013). *Cognitive Therapy for command hallucinations*. London, UK: Routledge.

Mersch, P. P., Emmelkamp, P. M., Bogels, S. M., & van der Sleen, J. (1989). Social phobia: Individual response patterns and the effects of behavioral and cognitive interventions. *Behavior Research and Therapy, 27*, 421–434. https://doi.org/10.1016/0005-7967(89)90013-2

Montgomery, G. H., David, D., DiLorenzo, T. A., & Schnur, J. B. (2007). Response expectancies and irrational beliefs predict exam-related distress. *Journal of Rational-Emotive and Cognitive-Behavior Therapy, 25*(1), 17–34. https://doi.org/10.1007/s10942-006-0029-y

Montgomery, G. H., David, D., Kangas, M., Green, S., Sucala, M., Bovbjerg, D. H., … Schnur, J. B. (2014). Randomized controlled trial of a Cognitive-Behavioral Therapy plus hypnosis intervention to control fatigue in patients undergoing radiotherapy for breast cancer. *Journal of Clinical Oncology, 32*(6), 557–563. https://doi.org/10.1200/JCO.2013.49.3437

Ogbuanya, T. C., Eseadi, C., Orji, C. T., Ohanu, I. B., Bakare, J., & Ede, M. O. (2017). Effects of Rational Emotive Behavior Coaching on occupational stress and work ability among electronics workshop instructors in Nigeria. *Medicine, 96*(19), e6891. https://doi.org/10.1097/MD.0000000000006891

Oltean, H. R., & David, D. (2018). A meta-analysis of the relationship between rational beliefs and psychological distress. *Journal of Clinical Psychology, 74*, 883.

Oltean, H. R., Hyland, P., Vallières, F., & David, D. O. (2017). An empirical assessment of REBT models of psychopathology and psychological health in the prediction of anxiety and depression symptoms. *Behavioural and Cognitive Psychotherapy*, 1–16. https://doi.org/10.1017/S1352465817000133

Onyechi, K. C. N., Onuigbo, L. N., Eseadi, C., Ikechukwu-Ilomuanya, A. B., Nwaubani, O. O., Umoke, P. C., … Utoh-Ofong, A. N. (2016). Effects of Rational-Emotive Hospice Care Therapy on problematic assumptions, death anxiety, and psychological distress in a sample of cancer patients and their family caregivers in Nigeria. *International Journal of Environmental Research and Public Health, 13*(9), 929. https://doi.org/10.3390/ijerph13090929

Papageorgiou, C., Panagiotakos, D. B., Pitsavos, C., Tsetsekou, E., Kontoangelos, K., Stefanadis, C., & Soldatos, C. (2006). Association between plasma inflammatory markers and irrational beliefs: The ATTICA epidemiological study. *Progress in Neuro Psychopharmacology and Biological Psychiatry, 30*, 1496–1503. https://doi.org/10.1016/j.pnpbp.2006.05.018

Sælid, G. A., & Nordahl, H. M. (2017). Rational Emotive Behaviour Therapy in high schools to educate in mental health and empower youth health: A randomized controlled study of a brief intervention. *Cognitive Behaviour Therapy, 46*(3), 196–210. https://doi.org/10.1080/16506073.2016.1233453

Sava, F., Yates, B., Lupu, V., Szentagotai, A., & David, D. (2009). Cost-effectiveness and cost-utility of Cognitive Therapy, Rational Emotive Behavior Therapy, And Fluoxetine (Prozac) in treating depression: A randomized clinical trial. *Journal of Clinical Psychology, 65*, 36–52. https://doi.org/10.1002/jclp.20550

Schnur, J. B., David, D., Kangas, M., Green, S., Bovbjerg, D. M., & Montgomery, G. M. (2009). A randomized trial of a Cognitive-Behavioral Therapy and hypnosis intervention on positive and negative affect during breast cancer radiotherapy. *Journal of Clinical Psychology, 65*, 443–455. https://doi.org/10.1002/jclp.20559

Şoflău, R., & David, D. O. (2017). A meta-analytical approach of the relationships between the irrationality of beliefs and the functionality of automatic thoughts. *Cognitive Therapy and Research, 41*(2), 178–192. https://doi.org/10.1007/s10608-016-9812-y

Szentagotai, A., & David, D. (2013). Self-acceptance and happiness. In M. Bernard (Ed.), *The strength of self-acceptance* (pp. 121–137). New York, NY: Springer.

Szentagotai, A., David, D., Lupu, V., & Cosman, D. (2008). Rational Emotive Therapy, Cognitive Therapy, and medication in the treatment of major depressive disorder: Theory of change analysis. *Psychotherapy: Theory, Research, and Practice, 4*, 523–538. https://doi.org/10.1002/jclp.20487

Szentagotai, A., & Freeman, A. (2007). An analysis of the relationship between irrational beliefs and automatic thought in predicting distress. *Journal of Cognitive and Behavioral Psychotherapies, 7*(1), 1–9.

Szentagotai, A., & Jones, J. (2010). The behavioral consequences of irrational beliefs. In D. David, S. J. Lynn, & A. Ellis (Eds.), *Rational and irrational beliefs in human functioning and disturbances* (pp. 75–97). Oxford: Oxford University Press.

Terjesen, M. D., Salhany, J., & Sciutto, M. J. (2009). A psychometric review of measures of irrational beliefs: Implications for psychotherapy. *Journal of Rational-Emotive & Cognitive-Behavior Therapy, 27*(2), 83–96. https://doi.org/10.1007/s10942-009-0093-1

Tiba, A., & Szentagotai, A. (2005). Positive emotions and irrational beliefs: Dysfunctional positive emotions in healthy individuals. *Journal of Cognitive Behavioral Psychotherapies, 5*, 53–72.

Trip, S., Vernon, A., & McMahon, J. (2007). Effectiveness of Rational-Emotive Education: A quantitative meta-analytical study. *Journal of Cognitive & Behavioral Psychotherapies, 7*(1), 81–93.

Ugwoke, S. C., Eseadi, C., Igbokwe, C. C., Chiaha, G. T., Nwaubani, O. O., Orji, C. T., … Onu, E. A. (2017). Effects of a Rational-Emotive Health Education Intervention on stress management and irrational beliefs among technical college teachers in Southeast Nigeria. *Medicine, 96*(31), e7658. https://doi.org/10.1097/MD.0000000000007658

Vîslă, A., Cristea, I. A., Tătar, A. S., & David, D. (2013). Core beliefs, automatic thoughts and response expectancies in predicting public speaking anxiety. *Personality and Individual Differences, 55*(7), 856–859. https://doi.org/10.1016/j.paid.2013.06.003

Vîslă, A., Flückiger, C., Grosse Holtforth, M., & David, D. (2016). Irrational beliefs and psychological distress: A meta-analysis. *Psychotherapy and Psychosomatics, 85*(1), 8–15. https://doi.org/10.1159/000441231

Vîslă, A., Grosse Holtforth, M., & David, D. (2015). Descriptive/inferential cognitive processes and evaluative cognitive processes: Relationships among each other and with emotional distress. *Journal of Rational-Emotive & Cognitive-Behavior Therapy, 33*(2), 148–159.

Wessler, R. L. (1982). Varieties of cognitions in the cognitively-oriented psychotherapies. *Rational Living, 17*, 3–10.

Woods, P. J., & Lyons, L. C. (1990). Irrational beliefs and psychosomatic disorders. *Journal of Rational Emotive & Cognitive Behavior Therapy, 8*, 3–21. https://doi.org/10.1007/BF01072091

Zettle, R. D., & Hayes, S. C. (1980). Conceptual and empirical status of Rational-Emotive Therapy. *Progress in Behaviour Modification, 9*, 125–166.

Chapter 6
Future Research Directions for REBT

Daniel O. David, Silviu A. Matu, Ioana R. Podina, and Răzvan M. Predatu

Introduction

Previous chapters have presented extensively the current status of Rational Emotive and Behavior Therapy (REBT) in terms of treatment efficacy and effectiveness, the scientific status of its theory, the validity of the assessment instruments derived from this approach, and other important topics. In order to understand the directions that both research and practitioners communities should be aiming for, in this chapter we will build on the key conclusions related to such topics as those enumerated, as they offer the current starting point for all future developments.

D. O. David (✉)
Department of Clinical Psychology and Psychotherapy and The International Institute for the Advanced Studies of Psychotherapy and Applied Mental Health, Babeş-Bolyai University, Cluj-Napoca, Romania

Department of Oncological Sciences, Icahn School of Medicine at Mount Sinai, New York, NY, USA
e-mail: danieldavid@psychology.ro

S. A. Matu
Department of Clinical Psychology and Psychotherapy and The International Institute for the Advanced Studies of Psychotherapy and Applied Mental Health, Babeş-Bolyai University, Cluj-Napoca, Romania
e-mail: silviu.matu@ubbcluj.ro

I. R. Podina
Laboratory of Cognitive Clinical Sciences, Department of Psychology, University of Bucharest, Bucharest, Romania
e-mail: ioana.podina@fpse.unibuc.ro

R. M. Predatu
Evidence-Based Assessment and Psychological Interventions Doctoral School and The International Institute for the Advanced Studies of Psychotherapy and Applied Mental Health, Babeş-Bolyai University, Cluj-Napoca, Romania

© Springer Nature Switzerland AG 2019
M. E. Bernard, W. Dryden (eds.), *Advances in REBT*,
https://doi.org/10.1007/978-3-319-93118-0_6

As a general guide for our discussion about what should be done from now on, we will use David and Montgomery (2011)'s framework for evaluating the scientific status of psychotherapies. This framework has been developed to assess the evidence base of a psychological intervention by taking into account two factors: (1) the research supporting the efficacy / effectiveness of the strategies and techniques making-up the treatment package for a psychological condition; and (2) the research supporting the theory on which the treatment package was developed. This framework has been now widely used for analyses and discussions about the evidence-based status of different psychological interventions (e.g., Beck, Freeman, & Davis, 2015). Although REBT has today many more applications than just mental health treatments, including educational and coaching interventions, preventions programs, and others, the framework can be extended to such applications for our discussion, as the main two questions that we ask are similar to those that we ask about psychotherapeutic interventions: (1) how is REBT theory helping us to understand the phenomena and the problems that we are confronted within these fields of applications; and (2) how effective are the procedures we have developed based on the REBT theory. According to this framework, the empirical support for both the intervention methods and the theory can be placed on one of three levels: (a) well supported; (b) preliminary or mixed data; and (c) strong evidence against it. By taking into account the level of evidence for both factors (support for the intervention package and support for the theory), any psychological intervention can be placed in one of nine categories, ranging from strong evidence against both the theory and the intervention package (Category IX; see David & Montgomery, 2011) to strong evidence for both the theory and the intervention package (Category I), as indicated by at least two well conducted studies, from two independent teams. Intermediate categories (Categories from VIII to II) imply that either the theory or the treatment package has not received enough empirical support. In our discussion of the future developments of REBT, we will analyze where REBT would be placed on this framework. Of course, a complete analysis would require an examination/analysis of every type of intervention (psychotherapeutic, educational, etc.), for any kind of problem (depression, sub-clinical issues, etc.), derived from REBT theory; however, this is beyond the scope of this chapter. Instead, we will make an overview of the support for the efficacy/effectiveness of REBT interventions and the theory of change, and make some specific analyses for those that are commonly reported in the literature. Future directions for research on theory and intervention development will be pointed for fields of applications that have been less explored at this point. These issues will be presented in the sections related to REBT interventions and the theory of change.

Our discussion about the future developments of REBT will also include reference to some emerging fields and topics in psychological and mental health sciences, such as genetics, brain imaging, automatic information processing, and technology. These advancements have important implications for understanding the human mind and behavior. REBT should carefully follow such developments and understand the relationship between its theory and the new concepts coming from these fields. Our discussion of these topics will also focus on how REBT could make use of the new knowledge and methods in order to promote scientific advances, to improve the efficacy / effectiveness of its interventions and increase the dissemination of evidence-based interventions. These issues will be presented in the sections related to fundamental research and integration with technology.

One of the final sections of the chapter will focus on using REBT as a possible platform for psychotherapy integration. We will discuss why REBT is a fruitful theoretical ground to do so, and we will analyze what is still needed to be done in order to reach such an integrative potential. REBT has also reached other fields of psychology, such as educational (e.g., Rational Emotive Education), organizational (e.g., Rational Managerial Coaching) and cross-cultural psychology (studying the impact of irrational beliefs at country-level, and their interaction with cultural variables). For example, the integration between REBT theory and cross-cultural methodology, by moving from individual-level analysis to group and country-level analysis, could have a major impact on society and policy making, providing sound explanations and practical tools for tackling social phenomenon, by investigating shared or country-level irrational beliefs. Some interesting work has been started following this track. We will present this and other possible avenues in other fields of psychology in the last section, before our concluding remarks.

The outline for this chapter is as follows:

I. Future directions for REBT interventions

   Process-based REBT interventions
   Meta-beliefs as a transdiagnostic factor
   Integration of REBT interventions with pharmacological interventions
   REBT interventions in psychopathology prevention and health promotion

II. Future directions for REBT theory of change

   Plausibility and theoretical coherence
   Research on a strong association and dose-response relationship
   Research aimed at demonstrating a cause-effect timeline
   Specificity
   Experimental manipulation and consistency
   Theory of change vs. theory of the disorder

III. REBT and fundamental research

   Neurobiological underpinnings
   Therapygenetics
   Distraction's new role in exposure
   Integration of REBT and Technology

IV. REBT as a platform for psychotherapy integration

V. REBT and other fields of psychology

   REBT and cross-cultural psychology
   REBT in educational and organizational settings

VI. Concluding remarks

Future Directions for REBT Interventions

To date, REBT interventions have been investigated in a series of randomized control trials which demonstrated that they are efficacious for a variety of mental disorders and conditions, such as depression, social anxiety, obsessive-compulsive disorder, child behavior problems and parental emotional distress, side effects of medical treatments for breast cancer, as well as psychotic symptoms (e.g., David, Cotet, Matu, Mogoase, & Stefan, 2018). Moreover, a series of meta-analysis, including a recent one, offer empirical support to claim that REBT treatments, in the form of psychotherapy, educational, or counseling interventions are indeed effective for a variety of conditions, regardless of clinical status, age of sample, and delivery format (e.g., David, Cotet, et al., 2018; Engels, Garnefski, & Diekstra, 1993). In addition, based on a number of studies, notable organizations promoting evidence-based psychological treatments, including the American Psychological Association (see Division 12's List of Research Supported Psychological Treatments), National Institute for Health and Clinical Excellence (see NICE's Guidelines) and Cochrane (see Cochrane Reviews) prescribed REBT for the treatment of various conditions, such as depression, conduct disorder, and parental distress (e.g., Szentagotai, David, Lupu, & Cosman, 2008).

However, research to date reveals a few shortcomings in REBT intervention research that need to be addressed in the future (David, Cotet, et al., 2018):

1. Future studies should pay more attention to current standards in methodological criteria (e.g., using randomized controlled trials, the use of more diverse samples of participants, assessment and diagnosis of mental disorders on a continuum).
2. More research is needed on the efficacy of REBT interventions with some psychiatric disorders and conditions – both transdiagnostic as well as disorder specific – that are not in the forefront of REBT research yet, such as eating disorders, bipolar disorders, and sleep disorders. In this way, future studies will provide further support that could move REBT from the status of *probably efficacious* to a *strong empirical support* status for different conditions and mental disorders.

Process-based REBT interventions In recent years, new paradigms have emerged for conducting research to understand and treat mental disorders. The U.S. National Institute of Mental Health (NIMH) Research Domain Criteria (RDoC; Insel, Cuthbert, Garvey, Heinssen, & Pine, 2010) and The Roadmap for Mental Health Research in Europe (ROAMER; Emmelkamp et al., 2014) are two major projects that advocate for a new way of classifying mental disorders based on their central endophenotypes. More specifically, these models suggest that, rather than approaching specific mental disorders, the focus should be on observable behavior and neurobiological processes that cross conventional diagnostic boundaries (i.e. transdiagnostic). As a result, this changes the targets of psychological treatments from disorder categories to transdiagnostic dysfunctions / processes, irrespective of a psychiatric diagnosis.

In light of these new research developments, more targeted, process-based REBT interventions are needed. Process-based REBT means that processes and procedures underlying REBT interventions, as well as their linkage are evidence-based and are used to reduce emotional problems and promote psychological well-being (e.g., Hayes & Hofmann, 2017). In this context, a focus on how REBT interventions can target and improve basic evidence-based processes that are not disorder specific, but transdiagnostic, is of crucial importance. In particular, future research on efficacy and effectiveness of REBT should conduct clinical trials that investigate the effect of interventions in samples that displays impairments and vulnerability in a specific transdiagnostic process (e.g., people with excessive catastrophic thinking), regardless of mental disorder diagnostic. Having in mind that REBT has initially focused on effectiveness studies examining mainly transdiagnostic outcomes (David, Cotet, et al., 2018), future research should reconsider these studies in the light of these new research paradigms and continue this trend in the future. However, the above does not suggest that there is no longer a need to improve our understanding and refine classic REBT treatments for specific mental disorders, including those which have proved to be highly effective. But, along with improvements in clinical trials that evaluate the efficacy of disorder-specific REBT interventions, future research should focus more on clinical trials that targets specific psychological processes.

Secondary/meta-beliefs as a transdiagnostic factor Another important concept in REBT with transdiagnostic relevance, that has been less investigated, is related to patients' reactions to initial symptoms (secondary disturbance). According to REBT theory (e.g., David, 2015), individuals experience various (A) negative and undesirable life events (e.g., failing an exam), which they interpret and further evaluate through rational or irrational beliefs (B). Irrational beliefs about life events (e.g., "Failing my exam means the end of the world for me") lead to (C) dysfunctional emotional, behavioral, and physiological reactions (i.e., a primary disturbance, such as being depressed about my failure). Once experienced, this (C) primary disturbance (i.e., being depressed about my failure) can further become an (A) undesirable internal event, which, if it is irrationally appraised (B; e.g., "Feeling depressed means I'm a failure"), can lead to secondary dysfunctional emotional, behavioral, and physiological reactions (C; i.e., secondary disturbances, such as being depressed about depression). In line with REBT theory, these secondary irrational beliefs/meta-beliefs and secondary disturbances/meta-reactions can be conceptualized as transdiagnostic factors that could maintain and amplify the primary symptoms of any disorder (e.g., amplifying and maintaining primary depression by secondary depression). Thus, more studies are needed to investigate the role of these secondary beliefs as a transdiagnostic factor. Also, future studies should examine the differential role of rational meta-beliefs vs. irrational meta-beliefs, as well as their impact on emotion regulation processes (e.g., suppression of emotions) and emotional responding. We suggest that this line of research could contribute to more efficient treatments, in terms of preventing the escalation and complication of primary clinical conditions, which is often the case, or preventing more severe relapses when the patients are confronted again with primary symptoms.

Integration of REBT interventions with pharmacological interventions Another avenue for future research should be the integration of REBT with pharmacological interventions. This integration may hold promise for higher efficacy of mental health treatments. To date, research has shown that a combination of REBT and medication is more effective than either REBT or medication alone for various disorders (e.g., dysthymic disorder; e.g., Wang, Jia, Fang, Zhu, Huang, 1999). Also, REBT has been shown to be an effective adjunct to pharmacotherapy for patients with schizophrenia (Shelley et al., 2001). However, in a recent clinical trial conducted on outpatients with major depression, REBT was as efficient as cognitive therapy and medication at the end of the treatment, and more efficient than medication at a 6-month follow-up on the Hamilton Rating Scale for Depression (David, Szentagotai, Lupu, & Cosman, 2008). Thus, these results encourage further research on establishing the exact boundaries between REBT and pharmacological interventions in treating patients with mental disorders. Given the complex etiologies of psychiatric conditions, it is very important to closely work with neighboring disciplines (e.g., medical sciences) to clearly delineate when, why, and how combined strategies of REBT and pharmacotherapy interventions can be beneficial, and when they are detrimental for patients' mental health. Increased knowledge in this area of research should pave the way for the development of more efficient interventions that rationally combine REBT and pharmacological interventions.

REBT interventions in psychopathology prevention and health promotion Currently, estimates suggest that approximately 1 in 5 adults in the U.S. (18.5%) experiences mental illness in a given year (National Institute of Mental Health [NIMH], 2015). Also, psychiatric disorders affect between 10% and 20% of children and adolescents worldwide (Kieling et al., 2011). Despite this alarming prevalence of mental disorders, as well as the subsequent personal, social, and economic burden, the focus in mental health has been primarily on treatment rather than prevention. In this context, developing evidence-based prevention and optimization strategies, in an effort to reduce the impact of mental disorders and improve human functioning, is highly important. REBT interventions are not only effective in the treatment of mental disorders, but also very promising in mental illness prevention, as well as in mental health promotion and human optimization. REBT principles and strategies have been applied in numerous domains, such as education (i.e., Rational Emotive Behavior Education, Rational Parenting Program), organizational settings (Rational Emotive Behavior Coaching), and optimization (life and business coaching, rational pastoral counseling, sports performance training). To date, there is significant evidence supporting the use of REBT prevention programs for reducing emotional distress in teachers, parents, pregnant women, as well as in dealing with disrupting behavior, gambling and other risk behaviors in children and adolescents (e.g., Gavița, David, Bujoreanu, Tiba, & Ionuțiu, 2012; Vernon & Bernard, 2006). Also, research has shown that REBT is efficient in optimization and in facilitating performance for workers, athletes, and college students (e.g., Palmer & Gyllensten, 2008).

Overall, REBT is an effective intervention for prevention of numerous problems in nonclinical and subclinical populations, as well as for optimization of diverse performance indexes in various domains. However, despite this large pool of applications, the main shortcoming in this area of research is that REBT as a prevention intervention has been less rigorously investigated. Thus, future research should focus on adopting a more theory-driven, programmatic research agenda with an increased focus on methodological rigor. Such intervention could be designed to address psychiatric disorders prevention and health promotion in diverse samples (i.e., children, adults) by targeting cognitive vulnerability and by cultivating rational beliefs as protective factors, using innovative and accessible delivery methods.

In sum, in order to provide more effective REBT interventions, there is a need of:

1. greater improvements in research methodologies, as well as an increased focus on conditions that were not in the forefront of REBT research yet;
2. more precisely targeted treatments on specific transdiagnostic deficits (e.g., excessive catastrophic thinking), irrespective of psychiatric disorder;
3. integration of REBT interventions with pharmacological interventions augmented by a strong collaborative work with other research fields (e.g., medical sciences);
4. adoption of a more theory-driven, programmatic research agenda on psychopathology prevention and health promotion with an increased focus on methodological rigor in these areas.

Last but not least, along with these developments for future research, a strong consideration of costs, cost-effectiveness, and cost-benefit of REBT treatments is mandatory. We emphasize that research on the efficacy and/or effectiveness of REBT treatments should be followed by the evaluation of (a) how expensive are the REBT treatments relative to other available interventions, (b) how easily are assimilated in real clinical practice, and (c) how their assimilation can be improved. We suggest that a continued effort to achieve these objectives is a sine qua non condition for further survival, augmentation, and development of REBT treatments.

Future Directions for REBT Theory of Change

In 2011, David and Montgomery introduced the notion that knowing why psychotherapy works – also known as a *mechanism of change* – is as important as gaining knowledge about its efficacy and both criteria should be considered when rating the evidence-based status of psychotherapy. REBT is the first form of CBT. However, its underlying mechanisms of change have not been fully empirically tested, especially in methodologically rigorous studies.

Kazdin (2007) suggested several requirements needed for demonstrating mechanisms of change. These requirements are briefly listed.

(a) *Plausibility or coherence* entails providing a theoretical explanation of how the mechanism of change works, how it causes the onset of a clinical problem or leads to therapeutic change; (b) S*trong association* between the psychotherapeutic (A) intervention and the hypothesized mediator of change (B), as well as between

(B) and therapeutic change (C); (c) *Gradient or a dose-response relationship* increases the plausibility of mechanism-outcome connection, however it does not imply causality; (d) *Demonstrating a timeline between cause/mechanism of change and outcome* is probably the most important criterion as changes in the mechanism should precede changes in the outcome, a clear statement of causality; (e) *Specificity* is a demonstration that only one alleged mechanism leads to therapeutic change; (f) *Experimental manipulation* requires experiments that manipulate the alleged mechanism with an impact on the outcome. (g) *Consistency* entails the replication of an observed result across studies.

With the help of the criteria evidenced by Kazdin (2007), we highlight in the following several avenues that require future investigation with regard to REBT's mechanism of change. Additionally, we accompany our critical review of the literature with a rating on each of the above criteria adapted to the current status of REBT research on mechanisms of change.

Plausibility and theoretical coherence With half a century of theoretical refinements, REBT irrefutably has a plausible and coherent theory with regard to mechanisms of change. However, given the progress of newer scientific fields, such as genetics and neuroscience, REBT's model of psychopathology and mental health will certainly have to expand in order to accommodate new research. So far, as argued in this chapter, such fundamental research is only in its early stages. However, researchers are already preparing more detailed models that envision a future contribution of genetics to the spectrum of rational/irrational beliefs (see the expanded ABC model; David, 2015). Testing the reliability of these models will be a priority in the nearby future.

Research on a strong association and dose-response relationship There is a handful of research supporting a link between irrational beliefs and emotional distress and even between REBT and therapeutic change. Moreover, some studies also indicate a dose-response relationship between the intensity of irrational beliefs and difficulty in recovering for psychopathology (David, Cotet, et al., 2018) or a directly proportional relationship to the magnitude of emotional distress (Vîslă, Flückiger, grosse Holtforth, & David, 2016).

On a larger scale, two recent meta-analyses found a moderate, but stable connection between irrational beliefs and emotional distress (Vîslă et al., 2016), as well as between REBT and therapeutic change (David, Cotet, et al., 2018). However, as these meta-analyses point out, there is far less research on the link between REBT and change in irrational beliefs, and even less on its link to rational beliefs. Hence, this is certainly an area where improvements, even numerically (i.e., more studies) could be made so as to allow a reliable overview of the literature.

Research aimed at demonstrating a cause-effect timeline Another issue that needs to be addressed in the future is that most efficacy and effectiveness studies continue to exclude the assessment of mechanisms of change from their design. A recent meta-analysis indicated that out of 68 REBT studies only half reported measures of rational and/or irrational beliefs at post-intervention, and less than 30 studies assessed these variables at follow-up (David, Cotet, et al., 2018). It is unclear how many of these studies measured rational and irrational beliefs during the intervention and ahead of the efficacy outcomes. The time of the assessment is of importance.

In any causality relationship where A determines B, irrational and rational beliefs should modify throughout the course of the therapy and ahead of the outcome (e.g., anxiety, depression, distress). To our knowledge, no randomized clinical trial on REBT investigated this temporal relationship between changes in mechanisms and changes in outcomes during therapy. Only in this manner can the mediation hypothesis of irrational beliefs be properly tested.

Research would also benefit more from longitudinal studies, which are currently scarce. Longitudinal designs would bring conclusive evidence regarding the etiopathogenetic role played by irrational beliefs in the development of psychopathology.

Specificity A study published in 2008 (Szentagotai et al., 2008) contrasted for the first time REBT and CT, measuring within the same experimental design therapeutic change alongside the mechanisms of change central to each form of therapy. The results indicated that REBT and CT affected both classes of cognitions (i.e., irrational beliefs and dysfunctional attitudes). If replicable, future research needs to provide an answer to the following question. To what extent are REBT's mechanisms of change particular to this form of therapy or shared with other forms of CBT? An overlap between seemingly different classes of cognition would demand a unified exploratory model of CBT.

Also connected to the issue of specificity, recent findings contradict the core CBT/REBT assumption that change in cognitions is a condition sine qua non for long-lasting therapeutic change or even that cognitions have to be explicitly challenged to elicit cognitive change (Emmelkamp et al., 2014). Hence, we are currently confronted with a "skepticism crisis" in CBT, but mainly in CT, and dismantling and component analysis designs are a good tool to investigate some of these lingering core questions.

Existing CT component analysis studies indicate that, surprisingly, cognitive techniques (i.e., cognitive restructuring) do not outperform behavioral techniques in the treatment of anxiety (e.g., Ougrin, 2011). Moreover, exposure therapy was found to be equally effective in promoting cognitive change as exposure plus cognitive therapy in participants with social anxiety, for instance (Powers, Sigmarsson, & Emmelkamp, 2008).

REBT needs to go through the same "skepticism crisis" as CT and undergo its first dismantling and component analysis studies so as to better clarify the specificity of its mechanisms of change.

Experimental manipulation and consistency Aside from the methodological improvements previously suggested, we believe that progress would also be attained if the number of experimental manipulation studies investigating the mechanism of change outside of the treatment package would numerically (but also qualitatively) increase. As Vîslă and collaborators pointed out (2016), current research on the link

Table 6.1 Ratings of the requirements needed for demonstrating REBT's mechanisms of change in research

Criteria for mechanisms of change	Ratings
Plausibility/coherence	+++
Strong association	++
Gradient	++
Experimental manipulation	++
Specificity	+
Consistency	+
Timeline	+

between irrational beliefs and emotional distress does not allow for a conclusion regarding a causal relationship. Out of a total of 83 studies, only 5 were experimental designs and assessed emotional distress before and after the manipulation of irrational beliefs. Hence, we need more empirically rigorous experimental designs. More importantly, we need experimental designs whose results are replicated in several trials.

Below, in Table 6.1, we render our rating on each of the above criteria with regard to the status of REBT research on the mechanism of change. As such, +++ stands for *optimal*, ++ for *relatively optimal*, and + for *suboptimal research.*

We argue that REBT's half a century of theoretical refinements rendered a plausible and coherent theory with regard to its mechanisms of change that can be rated as optimal. Criteria such as *strong association*, *gradient,* and *experimental manipulation* were rated as relatively optimal because there is more than one paper to provide evidence for each of these criteria, keeping in mind though that many of these studies have an inherent poor methodological quality. However, *specificity, consistency*, and *timeline* were rated as suboptimal because to our knowledge there are currently one or no publications to provide information to fit either of those criteria.

The above-cited research mainly reviewed irrational beliefs research. However, we would like to point out that irrespective of the above mentioned methodological requirement, rational beliefs research is lagging behind. As pointed out by a recent meta-analysis, out of 83 studies, only 5 studies investigated rational beliefs (Vîslă et al., 2016). This setback is a consequence of the fact that for many years rational beliefs were mistakenly conceptualized as low levels of irrational beliefs (David, 2015).

The in-depth study of rational beliefs and its psychological health model could become central to the newly developing field of *positive clinical psychology*. One example in this respect is the work of Oltean and collaborators (2017) which intertwined elements of positive psychology (i.e., satisfaction with life; SWL) with elements of clinical psychology (i.e., rational beliefs) to provide an explanatory model for anxiety and depression symptoms. Following SEM (i.e., structural equation modeling), the results indicated that rational beliefs explained 31% of the variance in SWL scores and the model on the whole – including rational beliefs – predicted 33% of the variance in self-reported anxiety and depression levels. Notably, preference beliefs were predictive of lower levels of anxiety/depressive symptomatology indirectly via unconditional acceptance and satisfaction with life. The authors concluded that "*integrating core concepts of positive psychology, into an evidence-based form of psychotherapy (REBT) could help to integrate the fields of clinical and positive psychology, leading to the development of more efficient and comprehensive clinical interventions*" (Oltean et al., 2017; p. 612). This will most likely be an important future direction for a comprehensive and interdisciplinary investigation of rational beliefs.

Theory of change vs. theory of the disorder The general framework of evidence-based psychotherapy that we have used throughout the chapter (David & Montgomery, 2011) brings to focus the mechanisms of change for a treatment package, but from a scientific point of view, there are some details that are worth being discussed. More specifically, we would like to point that a treatment might work by changing some hypothesized mechanisms, following the criteria above. However, if these mechanisms are not corresponding with the etiopathogenetic theory of the disorder, the positive result for the mechanisms of change of the treatment package might be elusive. Let us take a brief example, for depression and irrational/dysfunctional thinking. Even if REBT/CBT works for depression (empirical support for the treatment package) by changing these types of cognitions (empirical support for the mechanisms of change), if fundamental research shows that irrational/dysfunctional cognitions are not ethiopathogenetic factors, but are just another type of symptom, which when it is reduced has some secondary effect on mood as well, then, it would be more scientifically correct to say that REBT/CBT treatments are symptomatic. The intervention might actually work by accidentally engaging a yet unknown mechanism. Thus, it is important that REBT (and the broader field of CBT) focuses on the mechanisms of change of its treatment but also invest the required effort, in terms of fundamental research, to clarify the etiopathogenetic role of cognitive variables for mental disorders. This might require to build both specific modes of different disorders and to investigate transdiagnostic mechanisms (for an in depth discussion see also David, Matu, Mogoaşe, & Voinescu, 2016).

To sum up, rather than taking two steps forward, REBT research on mechanisms of change requires two steps backward to fundamental research and more rigorously designed studies. Improving the methodological quality of mechanism of change investigations with more experimental manipulations, timeline sensitive RCTs, and intricate component analysis and dismantling designs seem to be a good starting point in the future for good quality research and rigorous conclusions with regard to mechanisms of change. Fundamental research should also focus on investigating the etiopathogenetic nature of irrational beliefs.

REBT and Fundamental Research

REBT has always held that psychopathology originates from cognitive, emotional, behavioral, and biological "causes", "hence effective therapy needs to be heavily integrated and multimodal" (Ellis, 1997, p. 336). Currently, in REBT (and CBT) most of our empirical knowledge is at the *computational level* (i.e., the role of vulnerability factors in psychopathology) and most of our theoretical understanding is at the *algorithmic-representational* level (i.e., how cognitions are represented in our cognitive system). At present, we know too little about the *implementational level or the underlying genetic and neurobiological basis* especially of rational and irrational beliefs. Overall, REBT has lacked a strong link to experimental cognitive psychology, neuroscience, and genetics or at least until very recently.

Currently, REBT is ready to accommodate theoretically some of the most important findings in fundamental research, recognizing the relevance of the basic research input that genetics, neuroscience, or even cognitive experimental psychology can bring (David, 2015). In this respect, the ABC model underlying the REBT framework was recently extended to accommodate the genetic underpinnings of rational and irrational beliefs (David, 2015). Therefore, the extended ABC model theorizes that rational and irrational beliefs develop during ontogenesis, and both genetic and environmental (e.g., parenting) factors have important contributions to their development. Similarly, the model integrated in its conceptualization the notion of *bias* from experimental cognitive psychopathology arguing that general core rational and irrational beliefs are coded in the cognitive system as schemas and they bias the perception of the external events generating more specific rational and irrational beliefs. For more information on the extended ABC model we recommend David (2015).

Following this favorable trend, we suggest that translating some of the advances in fundamental research into psychotherapy research and clinical practice is a critical step to fine-tune and tailor REBT – and CBT in general – in the future. Namely, we pinpoint three significant modalities in which progress in fundamental research could push forward psychotherapy research and practice.

1. *Gaining knowledge on the neurobiological underpinnings of markers of psychopathology could modify current methods of therapeutic change assessment following REBT.* One such vulnerability marker central in REBT's framework is irrational beliefs. To our knowledge, there was only one study that was, however, distally focused on the neurobiological underpinnings of irrational beliefs alongside rational beliefs (Cristea et al., OHBM, 2011). This study used rational reevaluation strategies in response to negative contents, a particular form of emotional regulation called "functional negative reappraisal". As such, functional negative reappraisal was associated with increased activation in the precuneus, a brain area associated with self-mentalization. Although this study may inform future studies focused on the neurobiological basis of rationality/irrationality, the research investigated the neurobiological correlates of functional cognitive revaluation rather than those of rational/irrational beliefs. Therefore, a study in this respect is still needed.

In contrast to task-related functional imaging studies, such as the example above, a highly promising avenue of research is connected to the default mode network (DMN), a distributed network of brain regions that is task independent and active during rest, characterized by a high degree of functional connectivity (i.e., temporal correlations between brain regions). Researchers speculate that in the future DMN will play an important role in identifying vulnerability trait factors to psychopathology that are deep-seated in the brain's default mode of functioning (Raichle, 2015). Some research has already been done in this respect. One such example is the case of impulsivity, a trans-diagnostic susceptibility factor to psychopathology that underlies substance abuse, addictions, and impulse control disorders (e.g., Robbins, Gillan, Smith, de Wit, & Ersche, 2012). Recent research indicates that impulsivity is deep-seated in the brain's resting-state functional architecture, such as reward and pain/loss related areas (i.e., insula, putamen, and the caudate; Gentili et al., 2015).

We believe that the neurobiological peculiarities of irrationality either task-related or not, can be best investigated by contrast with rationality. We speculate that irrationality, due to its evolutionary basis, can recruit older subcortical regions of the brain, compared to rationality, which is supposed to be a newer acquisition of human thinking.

Though promising, current knowledge regarding the neurobiological underpinnings of vulnerability markers to psychopathology is in its early stages and its progress is most likely tied to the success of the Human Connectome Project or the BRAIN research initiative. Several questions still await clarifications: Are rational and irrational cognitions differently represented at the cerebral level?; As stable traits, are they reflected in the brain's default mode of functioning?; Given that REBT and CT indiscriminately affect both irrational beliefs and dysfunctional attitudes (Szentagotai et al., 2008), could we expect the same neural circuits to change in the case of REBT, as in the case of CT?

On the upside, gaining more knowledge on the vulnerability markers would entail also gaining more knowledge on the mechanisms of change given that in REBT cognitive markers of psychopathology overlap with mechanisms of change.

2. *Extending therapygenetics research could contribute to an individualized tailoring of REBT.* Currently, there are only a handful of studies investigating the genetic predictors of differential response to psychotherapy, a line of research known as *therapygenetics*. There are several mixed results in the field. One example is that of the low expression S allele, a common genetic variant (5-HTTLPR) of the serotonin transporter gene (i.e., SERT) that was in some studies associated with a positive response to CBT for adult depression (e.g., Eley et al., 2012), while in others it was non-significant (e.g., Landrø, 2014).

David and collaborators (David et al., 2016) argued that these mixed findings in therapygenetics could be the result of an erroneous exclusive focus on genetic markers of psychopathology instead of a focus on the genetic markers of mechanisms of change. In this respect, a recently published paper was the first to connect classical REBT mechanisms of change (i.e., irrational beliefs) to a functional genetic marker of psychopathology (i.e., COMT VAL^{158}Met) (Podina, Popp, Pop, & David, 2015). Interestingly, the targeted susceptibility variant (i.e., the Met allele) was significantly connected to irrational beliefs only when volunteers were in the average to high range of emotional distress indicating an epigenetic interaction. More research is needed to investigate whether such genetic susceptibility markers could interfere with the success of REBT in changing irrational beliefs and, hence, with its overall efficacy.

These findings provide all the more reason to pursue a fundamental research approach. In the future, these susceptibility markers will be known from the assessment phase and treatment could be personalized accordingly. Knowing who might benefit the most from REBT based on the genetic makeup could save money and time resources and provide on point interventions to individuals that are likely to benefit from them.

3. *Translating advances in recent fundamental and clinical research could enhance and/or update current REBT practice and applied research.* Despite its claim as being scientifically based, current REBT manuals are not entirely consistent with recent fundamental and clinical research. We present three mainstream and separate lines of research with plenty of evidence which – if inserted in clinical practice – could enhance or at least bring up to date existing REBT (and CBT) manuals. These examples are highly relevant for the progress of REBT/CBT in anxiety where – as argued by Emmelkamp and collaborators (2014) – fundamental research contributed the most to the tailoring of the treatment of psychopathology.

   (a) ***Distraction's new role in exposure.*** Exposure is a valuable technique in REBT, as well as in CBT overall. For more than three decades researchers and clinicians alike disagreed over the consequences of diverting attention away from threat during exposure. This is one important reason for which exposure is rarely performed unguided by a therapist. However, the most recent results, including a meta-analysis, indicate that distraction during exposure is less detrimental than previously believed especially in specific phobia (Podina, Koster, Philippot, Dethier, & David, 2013). Depending on the nature of the distractor (e.g. interactive distraction), exposure with distraction outperformed exposure with attention focus with no indication of symptom return. Similarly, meta-analyses extended to other safety behaviors could not provide compelling evidence supporting the removal of safety behaviors during exposure (Meulders, van Daele, Volders, & Vlaeyen, 2016).

   From a theoretical and clinical standpoint, the role played by distraction in exposure therapy for specific phobia, especially, should be radically reconsidered. Furthermore, such results enable self-help REBT/CBT programs where exposure exercises are performed in a self-guided matter. Moreover, it simplifies current clinical protocols for exposure that are highly employed in REBT and CBT for anxiety.

   (b) ***Post-retrieval extinction – an alternative to the exposure component of REBT.*** An exciting and more recent discovery is that fear memories are not read-only, as it has been previously thought, but are liable to change and update with each retrieval (Schiller et al., 2010). Therefore, an alternative to standard extinction emerged, called *post-retrieval extinction* (Schiller et al., 2010). This technique entails that in a brief interval of time of 10 min up to 1 hour following threat reminders memories become unstable and fear memories can be updated with non-threatening information via extinction training. As a result of this procedure, fear responses are no longer trigerred (i.e., Schiller et al., 2010, pp. 49). Post-retrieval extinction has been obtained through pharmacological means (Brunet et al., 2008) and more recently through non-invasive procedures in humans (Schiller et al., 2010).

A recent meta-analysis on sixty-three comparisons examining post-retrieval extinction for preventing the return of fear in humans identified a significant small-to-moderate effect size in reducing the return to fear (Kredlow, Unger, & Otto, 2016). These findings are highly important since any form of psychotherapy, REBT included, is plagued by considerable rates of symptom return depending on the addressed form of psychopathology. REBT and CBT research alike should not miss this research opportunity in order to upgrade its behavioral strategies (i.e., exposure) for dealing with phobias.

(c) ***Attention bias modification's (ABM) Augmenting Effects on REBT.*** ABM is a relatively novel intervention pertaining to experimental cognitive sciences and developed to adjust exaggerated attention to threat (attention bias; AB), which is a highly researched risk factor for psychopathology (e.g., Amir, Beard, Burns, & Bomyea, 2009). ABM was added to REBT parenting programs where it was used to reduce the negative attention bias of the parents and help them to pay attention to their children's positive behaviors and reinforce them. The existing are favorable in this respect (David, Capris, & Jarda, 2017).

There are studies which suggest that ABM may also be an alternative to boosting the efficacy of exposure within an REBT/CBT treatment package for anxiety (Najmi & Amir, 2010). The combination between ABM and exposure could be highly efficient for individuals that are both vigilant and avoidant; their early vigilance may heighten anxiety, while their attentional avoidance may help preserve fear. Hence, attention training may be an optimal solution for reducing vigilant response, while exposure therapy could be used for altering the attentional avoidance.

While the adjunct effects of ABM to CBT are promising irrespective of age and mode of delivery, ABM techniques require several clarifications of their own, starting from their underlying mechanisms of change to alternative and more reliable methods of assessing attention bias. Nevertheless, ABM seems to extract the maximum of therapeutical benefits in the initial stages of therapy and its augmenting effects on REBT/CBT should be further investigated so it can be successfully integrated within the cognitive-behavioral framework.

Given the continuous progress made in fundamental research, our list of the most relevant lines of research that are important for REBT's advancement is far from exhaustive. Nevertheless, we argue that it is highly important to sustain strong ties between fundamental research and psychotherapy research and practice. The history of psychology evidences that most of the progress in the treatment of psychopathology was made when the intervention was closely molded onto fundamental research. CBT for anxiety has evolved due to the numerous fundamental studies that clarified the neurobiological underpinnings of behavioral components, such as exposure. Moreover, efforts should be made to incorporate the diversity of multimodal findings in order to develop a common overarching integrative framework in REBT/CBT.

Integration of REBT and Technology

REBT has already been successfully integrated with some of major technological developments in the last decades, ranging from internet and mobile-based mental health interventions, to virtual reality (VR) and robotic-based therapeutic applications. Also, the scope of these tools has been wide, from prevention, increasing the quality of life in non-clinical populations, to interventions for patients meeting a diagnostic criteria, for both children and adults. Such applications have several potential advantages over the classical means of delivering mental health services, such as increasing accessibility (e.g., internet-based interventions can be accessed from virtually everywhere there is an internet connection and services provision does not depend on whether there is a clinician in the close proximity of the patient), reducing the cost (e.g., guided internet or mobile-based interventions do not require a therapist to closely follow each step of the patient; their input is required only for feedback on progress or in critical moments, and thus this will reduce the time and costs for each case), or making them more appealing to users (e.g., exposure in virtual reality might be more appealing for patients than real life exposure; Garcia-Palacios, Botella, Hoffman, & şi Fabregat, 2007).

We will briefly present here some of the most relevant integrations of REBT with these technological developments. For example, David and David (2013) have developed the PsyPills mobile-app (https://itunes.apple.com/us/app/psypills/id589004229?mt=8), which guides users from the general population in identifying their irrational beliefs, challenging them, and adopting more rational alternatives, in order to change negative dysfunctional emotions into functional ones. Another example is the DCombat application (Giosan et al., 2017; http://dcombat.net/en/), also a mobile-based tool, which aims at reducing depressive symptoms, up to a moderate degree, by incorporating REBT techniques, among other CBT components, in an interactive application, with minimum supervision from a therapist. DCombat is currently undergoing a rigorous testing of its efficacy, in a robust RCT (see Giosan et al., 2017). The *RE*Think game (http://rethink.info.ro/index.html) is another example of integrating REBT theory and technology in a game scenario for children and adolescents, in order to prevent emotional disorders. RETMAN, the main positive character from the game' story line represents a modern reinterpretation of the RETMAN superhero from the comics developed by the Institute for Rational Living in the 70's (Merrifield & şi Merrifield, 1979). The results from a rigorous trial testing the efficacy of the *RE*Think therapeutic game (David, Cardoş, & Matu, 2018) showed that indeed vulnerability for emotional disorders, such as depression, might be reduced by playing the mobile-based game.

Some example related to virtual-reality is the Help4Mood computerized system (http://help4mood.info/site/default.aspx), designed to assist patients that are recovering from depression, or have recovered and the system helps them prevent future relapses. This system includes an interactive avatar which assesses depressive symptoms and guides the patient through a CBT self-help protocol, which includes REBT content and techniques related to restructuring irrational beliefs, among other modules, such as behavioral activation and relaxation, which are not exclusively specific to REBT. The small-scale trial testing its efficacy and acceptability (Burton et al., 2016) shows some positive results but more research is needed to prove its evidence-based status.

Some pilot work has been also made on robot-based interventions, such as the Robo-RETMAN (David, David, & Vanderborght, 2013), a robotic action figure, developed to teach preschool and primary school children, in a simple and game-like interaction, some basic emotion regulation skills, based on rational thinking, in order to prevent the development of emotional disorders. More research is needed to prove its preventive potential.

As one can see, REBT has already penetrated the emerging fields that stem from the integration between psychotherapy and technological tools, but most of the applications and the most robustly documented ones are related to internet and mobile-based applications. These ones have also known a strong development in the CBT field in general and today there are meta-analyses providing compelling evidence that such interventions are not only easy accessible, but they are also effective for a variety of mental health problems, especially emotional ones (e.g., Andersson, Cuijpers, Carlbring, Riper, & Hedman, 2014). However, REBT applications such as those presented above have not reached yet the desired evidence-based status, as more consistent studies testing their efficacy / effectiveness are still undergoing or are needed. Moreover, as we have presented above, internet and mobile-based applications' strong point is related to their increased cost-effectiveness, which is a claim that requires more empirical support. Future research could extend the spectrum of problems than can be approached through internet and mobile technology (e.g., broadening their focus to include more diagnostic categories or taking a transdiagnostic approach) but should also focus on testing their efficacy in rigorous studies (e.g., RCTs), as well as their effectiveness and cost-effectiveness in real life conditions. Such developments could have a major impact on disseminating REBT theory and practice, as well as having a needed contribution to reducing the overall burden of mental disorders that we are now confronted with. Also, staying close to our general framework of evidence-based psychotherapy, from a theory perspective, more work is needed to clarify if internet and mobile-based interventions work by engaging the same mechanisms as classical interventions. Although the theory predicts that the same cognitions should be responsible for developing psychological problems, we need empirical studies to investigate if indeed the mechanisms of change are similar. This is also true for the general CBT field, not only for REBT. Work has already started on this topic (e.g., Mogoaşe, Cobeanu, David, Giosan, & Szentagotai, 2017) but more consistent research is needed. Also, the criteria that should be met by a construct in order to be called a mechanism of change, as those described in the previous section, should also apply for online and mobile interventions.

Much more work is needed on the integration with VR. The potential of this technology to offer an ecological and controllable environment for both assessment and intervention has still to be exploited (see David, Matu, & David, 2013). Much of the psychotherapy research with VR has focused on exposure for anxiety disorders, but more could be done. For example, same anxiogenic environments could be used as primers for eliciting real time appraisals containing irrational beliefs. Moreover, the patient could also be taught how to challenge these beliefs as they emerge and practice rational alternatives while confronted with the same stimuli. This might improve the assessment of irrational beliefs, but it might also improve the efficacy of exposure and / or cognitive restructuring techniques. Same rationale could be applied to assess and restructure irrational beliefs relevant for other symptoms, such as eating disorders, paranoid ideation, addictions, or any other symptom that could be associated with a stimulus that can be represented in VR. Such studies could impact both the practice of REBT, but also the fundamental research, as it could allow to study the impact of irrational beliefs in very controlled, yet ecological conditions (for an in depth discussion see David et al., 2013).

The integration of REBT with robotic-based agents is also a promising endeavor that should be explored in more depth by future research. Robots could undertake some of the practitioners' tasks that are not mandatory for the treatment success, but they could facilitate it, (as a robotic assistant; for a detailed discussion on the possible roles of robotic agents in psychotherapy see David, Matu, & David, 2014). These activities could be related to any of the roles of the practitioner, be it assessment, treatment, prevention, or mental health promotion (e.g., by monitoring the mood of the patient during the week with simple daily questions, or by reminding the patient about daily exercises). Sometimes, the robot could actually perform all of the therapeutic tasks (a robo-therapist), by conducting assessment, prevention or intervention, without the direct presence of the therapist (e.g., the avatar from the Help4Mood project), although such developments depend to a great extent on the advancements in artificial intelligence. The robot might even improve the efficacy of the intervention (as a mediator of the intervention; see David et al., 2014), such as it has been hypothesized for behavioral treatments in the case of children with autism spectrum disorders (e.g., Pop, Pintea, Vanderborght, & David, 2014), but it is not clear now how this role might be played for REBT treatments. The robotic agents could facilitate the dissemination and extension of REBT interventions in places where the practitioners do not have regular access, such as in the homes of the patients. The integration of robotic agents in services delivery offers many new possibilities that should be explored by future research.

REBT as a Platform for Psychotherapy Integration

Even though efficient evidence-based treatments (EBT) are available, it is estimated that more than a half of patients with any mental disorder fail to receive an EBT treatment due to lack of accessibility and poor dissemination (Wang et al., 2005).

Also, even if patients with mental disorders manage to access EBT, a large number of them are not treatable, given the fact that numerous patients do not respond to treatment, and a significant percentage of those who respond relapse (Steinert, Hofmann, Kruse, & Leichsenring, 2014). Moreover, in the last decade, many of the trials investigating the efficacy of new psychological treatments have moved from superiority designs (i.e., aimed at evidencing that a new treatment is better than an already established one) to equivalence and/or to non-inferiority designs (i.e., aimed at evidencing that a new treatment is at least as equally effective as an already available treatment), while the competitive advantages of different treatments focus now on issues such as duration, dropout rate, costs, or the complexity in training the therapists that deliver the new treatment. Although such improvements are still valuable, the clinical field does not bring any therapeutic innovations that can significantly improve the efficacy of psychological interventions for mental disorders. There were expectations that the advancements in neurosciences and genetics might change this state of affairs, by leading to new treatments developed via translational research, but these expectations have not been fulfilled until now (David, Matu, et al., 2016).

Another possibility to move the field forward in this context, is to go beyond the traditional framework of having different psychotherapy schools, which has dominated CBT as well, each of these school promoting their specific theories and practices, to a more integrative and multimodal framework, in which the scientific advancement and the development of more effective treatments become the main focus, regardless of the allegiance to any of the schools of thought. The pressure coming from the health system which is overwhelmed by the increasing burden of mental disorders and the competition with psychiatric treatments are factors that will probably contribute to such a shift. In such an integrative framework, different schools of therapy will likely become different clinical strategies within a more coherent field of psychotherapy.

Given its transdiagnostic approach of psychological problems and its reliance on the ABC model as a guide for understanding and treating mental disorders, REBT might act as a theoretical platform for integrating the competing CBT and EBT approaches within the clinical field. In fact, since its beginning, Albert Ellis designed and presented this model as a super-theory that can integrate various micro-theories related to mental disorders (Ellis, 1997). Moreover, REBT might also accommodate the new translational developments related to the role of genetic factors, automatic information processing, and neuroscience (see also the previous section on this topic). Recent theoretical developments in REBT (David, 2015; David, Matu, et al., 2016) have presented how the ABC model can be extended to act as a transdiagnostic framework that can integrate various underlying cognitive mechanism, coming from different CBT schools, that can explain the development and the maintenance of mental disorders, while also taking into account genetic factors, brain and molecular changes. The extended ABC model also assumes the cognitive mediation hypothesis, which states that the emotional, behavioral and psychophysiological consequences are not a direct consequence of life events, but rather are result of the cognitive information processing. At this level, the model first differentiates between conscious (i.e., different types of cognitions and cognitive biases that a patient can become aware of) and unconscious information processing (i.e., classical conditioning, implicit expectancies and associations). Conscious information processing can be further analyzed in terms of its (1) content, which can take the form of (a) appraisals/irrational beliefs or could take the form of (b) description and inferences, or could be analyzed in terms of (2) specificity of content, which can reflect (a) general cognitive structures, such as schemas and core beliefs, or (b) situationally specific cognitions, taking the form of automatic thoughts. Cognitive biases might be represented as the processes through which general beliefs and cognitions alter the content of specific beliefs related to a certain life event. Genetic factors and neurobiological processes might have an independent impact on the dynamics of information processing (e.g., by acting as vulnerabilities towards developing a cognitive bias) or they might in fact be descriptions of the same phenomenon at a different level of analysis. The nature of these complex relationships is still to be elucidated by future research (for more details see David, Matu, et al., 2016). However, we have exemplified how the theoretical foundations of REBT could in fact accommodate most of the constructs that have been put forward by different clinical school and by fundamental research in order to explain mental disorders and their treatment. Probably, each of the CBT schools can accommodate their specific constructs within this integrative framework, as well as the therapeutic techniques they propose for tackling them. In order to achieve this integrative potential, more research is needed, both fundamental and clinical, in order to empirically test all of the links and the relationship described in the model, as well as its utility to generate effective treatments.

In sum, REBT theory could serve as a platform for psychotherapy integration by using the ABC model as a transdiagnostic framework that can accommodate various underlying mechanism involved in mental disorders. This integrative theory can further generate multimodal interventions which can be tested using the evidence-based criteria.

REBT and Other Fields of Psychology

REBT and cross-cultural psychology REBT theory predicts that irrational and inflexible beliefs will act as vulnerabilities and will be associated with poor functioning and distress. This prediction has received extensive empirical support at individual-level. However, this prediction could also be extended to groups of individual, be them smaller or larger. If distorted and irrational beliefs are shared by a large community, such as the population of a country, then it would be expected that the community as a whole will have a poorer functioning as compared to other communities that do not share such beliefs. Beck (1999) has speculated that dysfunctional beliefs from CBT models could be used to understand large scale negative social phenomenon, such as violence, war and other destructive behaviors. However, this hypothesis has not been tested until recently. Using the REBT/CBT definition of an irrational / dysfunctional belief as a cognition that does not reflect reality, David and his collaborators (David, Matu, David, & Terracciano, 2017) measured the "irrational beliefs" of 47 countries as a cognitive discrepancy index between how the citizens of a specific country perceive their own personality (the personality of the average person from that country) and how they actually are, based on standardized instruments assessing personality traits (the average country score on each trait). The discrepancy index was calculated by contrasting the data related to the Revised NEO Personality Inventory (NEO-PI-R; Costa Jr. & McCrae, 1992) with the data from the National Character Survey (Terracciano et al., 2005), describing the personality of a typical individual from a given country on the same dimensions as the NEO-PI-R model. Results have confirmed the predictions form the REBT/CBT theory, showing that higher country-level discrepancy scores were associated with lower country-level development, lower life satisfaction, and increased levels of conflict and violence. Another study now being under peer-review (Bartucz & David, submitted) used irrationally phrased items from international databases (i.e., the World Values Survey; http://www.worldvaluessurvey.org/wvs.jsp) and showed that higher country-irrationality was related to lower levels of autonomy, human development and economic prosperity. An undergoing study by the same time now collects data with standardized instruments for assessing irrationality from several countries across the globe and similar country-level analyses could be soon conducted using reliable measures of irrational beliefs.

This line of research could be ground breaking for REBT and CBT in general, as it would allow the extension of the theory and applications to a new level, namely analyzing communities and countries and have an impact on policy making. Much research is needed to replicate the initial results, to look at temporal dynamics between the emergence of irrational beliefs and changes in country-level functioning (which would allow to explore the plausible causality role of such beliefs, as it is predicted by the model), and extend to other relevant outcomes (e.g., attitudes towards foreigners, responses to critical events, etc.). Research should also look at the social mechanisms that contribute to the developments of such beliefs. Also, another important line of cross-cultural research would be to investigate how culture might moderate the impact of irrationality on both individual and country level outcomes. Some interesting findings from genetics show that the impact of genetic vulnerabilities on mental health might be lowered in some cultures that have collectivistic traits (Chiao & Blizinsky, 2009).

REBT in educational and organizational settings REBT has been used extensively to promote mental health among children and adolescence, by teaching children the REBT principles for a healthy emotional life (e.g., Ellis & Bernard, 2006), in the form of Rational Emotive Education (e.g., Vernon & Bernard, 2006), or by teaching parents how to promote mental health in children and helping themselves overcome the distress of the parental role, in the form of Rational Positive Parenting (David & DiGiuseppe, 2016). Available reviews (e.g., David, Capris, & Jarda, 2017) support the efficacy / effectiveness of these interventions and the observed effects are similar with those for psychotherapeutic interventions. However, the field needs more studies of better quality and long term monitoring of the effects, in order to prove the value of these interventions in favoring long term healthy development and preventing the development of mental disorders.

REBT has long been used as an organizational intervention to promote distress management in managers and employees and has been proved to be cost effective (Klarreich, DiGiuseppe, & DiMattia, 1987). Also, REBT has followed the recent developments in organizational and managerial coaching and such services are now available and have been proved to work for both specific outcomes relevant for REBT (e.g., cognitive vulnerabilities expressed as irrational beliefs), but also for improving managerial coaching skills and other organizational outcomes (e.g., team satisfaction). As coaching field continues to develop, REBT researchers and practitioners should work on developing and testing the efficacy / effectiveness of such interventions, as well as looking at the mechanisms of change, in order to offer theoretically sound and evidence-based services that cover the increasing requests from the market.

Concluding Remarks

Over the past decade, great progress has been made in developing REBT as an evidence-based psychotherapy. Currently, REBT has a consistent empirical support, reaching international guidelines as a recommended evidence-based intervention for some conditions (e.g., depression). It is highly important to continue to improve upon current REBT treatments, with an emphasis on disorders that have been less investigated (e.g., eating disorders), as well as with an increased focus on methodological rigor such as using well designed RCTs to prove the efficacy of the treatments. However, a strong point is that REBT has been developed as a transdiagnostic treatment. Thus, reconsidering past studies in light of new research paradigms and initiatives, such as RdoC and ROAMER, could provide a substantial competitive advantage for the psychological research of mental disorders.

Another challenge for REBT research over the next years will be to continue to empirically test and expand the knowledge base regarding the mechanisms of change underlying its efficacy. More experimental manipulations, timeline sensitive RCTs, component analysis and dismantling designs are required to elucidate these mechanisms. The integration with developments in basic science should also become a priority for researchers, as these findings might prove the key for improving the efficacy and effectiveness of existing treatments. The integration with technological developments has been proven to be successful for internet and mobile-based application. However, more rigorous studies are needed to promote these applications as a viable alternative to classical interventions. Also, future studies should focus more on the integration with VR and with robotic technology. Finally, as we have discussed in the last section, REBT has a strong potential for acting as a platform for psychotherapy integration, accommodating the constructs and techniques proposed by different CBT schools in a unitary framework that can be used as the foundation for more effective multimodal treatments. Research should focus on empirically testing this potential (a) by investigating the relationship between REBT constructs and other constructs coming from other CBT schools, and (b) by clarifying the nature of the interaction between irrational beliefs, genetic factors and brain activity. We suggest that this integrative and multimodal approach represents a step forward in REBT research that could promote REBT as a best-practice, especially due to: (a) a better understanding of psychological mechanisms with relevance for psychopathology and mental health, stemming from fundamental research within a multi-level approach of human mind (i.e., from genes and molecules to society and culture) (b) a more comprehensive theory-driven case conceptualization leading to more personalized psychological interventions and protocols.

Progresses have also been made in integrating REBT with other fields of psychology, such as cross-cultural research, education and parenting, and organizational counseling and coaching. Both educational and organizational interventions have a long tradition in REBT, but more quality research is needed here to affirm their evidence-based status and to gain an important competitive advantage over other services that are already available on the market. Research on cross-cultural psychology has the potential to contribute to policy making and large scale societal change. We suggest that this line of research could be an important avenue for future research that would help to further promote REBT both at the level of theory and practice.

References

Amir, N., Beard, C., Burns, M., & Bomyea, J. (2009). Attention modification program in individuals with generalized anxiety disorder. *Journal of Abnormal Psychology, 118*(1), 28.

Andersson, G., Cuijpers, P., Carlbring, P., Riper, H., & Hedman, E. (2014). Guided Internet-based vs. face-to-face cognitive behavior therapy for psychiatric and somatic disorders: a systematic review and meta-analysis. *World Psychiatry, 13*(3), 288–295.

Beck, A. T. (1999). *Prisoners of hate: The cognitive basis of anger, hostility, and violence*. New York, NY: Harper Collins.

Beck, A. T., Freeman, A., & Davis, D. D. (Eds.). (2015). *Cognitive therapy of personality disorders*. New York, NY: Guilford Publications.

Brunet, A., Orr, S. P., Tremblay, J., Robertson, K., Nader, K., & Pitman, R. K. (2008). Effect of post-retrieval propranolol on psychophysiologic responding during subsequent script driven traumatic imagery in post-traumatic stress disorder. *Journal of Psychiatric Research, 42*(6), 503–506.

Burton, C., Szentagotai Tatar, A., McKinstry, B., Matheson, C., Matu, S., Moldovan, R., … Serrano Blanco, A. (2016). Pilot randomised controlled trial of Help4Mood, an embodied virtual agent-based system to support treatment of depression. *Journal of Telemedicine and Telecare, 22*(6), 348–355.

Chiao, J. Y., & Blizinsky, K. D. (2009). Culture–gene coevolution of individualism–collectivism and the serotonin transporter gene. *Proceedings of the Royal Society of London B: Biological Sciences*. rspb20091650.

Costa, P. T., Jr., & McCrae, R. R. (1992). *Revised NEO Personality Inventory (NEO-PI-R) and NEO Five-Factor Inventory (NEO-FFI) Professional Manual*. Odessa, FL: Psychological Assessment Resources.

Cristea, I., Gentili, C., Ricciardi, E., Rota, G., Bonino, D., David, D., Pietrini, P., & Guazzelli, M. (2011). Brain correlates of rational and irrational beliefs: an fMRI study of cognitive reappraisal. Poster presentation at the Organization for Human Brain Mapping, Quebec.

David, D. (2015). Rational emotive behavior therapy (REBT). In R. L. Cautin & S. O. Lilienfeld (Eds.), *Encyclopedia of clinical psychology*. New Jersey: Wiley-Blackwell.

David, D., Cotet, C., Matu, S., Mogoase, C., & Stefan, S. (2018). 50 years of rational-emotive and cognitive-behavioral therapy: A systematic review and meta-analysis. *Journal of Clinical Psychology, 74*(3), 304–318.

David, D., Gherman, A., Podina, I., Mogoaşe, C., Sucală, M., & Voinescu, B. (2016). The added value of CBT in the genetic counseling process: concept development, state of the art and new directions. *Journal of Rational-Emotive & Cognitive-Behavior Therapy, 34*(4), 310–331.

David, D., Matu, S., Mogoaşe, C., & Voinescu, B. (2016). Integrating cognitive processing, brain activity, molecules and genes to advance evidence-based psychological treatment for depression and anxiety: From cognitive neurogenetics to CBT-based neurogenetics. *Journal of Rational-Emotive & Cognitive-Behavior Therapy, 34*(3), 149–168.

David, D., Matu, S. A., & David, O. A. (2013). New directions in virtual reality-based therapy for anxiety disorders. *International Journal of Cognitive Therapy, 6*(2), 114–137.

David, D., Matu, S. A., & David, O. A. (2014). Robot-based psychotherapy: Concepts development, state of the art, and new directions. *International Journal of Cognitive Therapy, 7*(2), 192–210.

David, D., Matu, S. A., David, O. A., & Terracciano, A. (2017). The role of cognitive discrepancy between perception of national character and personality in the functioning and adaptation of 46 Countries: An exploratory study. *Cross-Cultural Research, 51*, 412.

David, D., & Montgomery, G. H. (2011). The scientific status of psychotherapies: A new evaluative framework for evidence-based psychosocial interventions. *Clinical Psychology: Science and Practice, 18*(2), 89–99.

David, D., Szentagotai, A., Lupu, V., & Cosman, D. (2008). Rational emotive behavior therapy, cognitive therapy, and medication in the treatment of major depressive disorder: a randomized clinical trial, posttreatment outcomes, and six-month follow-up. *Journal of Clinical Psychology, 64*(6), 728–746.

David, O. A., Capris, D., & Jarda, A. (2017). Online coaching of emotion-regulation strategies for parents: Efficacy of the online rational positive parenting program and attention bias modification procedures. *Frontiers in Psychology, 8*, 500.

David, O. A., Cardoş, R. A., & Matu, S. (2018). Is REThink therapeutic game effective in preventing emotional disorders in children and adolescents? Outcomes of a randomized clinical trial. *European child & adolescent psychiatry*. Advanced online publication. doi: 10.1007/s00787-018-1192-2

David, O. A., & David, D. (2013). The "PsyPills" app: Emerging modalities for applying CBT in real life. In *Poster presented at the 43rd Annual Congress of the European Association for Behavioral and Cognitive Therapies*. Marrakech, Marocco.

David, O. A., David, D., & Vanderborght, B. (2013, September). *The efficacy of the RETMAN robot versus cartoons in helping children manage exam anxiety*. Paper presented at the 43rd Annual Congress of the European Association for Behavioral and Cognitive Therapies, Marrakech, Morocco.

David, O. A., & Digiuseppe, R. (2016). *The rational positive parenting program*. New York, NY: Springer International Publishing.

Eley, T. C., Hudson, J. L., Creswell, C., Tropeano, M., Lester, K. J., Cooper, P., … Uher, R. (2012). Therapygenetics: the 5HTTLPR and response to psychological therapy. *Molecular Psychiatry, 17*(3), 236.

Ellis, A. (1997). Extending the goals of behavior therapy and of cognitive behavior therapy. *Behavior Therapy, 28*(3), 333–339.

Ellis, A., & Bernard, M. E. (Eds.). (2006). *Rational emotive behavioral approaches to childhood disorders: Theory, practice and research*. Boston, MA: Springer.
Emmelkamp, P. M., David, D., Beckers, T., Muris, P., Cuijpers, P., Lutz, W., … Berking, M. (2014). Advancing psychotherapy and evidence-based psychological interventions. *International Journal of Methods in Psychiatric Research, 23*(S1), 58–91.
Engels, G. I., Garnefski, N., & Diekstra, R. F. W. (1993). Efficacy of rational-emotive therapy: A quantitative analysis. *Journal of Consulting and Clinical Psychology, 61*(6), 1083–1090.
Garcia-Palacios, A., Botella, C., Hoffman, H., & Şi Fabregat, S. (2007). Comparing acceptance and refusal rates of virtual reality exposure vs. in vivo exposure by patients with specific phobias. *Cyberpsychology & Behavior, 10*(5), 722–724.
Gaviţa, O. A., David, D., Bujoreanu, S., Tiba, A., & Ionuţiu, D. R. (2012). The efficacy of a short cognitive–behavioral parent program in the treatment of externalizing behavior disorders in Romanian foster care children: Building parental emotion-regulation through unconditional self-and child-acceptance strategies. *Children and Youth Services Review, 34*(7), 1290–1297.
Gentili, C., Cristea, I.A., Podina, I.R., David, D., Vanello, N., & Pietrini, P. (2015). *Caudate resting state activity predicts impulsivity performance in subsequent Balloon Analogue Risk Task*. Poster presentation at the Organization for Human Brain Mapping, Honolulu, Hawaii.
Giosan, C., Cobeanu, O., Mogoaşe, C., Szentagotai, A., Mureşan, V., & Boian, R. (2017). Reducing depressive symptomatology with a smartphone app: study protocol for a randomized, placebo-controlled trial. *Trials, 18*(1), 215.
Hayes, S. C., & Hofmann, S. G. (2017). The third wave of cognitive behavioral therapy and the rise of process-based care. *World Psychiatry, 16*(3), 245–246.
Insel, T. R., Cuthbert, B. N., Garvey, M. A., Heinssen, R. K., & Pine, D. S. (2010). Research Domain Criteria (RDoC): Toward a new classification framework for research on mental disorders. *American Journal of Psychiatry, 167*(7), 748.
Kazdin, A. E. (2007). Mediators and mechanisms of change in psychotherapy research. *Annual Review of Clinical Psychology, 3*, 1–27.
Kieling, C., Baker-Henningham, H., Belfer, M., Conti, G., Ertem, I., Omigbodun, O., … Rahman, A. (2011). Child and adolescent mental health worldwide: evidence for action. *The Lancet, 378*(9801), 1515–1525.
Klarreich, S. H., Digiuseppe, R., & Dimattia, D. J. (1987). Cost effectiveness of an employee assistance program with rational-emotive therapy. *Professional Psychology: Research and Practice, 18*(2), 140–144.
Kredlow, M. A., Unger, L. D., & Otto, M. W. (2016). Harnessing reconsolidation to weaken fear and appetitive memories: A meta-analysis of post-retrieval extinction effects. *Psychological Bulletin, 142*(3), 314.
Landrø, N. I. (2014). Towards personalized treatment of depression: A candidate gene approach. *Scandinavian Journal of Psychology, 55*(3), 219–224.
Merrifield, C., & Şi Merrifield, R. (1979). *Call me RetMan and have a ball*. New York, NY: Institute for Rational Living.
Meulders, A., Van Daele, T., Volders, S., & Vlaeyen, J. W. (2016). The use of safety-seeking behavior in exposure-based treatments for fear and anxiety: Benefit or burden? A meta-analytic review. *Clinical Psychology Review, 45*, 144–156.
Mogoaşe, C., Cobeanu, O., David, O., Giosan, C., & Szentagotai, A. (2017). Internet-based psychotherapy for adult depression: What about the mechanisms of change? *Journal of Clinical Psychology, 73*(1), 5–64.
Najmi, S., & Amir, N. (2010). The effect of attention training on a behavioral test of contamination fears in individuals with subclinical obsessive-compulsive symptoms. *Journal of Abnormal Psychology, 119*(1), 136.
National Institute of Mental Health. (2015). Any Mental Illness (AMI) Among U.S. Adults. Retrieved from https://www.nimh.nih.gov/health/statistics/prevalence/any-mental-illness-ami-among-us-adults.shtml

Oltean, H. R., Hyland, P., Vallières, F., & David, D. O. (2017). An empirical assessment of REBT models of psychopathology and psychological health in the prediction of anxiety and depression symptoms. *Behavioural and cognitive psychotherapy, 45*(6), 600–615.
Ougrin, D. (2011). Efficacy of exposure versus cognitive therapy in anxiety disorders: systematic review and meta-analysis. *BMC Psychiatry, 11*(1), 200.
Palmer, S., & Gyllensten, K. (2008). How cognitive behavioural, rational emotive behavioural or multimodal coaching could prevent mental health problems, enhance performance and reduce work related stress. *Journal of Rational-Emotive & Cognitive-Behavior Therapy, 26*(1), 38–52.
Podina, I., Popp, R., Pop, I., & David, D. (2015). Genetic correlates of maladaptive beliefs: COMT VAL 158 MET and irrational cognitions linked depending on distress. *Behavior Therapy, 46*(6), 797–808.
Podina, I. R., Koster, E. H., Philippot, P., Dethier, V., & David, D. O. (2013). Optimal attentional focus during exposure in specific phobia: a meta-analysis. *Clinical Psychology Review, 33*(8), 1172–1183.
Pop, C. A., Pintea, S., Vanderborght, B., & David, D. (2014). Enhancing play skills, engagement and social skills in a play task in ASD children by using robot-based interventions. *Interaction Studies, 15*(2), 71–91.
Powers, M. B., Sigmarsson, S. R., & Emmelkamp, P. M. G. (2008). A meta-analytic review of psychological treatments for social anxiety disorder. *Interational Journal of Cognitive Therapy, 1*, 94–113.
Raichle, M. E. (2015). The brain's default mode network. *Annual Review of Neuroscience, 38*, 433–447.
Robbins, T. W., Gillan, C. M., Smith, D. G., de Wit, S., & Ersche, K. D. (2012). Neurocognitive endophenotypes of impulsivity and compulsivity: towards dimensional psychiatry. *Trends in Cognitive Sciences, 16*(1), 81–91.
Schiller, D., Monfils, M. H., Raio, C. M., Johnson, D. C., Ledoux, J. E., & Phelps, E. A. (2010). Preventing the return of fear in humans using reconsolidation update mechanisms. *Nature, 463*(7277), 49.
Shelley, A. M., Battaglia, J., Lucey, J., Ellis, A., Opler, L. A., & Center, B. P. (2001). Symptom-specific group therapy for inpatients with schizophrenia. *Einstein Quarterly Journal of Biology and Medicine, 18*(1), 21–28.
Steinert, C., Hofmann, M., Kruse, J., & Leichsenring, F. (2014). The prospective long-term course of adult depression in general practice and the community. A systematic literature review. *Journal of Affective Disorders, 152–154*, 65–75.
Szentagotai, A., David, D., Lupu, V., & Cosman, D. (2008). Rational emotive behavior therapy versus cognitive therapy versus pharmacotherapy in the treatment of major depressive disorder: Mechanisms of change analysis. *Psychotherapy: Theory, Research, Practice, Training, 45*(4), 523.
Terracciano, A., Abdel-Khalek, A. M., Adam, N., Adamovova, L., Ahn, C. K., Ahn, H. N., … Meshcheriakov, B. (2005). National character does not reflect mean personality trait levels in 49 Cultures. *Science, 310*, 96–100.
Vernon, A., & Bernard, M. E. (2006). Applications of REBT in schools: Prevention, promotion, intervention. In A. Ellis & M. E. Bernard (Eds.), *Rational emotive behavioral approaches to childhood disorders: Theory, practice and research* (pp. 415–460). Boston, MA: Springer.
Vîslă, A., Flückiger, C., Grosse Holtforth, M., & David, D. (2016). Irrational beliefs and psychological distress: a meta-analysis. *Psychotherapy and Psychosomatics, 85*(1), 8–15.
Wang, C., Jia, F., Fang, R., Zhu, Y., & Huang, Y. (1999). Comparative study of rational-emotive therapy for 95 patients with dysthymic disorder. *Chinese Mental Health Journal, 13*, 172–183.
Wang, P. S., Lane, M., Olfson, M., Pincus, H. A., Wells, K. B., & Kessler, R. C. (2005). Twelve-month use of mental health services in the United States: Results from the national comorbidity survey replication. *Archives of General Psychiatry, 62*(6), 629–640.

Chapter 7
Rational Emotive Behaviour Therapy and the Working Alliance

Windy Dryden

Introduction

In this chapter, I will consider the working alliance in REBT. As this concept makes clear, therapist and client have work to do and they are encouraged to become allies while doing this work. As we shall see the concept of the 'working alliance', is broader than that of the 'therapeutic relationship'. Historically, in published work in REBT, the relationship between therapist and client in REBT has not been emphasized as a therapeutic ingredient, even though it is generally regarded as important to, but not necessary for, therapeutic change. One of the reasons that the therapeutic relationship has not received much attention in the REBT literature is that it has usually been seen as synonymous with the bond between therapist and client and Ellis (in Dryden, 1997) always warned REB therapists to guard against developing an overly warm bond with their clients, for fear of exacerbating the latter's dire need for love and approval. However, the therapeutic bond is but one of four components of the working alliance between client and therapist that can be examined in REBT. The other domains are goals, views and tasks. In this chapter then I will consider issues to which REB therapists need to attend in each of the four alliance components.

In the same year as Beck, Rush, Shaw, and Emery (1979) published 'Cognitive Therapy of Depression', a paper by Ed Bordin (1979) was published in the journal, 'Psychotherapy: Theory, Research and Practice'. This article served to alert therapists across the psychotherapeutic spectrum of the importance of the working alliance in the practice of psychotherapy. Broader than the concept of the therapeutic relationship, the working alliance, as conceptualised by Bordin in his 1979 paper, was comprised of three components: bonds, goals and tasks. Almost 20 years later, I added a fourth component which I call 'views' (Dryden, 2011). Table 7.1 provides a brief definition of each of these four components. In what follows, I will attempt

W. Dryden (✉)
Goldsmiths University of London, London, UK

© Springer Nature Switzerland AG 2019

M. E. Bernard, W. Dryden (eds.), *Advances in REBT*,
https://doi.org/10.1007/978-3-319-93118-0_7

Table 7.1 Brief definitions of the four components of the working alliance

Bonds refer to the interpersonal connectedness between the therapist and client
Views refer to the understandings that both participants have on salient issues
Goals refer to the purpose of the therapeutic meetings
Tasks refer to the procedures carried out by both therapist and client in the service of the latter's goals

to show how these components illuminate important aspects of the therapeutic relationship in REBT. Before I do, I wish to stress that while I will be discussing these components separately, they are, in fact, very much inter-related.

Bonds

When the bond between REB therapist and client becomes a focus for consideration, certain concepts become salient.

The 'Core Conditions'

Albert Ellis, the founder of REBT, gave a paper at a workshop on psychotherapy held by the American Academy of Psychotherapists in Madison, Wisconsin in 1957, critiquing Rogers' (1957) paper on the necessary and sufficient conditions for therapeutic personality change. In this paper, which was later published, Ellis (1959) advanced the argument that the conditions articulated by Rogers in his 1957 paper – three of which have come to be known as the 'core conditions' in the field of psychotherapy (empathy, respect and genuineness) – may well be desirable, but are not necessary for therapeutic change to occur. He went on to outline, in his paper, that what the effective REB therapist needs to do, in addition to providing these desirable core conditions, is to adopt a highly active-directive stance and encourage clients to identify, challenge and change the irrational ideas which lie at the source of their psychological disturbances and to act and think in accord with their alternative rational ideas. While the language may have changed and softened over the years, this accurately encapsulates Ellis's view up to the time of his death in 2007 with one exception.

This exception concerns therapist warmth. Ellis's position on the place of therapist warmth in psychotherapy – and not just in REBT – was that while clients appear to value this condition, it may serve to reinforce their dire need for approval and lead them to become more rather than anxious about the possible future loss of approval, not only from their therapist, but from others in general (see Ellis in Dryden, 1997). A study carried out by DiGiuseppe, Leaf, and Linscott (1993) discovered that Ellis did, in fact, practise as he preached on this point. The researchers found that clients of Ellis perceived him as less warm and intimate than did clients of other REBT therapists. In other words, Ellis de-emphasized being warm with his clients while other REBT therapists did not do this with their own clients. This latter point is a salutary lesson to those who think that all REBT therapists develop relationships with their clients in the manner of Albert Ellis.

While the ‘core conditions’ are seen as important, but neither necessary nor sufficient for therapeutic change to occur in REBT, from a working alliance perspective, a more complicated picture is found that reflects recent research on the issue (Beutler et al., 2004) and which shows that such core conditions are often important for most but not for all clients. The implications for the REB therapist are that they need to emphasize certain conditions with some clients and to de-emphasize other conditions with other clients in order to establish the most productive and idiosyncratic therapeutic bond with each individual client. An example of this is shown in the following vignette.

> Larry felt very uncomfortable when his REB therapist displayed warmth in trying to understand things from his perspective. His therapist noticed this and brought this up at the end of a one of their sessions. Larry admitted that when his therapist showed warmth it reminded him of his mother’s intrusiveness and he really didn’t like it. The therapist took this issue to supervision and discussed two options with their supervisor: to explore this response with Larry or to deliver empathy in a more matter of fact manner. The therapist decided to raise these two possible strategies with the client and be guided by his decision. Larry did not want to explore his response to the perceived intrusiveness of the therapist’s warmth. He did not like it and that was that. His therapist decided to implement the ‘matter of fact’ form of empathy and in subsequent feedback sessions, Larry reported that he had noticed this change and found it more helpful.

This vignette shows a number of important points:

- The therapist uses their observational skills to identify a possible area of client interpersonal discomfort
- The therapist then raises it with the client in the feedback section at the end of the session to find out more about it
- The therapist discusses two ways forward with the client (after discussing it with their supervisor) and goes along with the client’s decision on this matter. If the therapist had favored the other approach, they would have given a rationale for it, but still abided by the client’s ultimate decision after discussion. To do otherwise would be to pose a threat to the working alliance

The feedback section of REB therapy sessions emerged from cognitive therapy and is discussed in Beck et al.’s (1979) seminal text. It is an aspect of what I call the “reflection process” (Dryden, 2011) where the therapist and client stand back from the “therapeutic action” to reflect on it. This standing back involves both therapist and client entering into an “observing ego” state of mind. When they are fully involved in that action, they are in an “experiencing ego” state of mind.

Interactive Style

The second area relevant to the therapeutic bond concerns work that has been done on the interactive styles of both therapist and client. In REBT, the preferred interactive style is where the two participants are actively collaborating in working with the cognitive-behavioural elements of the client's problems. However, not all clients can collaborate with the REB therapist or find this collaboration helpful as shown in the following vignette

> Melanie sought REBT, but had a problem working in a collaborative way with her therapist. She felt that her therapist knew what her irrational beliefs were and thus they should just come out and say it rather than "beating around the bush" with the Socratic approach. Melanie directly told the therapist to be straight with her and tell her what they thought her beliefs were rather than working gently to discover what they were. Her therapist discussed this in supervision and adjusted their style accordingly, stopped using Socratic questioning and was more didactic and declarative in their interventions. Melanie found this "up front" approach much more to her liking and was able to put into practice much of what her therapist directly suggested. She openly rejected the therapist's other suggestions and the therapist accepted such statements as Melanie's preferences for bluntness in relationships.

Adopting an interactive style that does not reinforce a client's problems/issues When two people come together in any interpersonal setting, their interactive styles may mesh or jar. Just because such styles may mesh should not necessarily be taken as a sign that effective therapy is taking place. For, what may mesh may be unproductive. While some therapists value the principle of therapist-client collaboration, there is a danger that, in some cases, such collaboration where the therapist is active may "pull" for client passivity. If a client becomes passive this may in turn "pull" for greater therapist activity and a vicious cycle may be established which may mirror and reinforce the client's passivity issues in their everyday life. Effective REB therapists are aware of the dangers of adopting an interactive style that reinforces their clients' problems or issues and guard against doing this. In addition to high levels of therapist activity with a passive client, the following are two examples of therapist interactive styles that may particularly reinforce a client's problems or issues.

Therapist directiveness with a client who is highly reactant A client who is highly reactant has an adverse reaction to actual or perceived attempts to influence them. Given this tendency, the therapist needs to emphasize client choice more than usual. Failure to do this may lead the client to leave therapy as a way of preserving their autonomy.

Therapist humor with a client who uses humor as a defence It is well known that people can use humour as a way of defending themselves against their emotional pain and from dealing with their problems in an effective manner. If the therapist employs humor with such a client, they may unwittingly reinforce this tendency. When it helps strengthen a defence, it is often introduced by the client themself and in this case, the therapist needs to respond without joining the client's levity. When humour is effective, it helps promote change particularly in disputing irrational beliefs (see below).

Styles of disputing irrational beliefs DiGiuseppe (1991) has discussed a number of therapist styles that can be employed in disputing or examining clients' irrational beliefs. Socratic questioning is the preferred style in REBT, but there are times when this questioning style does not yield therapeutic benefit for the client (see the above vignette). As DiGiuseppe (1991: 183) notes "Some clients of limited intelligence, limited creativity or extreme emotional disturbance may not come up with an appropriate answer to a Socratic question". He goes on to say that letting them suffer because they do not respond well to this interpersonal style of questioning may not be ethical. Thus, the REB therapist should persist with a particular style for a reasonable amount of time before switching to another style of questioning. DiGiuseppe (1991) outlines the following alternatives to Socratic questioning:

A didactic style Here points are made declaratively and the therapist then checks the client's understanding of and response to the point made.

A metaphorical style Here points are made with reference to a metaphor, story, analogy or parable. The main advantage of this style is that it increases the memorability of the point if the client can resonate to the method used (Blenkiron, 2010). Again, the therapist needs to check the client's understanding and response to the point expressed in the method used.

A humorous style Much has been written on the role of humor in psychotherapy (e.g. Lemma, 1999). With certain clients, humor can facilitate the working alliance and helps them to take themselves seriously, but not too seriously and thus encourages them to put their life situation into a healthier perspective (Ellis, 1977). However, with other clients, humor may either increase their tendency to defend themselves against psychological pain by the use of minimisation or leave them with these sense that the therapist is ridiculing them. Getting client feedback on the therapist's use of humor is, therefore, critical.

To DiGiuseppe's list, I would add:

A self-disclosing style While psychodynamic therapists strive to be neutral and anonymous in their encounters with most clients, REB therapists are more prepared to be reveal personal information about themselves. Thus, self-disclosure may be a powerful way of encouraging clients to re-evaluate dysfunctional schema or irrational beliefs and provide one way of dealing with their problems (Dryden, 1990). For example, I sometimes use a personal example of how I overcame my anxiety about stammering in public. I disclose that I used to believe "I must not stammer." I stress that this belief increased rather than diminished my anxiety. I then show how I questioned this irrational belief by proving to myself that there was no evidence to support it, then changed it to the following rational belief: "There is no reason why I must not stammer. If I stammer, I stammer. That's unfortunate, but hardly awful." I then describe how I pushed myself to put this rational belief into practice while speaking in public and finally outline the productive effects that I experienced by doing so.

The above is an example of the coping model of therapist self-disclosure where the therapist says, in effect, "I used to have this problem, but this is what I did to overcome it. This contrasts with a mastery model of therapist self-disclosure where the therapist discloses that they have never experienced a problem similar to their client's because they have always held rational beliefs about the issue at hand. The mastery model tends to accentuate the differences between the therapist and their client and, in my experience, is less productive than the coping model in encouraging clients to re-evaluate their own irrational beliefs. However, some clients will not find either model useful. If this is the case, it is best to avoid self-disclosure as a disputing style and use another style instead. As elsewhere, gaining client feedback on the use of therapist self-disclosure is crucial.

This section on interactive style shows the importance of the therapist demonstrating interpersonal flexibility in REBT. However, this needs to be done genuinely and putting on an act for a client may not be immediately noticed, but it will be discerned eventually with deleterious effects on the working alliance. Arnold Lazarus (1993) has argued elegantly that an effective therapist needs to be an "authentic chameleon". In this context, being able to modify one's interpersonal style from patient to patient, but to do so authentically.

The Bonds of Influence

In the 1980s, work emerging from social psychology in North America suggested that it was useful to consider the therapeutic relationship as an interpersonal setting where influence takes place (Dorn, 1984). While I will consider how REB therapists influence their clients, it is more accurate to say that clients allow themselves to be influenced by their therapists. They do so for three major reasons:

(i) Because they like their therapist or find them *attractive* in some way.
(ii) Because they find their therapist *trustworthy*.
(iii) Because they are impressed by their therapist's *credibility* as a therapist. This may include the therapist's expertise, experience and/or credentials. It may also be because they think the therapist knows what they are talking about because they have had personal experience of the problem(s) for which the client is seeking help.

Taking this framework, it is possible to ask clients the following question as part of the initial phase of therapy. "Are you most likely to listen to your therapist and give credence to what they have to say, if you like the person, if you trust the person or if the person appears to know what they are talking about?" and be guided by their answer in thinking about how to best influence them. My view is that REB therapists should endeavor to meet their clients' preferences on this matter to the extent that they are able to do so genuinely and to the extent that it is helpful for their clients for them to do so.

My own experience as a REB therapist, trainer and supervisor is that some clients may listen to and allow themselves to be influenced by therapists whom they like, but who do not show expertise, and others may listen to and allow themselves to be influenced by those who are expert, but whom they may not like. However, few clients will listen to therapists whom they do not trust, although they may like them or be impressed by their credentials.

Transference and counter-transference
The final area which is relevant to the bond between REBT therapist and client relates to the concepts of transference and counter-transference. Although these concepts have been derived from psychoanalytic approaches to psychotherapy (see Jacobs, 2010) and their very mention has a negative effect on many REBT therapists, my position is that it is the phenomena to which the terms point that are more crucial than the use of terms themselves. The terms point to the fact that both clients and therapists bring to the therapeutic relationship tendencies to perceive, feel and act towards another person which are influenced by their prior interaction with significant others. These tendencies can and often do have a profound influence on the development and maintenance of the working alliance. Working with transference in REBT/CBT is considered by Miranda and Andersen (2007) among others and the issue of counter-transference in REBT has been discussed by Ellis (2002).

Miranda and Andersen (2007) present a social-cognitive model of transference that has relevance for how REB therapists can deal with this issue. They suggest that the therapist ask the client to name and describe significant others with special reference to facets of their interpersonal relating. Once these representations have been identified the therapist can see when these are activated in the therapeutic relationship and the client can be helped to see the link between the present response to the therapist and the representations of significant others. Particular cues in the therapist's behaviour need to be identified with the help of the client. My own recommendation to the therapist is to apologise for any unintended sensitivity since this does help the client to process transferential experiences. Once this has ben done the therapist can help the client to identify and dispute any irrational beliefs that underpin any disturbed response to the therapist's behavior and also to the past behavior of the significant other(s).

Ellis (2002) identified unhelpful therapist irrational beliefs which render REB therapists to experiencing an unhelpful counter-transference response (e.g. need for approval, intolerance and emotional inhibition). Self-acceptance, self-compassion and humility are important if therapists are to acknowledge anti-therapeutic reactions to clients and the irrational beliefs on which they are based. REB therapists are particularly vulnerable to feeling ashamed of having such reactions (which lead them not to admit their existence even to themselves) particularly if they have irrational beliefs about being an REB therapist (e.g. "Because I am an REB therapist, I absolutely should not have negative reactions to my patients").

Having considered the bonds of REBT in the next sections, I will consider a component the alliance that I introduced (Dryden, 2011): views.

Views

The second component of the expanded model of the working alliance is called 'views (Dryden, 2011). These refer to the understandings that the therapist and the client have on such relevant issues as:

- The nature of the client's psychological problems
- How the client's problems can best be addressed
- The practical aspects of therapy

The Therapist's Views

REB therapists are obviously influenced by REB theory when they come to understand the nature of their clients' problems. Thus, in REBT the role of irrational beliefs is emphasized in psychological disturbance and these irrational beliefs are formulated in precise ways (i.e. rigid beliefs, awfulising beliefs, discomfort tolerance beliefs and devaluation beliefs) with the same irrational beliefs being deemed to be present across diagnoses (Dryden, 2015). It may be assumed that two different therapists working within REBT may have the same views of a client's problem. However, this is not necessarily the case. For example, Albert Ellis and I formulated the same client's problem differently in a single session intervention with that client (see Robb, 2010).

REB therapists' views of how to help clients with their problems stem logically from how they conceptualize these problems. This involves helping clients to stand back and dispute their irrational and rational beliefs and then act in ways that are consistent with and support the latter so that that can respond to adversities with a set of flexible and non-extreme beliefs rather than a set of disturbance-creating rigid and extreme beliefs.

The Client's Views

Clients also come to REBT with some idea of what determines their problems and how best their therapist can help them. Such ideas may be well informed and accurate as in the case of a person who has read about REBT, has sought an REB therapist because they have resonated with it and has a clear idea of what to expect. On the other hand, the ideas that potential clients may have about REBT may be inaccurate. This often happens when they have been referred for REBT, but have been told very little about what it is. When this is the case, therapists need to address the issue, explain clearly what REBT is and respond to any misconceptions that clients have about it. These misconceptions are also present in clients' doubts, reservations misconceptions about REBT concepts and practices and need to be identified and corrected.

Effective Therapy Occurs When the Client's Views Are Similar to the Therapist's

Working alliance theory holds that when a client's views are similar to their therapist's on the above issues then therapy is more likely to be effective than when such views are different. When they are different these differences need to be acknowledged and openly discussed. Effective REBT therapists are good at explaining REBT in a way that resonates with clients and, in particular, elicit instances when clients have changed unhelpful beliefs in other areas of their life with positive effect. Helping such clients to see that they have, in fact, used the principles of REBT in their own lives encourages them to see the relevance of REBT to their own problems and facilitates their engagement with this approach.

However, some potential clients are steadfast in their opposition to REBT and these clients should be referred to other therapies that better match their views on what determines their problems and how these can best be addressed as shown in the following vignette:

> Many years ago when I worked in Birmingham, a man rang me and asked me if I practised an approach to therapy known as RT. REBT was originally known as rational therapy (RT) and I thought that the man was referring to REBT but in its earliest form. On that misunderstanding, I agreed to see him. However, it soon transpired that he was seeking Reichian therapy (RT), a body-work oriented therapy, very different from REBT, an approach which he said was 'intellectual clap-trap' after I explained the nature of REBT to him. Consequently, I referred him to a local Reichian therapist that I knew. I heard later that he found Reichian Therapy (RT) very helpful.

The Contributions of Therapist and Client to REBT

Both client and therapist have roles and responsibilities to carry out to harness the power of REBT. To this end, it is important that both participants understand what their respective contributions are to the process of REBT and agree to make them. I will discuss the task component of the working alliance later in the chapter; here I am focusing on the duo's *views* of these roles and responsibilities.

The client's contribution to REBT The client contributes to the success of REBT by understanding that they have an active part to play in the process and agree to do the following

Be honest It is important that the client is honest with the therapist about the nature of the problem(s) for which they are seeking help. Because of the nature of the client's problem(s) and difficulties, it may be difficult for them to be honest right from the start and their honesty will be, in part, facilitated by their experience of the therapist as a trustworthy and understanding source of help.

Client honesty not only involves the disclosure of problems, it also involves the client giving their honest views concerning what they think may be helpful and not helpful about addressing their problems and giving the therapist sincere feedback about what is useful and perhaps not so useful about the therapist's contribution to REBT.

Set goals
Once the client has disclosed their problems, with the therapist's help they need to set goals since therapy is a purposeful activity. I will discuss this issue more fully in the next section.

Be open to the therapist's input
It is important that the client is open to the therapist's points and frameworks. Such openness should be accompanied by the client adopting a healthy questioning approach and to give their honest views as noted above. The client should ideally neither uncritically accept what the therapist says, nor immediately reject it if it does not fit what they are looking for

Carry out negotiated tasks
No matter how skilled the REB therapist is, unless the client agrees to carry out negotiated tasks in the service of their goals, they will derive little lasting benefit from REBT. This is perhaps the client's most important contribution to REBT. Of course, they may experience difficulty in implementing these tasks, in which case they need to be honest about such difficulty with their therapist so that the latter can address it with them.

The Therapist's Contribution to REBT

Here is a summary of the therapist's parallel contribution with respect to the client's contribution. Thus, the therapist should ideally:

- Encourage the client to express their honest views concerning their problem(s), possible ways of addressing the problem(s) and other matters related to the person's therapy.
- Help the client set meaningful goals
- Show that they value the client expressing their views concerning understanding and addressing their problem(s) and other relevant therapeutic matters and take their views very seriously. The client's past successful attempts to deal with similar problems should be identified and integrated into the treatment plan where appropriate
- Encourage the client to carry out their tasks, help them anticipate and deal with (i) potential obstacles to their execution and (ii) any actual obstacles that they encounter

Goals

The third component of the working alliance – goals – pertains to the objectives both client and REB therapist have for coming together. They are therefore the raison d'etre of therapy. Bordin (1979) argued that a good therapeutic outcome is facilitated when the therapist and client agree what the client's goals are, and agree to work toward the fulfilment of these goals. Thus, Bordin was concerned basically with outcome goals. The working alliance is threatened when either explicitly, or perhaps more commonly implicitly, the therapist and client have different outcome goals in mind for the client. These threats are minimised in REBT because goal setting is made explicit. REB therapists increase their chances of helping clients to reach their goals when both agree to pursue goals that are:

- Within clients' direct control to achieve;
- Realistic and achievable;
- Set by the clients themselves;
- Positively stated;
- Clearly stated;
- Uncontaminated by psychological disturbance;
- Based on the present state of clients (e.g. an overcoming-disturbance goal when clients are disturbed; a personal development goal when they are not);
- Set to reflect the amount of effort clients are prepared to make to achieve the goals.

It is important for the REB therapist to bear in mind that the client's goals may change during the therapeutic process and thus the therapist needs to check periodically on the current status of their client's goals.

Problems with Goals and How REB Therapists Deal with them

REB therapists are likely to encounter a number of problems with clients' goals. In what follows, I list the most common problems and how REB therapists respond to them.

The client expresses goals in vague terms Here the REB therapist will help the client to specify their goals as clearly as possible so that they are achievable.

The client sets goals that involve changes in other people or life events Here, the REB therapist renegotiates these goals so that their achievement falls within the client's power. The therapist shows the client that while they are in control of attempts to influence the other to change, they are not in control over the outcome of these influence strategies.

The client sets unrealistic goals When a client disturbs themself about adversity, they will often nominate goals that involve them feeling a less intense version of the disturbed emotion or indifference. When this happens, the REB therapist helps the client to see that both of these are unrealistic. The first still involves the client experiencing a disturbed emotion, albeit with decreased intensity and the second is predicated on the notion that it is possible for the client to convince themself that they don't care about something that, in reality, they do care about. Having done this the therapist helps the client to set a healthy negative emotion as a goal and that this is a realistic and constructive response to the adversity.

The client sets goals that are not comprehensive Psychological disturbed responses to adversities are emotional (negative in tone and unhealthy in effect), behavioral (unconstructive) and cognitive (highly distorted and skewed to the negative). Therefore, when the client sets only an emotional goal, only a behavioural goal or less frequently only a cognitive goal, they are not being comprehensive in their goal-setting. When the REB therapist helps their client set comprehensive goals these include emotional, behavioral and cognitive goals, all three together. As noted above emotional goals in response to emotions are negative in tone, but healthy in effect, behavioral goals are constructive and cognitive goals are realistic and balanced.

The client expresses goals that are based on their disturbed feelings, attitudes or behaviour When this happens the REB therapist will provide a rationale so that the client's disturbance is dealt with first before setting concrete goals.

Tasks

The final component in this view of the working alliance pertains to tasks – activities carried out by both REBT therapist and client that are goal-directed in nature. REBT is an approach that is rich in its use of techniques. However, when an alliance perspective on tasks is taken, the slant is different from one which emphasizes the content of such tasks and several issues become salient. From this perspective, effective REBT occurs when:

- The client understands the nature of the therapeutic tasks that they are being called upon to execute.
- The client sees the instrumental value of carrying out these tasks i.e. that doing so will help him to achieve their outcome goals.
- The client has the ability to carry out the therapeutic tasks required of them. If the client lack this ability then no amount of skill training will help them acquire it
- The client has the skills to carry out the therapeutic tasks required of them. If they lack the skills then the therapist should help them to acquire them before expecting them to execute the tasks

- The client has the confidence to execute the task.
- The task has sufficient therapeutic potency to facilitate goal achievement.
- The client understands the nature of their REB therapist's tasks and how these relate to their own
- The REB therapist has sufficient skill in implementing their tasks and in ensuring that the client can carry out his tasks as detailed above.

Negotiate 'homework' tasks
It is generally agreed that REBT/CBT is more effective when therapist and client negotiate agreed 'homework' tasks and that clients carry these out between sessions. From a working alliance perspective, the following is important. The REB therapist is advised to:

Negotiate tasks, don't assign them unilaterally I prefer the term 'task' to the term 'assignment' when discussing what a client is going to do for homework because the term 'assignment' means that something is assigned to the client to do while the term 'task' does not have this connotation. Thus, the REB therapist negotiates a task with the client and does not assign it to the person. The more the client is a party to the generation of the task, the more likely it is that they will do it (Kazantzis, Whittington, & Dattilio, 2010).

Take time to negotiate a task Homework tasks are usually negotiated at the end of the therapy session and enough time needs to be devoted to the negotiation process if the client is to do the task and gain benefit from it.

Ensure that the task is related to the work done in the therapy session A good homework task follows logically from what is discussed in a therapy session rather than be unrelated or peripherally related to the session focus.

Help the client to see the purpose of the agreed task The purpose of an effective homework task is ideally to provide the client with the opportunity to face a relevant adversity while rehearsing the person's rational beliefs and without the use of safety-seeking procedures (both behavioral and cognitive) designed to help the person avoid the adversity or keep themself safe if they cannot avoid it. The main problem with these procedures, which are often subtle in nature, is that they prevent the client from facing the adversity fully and thus from processing it in healthy ways. Consequently, it is important for the therapist to help the client identify their routinely used safety-seeking procedures and to encourage them to drop their use while carrying out homework tasks.

Ensure that the client has the skills or capability of doing the task If the client does not have the skills to carry out a homework task, and they can be taught these skills by the therapist quite easily, then the therapist should do this and then negotiate the task. However, if the skill is more complex and will take a while to be taught and acquired or the client lacks the capability to carry out the task then another task should be considered, especially in brief REBT (see Chap. 9).

Encourage the client to face the adversity whenever possible and to use the 'challenging, but not overwhelming' principle while doing so (Dryden, 1985) This states that the client should face an adversity when is challenging for them to do so, but not if is overwhelming for them. If the task is too easy then it has little therapeutic value, but if it is too difficult, then the person will not do it and may become discouraged with therapy.

Attend to the specifics when negotiating a task An effective homework task is one where the person carries out a specific task on a specific number of occasions in specific situations, at specific times. Consequently, the therapist should encourage the client to use the concept of 'specificity' while negotiating homework tasks.

Suggest that the client makes a written note of the negotiated homework task Rather than commit the negotiated task to memory, the client is more likely to remember it if they make a written note of it in a place to which they have ready access (e.g. a frequently consulted diary, in a notebook or on a smartphone).

Problem-solve any obstacles to task completion With homework negotiation, it is better to be forewarned than forearmed. Consequently, the therapist should ask the client to identify potential obstacles to task completion and to find ways of dealing with these to prevent them from becoming actual obstacles.

Suggest that the client uses imagery rehearsal in the session and between sessions Before carrying out the task 'in the field', as it were, the therapist can suggest that the client picture themself facing the adversity, acting constructively and holding in mind the rational beliefs that they wish to develop. This can be done first in the therapy session and later outside the session, but before the client carries out the task, in reality.

Review Homework Tasks

Unless there is a good reason not to, it is important that the REB therapist reviews the client's homework task at the beginning of the following session. Not reviewing this task communicates implicitly to the client that homework tasks are not important. When reviewing homework tasks with a client, it is advised that the REB therapist:

Discover what the person actually did for homework Ensure that the client did the task as agreed and explore and, if necessary, respond to any modifications that they made to the task.

Evaluate success by the client's efforts and behavior on the task rather than its outcome Thus, if a client agreed to assert themself with one person a day, then, if they did this, it was a success no matter how the other people responded to them.

Respond to the client's failure to carry out the task with empathy It is important that the therapist assesses and responds to the client's failure to initiate or complete the task with understanding and not censure. This will encourage the client to be honest about the reasons for task non-completion.

Respond to the client's routine failure to carry out homework tasks When a client routinely fails to do homework tasks, it is useful to use REBT's 'Situational ABCDEFG' framework to help them deal with any emotional-based obstacles to task completion.

Capitalize on the client's success It is important that the therapist help the client to articulate what they learned from doing the task and capitalize on their success by encouraging them to generalize that learning.

Teaching Clients the Tasks of REBT

REBT can be seen as a psycho-educational approach to therapy and as such, clients can be taught the skills of REBT assessment of intervention as an aid to more formal therapy and to help them become their own REBT therapists. There are several texts that help clients to learn these skills in a step-by-step manner (e.g. Dryden, 2001).

The Four Components of the Working Alliance Are Interrelated

So far, I have dealt with the four components of the working alliance in REBT – bonds, views, goals and tasks – as if they were separate. In reality, however, they are interrelated. Let me close by exemplifying this point.

- Successful structuring of therapist and client *task* behavior in the therapy process can help to strengthen the initial *bond* between counsellor and client and serve to clarify the client's *goals*.
- Skilful responding to a client's early test of trust in the therapy relationship can free the client to engage more deeply in the therapy process and will help to deepen the *bond* between therapist and client. It will also enable the client to concentrate on his own *task* behaviour.
- Sensitive and effective handling of client reluctance will increase the likelihood that the 'reluctant' client will commit himself to the therapy process and set *goals* that are relevant to himself rather than to any coercive third party.
- Selecting *tasks* that meet a client's predominant pattern of dealing with the world encourages the therapist to speak the client's 'language' and serves to strengthen the therapeutic *bond* by helping the client feel understood in the *task* domain of the alliance.

- Meeting a client's expectations for therapy early in the relationship helps to establish a solid relationship (*bond*) into which appropriate challenges (*tasks*) can be introduced in the middle stages of the work to facilitate client change.
- Becoming aware and handling sensitively so-called transference phenomena mitigates the development of self- and relationship-defeating patterns in therapy process and helps clients achieve their *goals* more effectively.
- When clients experience obstacles to change, their therapists can help them to use the four component model of the working alliance as a framework to identify the source or sources of the obstacle. Even if the obstacle has its origin in one component of the alliance, it may affect other components. Once the source of the obstacle has been located, possible intervention strategies based on this understanding can be discussed and implemented.
- Skilful handling of the termination process and the client's attempts to terminate therapy prematurely consolidates the client's progress towards *goal* attainment and helps to bring the *bond* to a mutually satisfying end.

In this chapter, I have shown how the 'four component' framework of the working alliance can be used to increase the effectiveness of REBT. As shown above, it can also be used as a way of understanding obstacles to change and while a full discussion of this issue is beyond the scope of this chapter, Safran and Muran (2000) have addressed this in their important text which I recommend as further reading.

References

Beck, A. T., Rush, A. J., Shaw, B. F., & Emery, G. (1979). *Cognitive therapy of depression*. New York: Guilford Press.

Beutler, L. E., Malik, M., Alimohamed, S., Harwood, T. M., Talebi, H., Noble, S., & Wong, E. (2004). Therapist variables. In M. J. Lambert (Ed.), *Bergin and Garfield's handbook of psychotherapy and behavior change* (5th ed., pp. 227–306). New York: Wiley.

Blenkiron, P. (2010). *Stories and analogies in cognitive behaviour therapy*. Chichester: John Wiley & Sons.

Bordin, E. S. (1979). The generalizability of the psychoanalytic concept of the working alliance. *Psychotherapy: Theory, Research and Practice, 16*, 252–260.

DiGiuseppe, R. (1991). Comprehensive cognitive disputing in rational-emotive therapy. In M. Bernard (Ed.), *Using rational–emotive therapy effectively* (pp. 173–195). New York: Plenum.

DiGiuseppe, R., Leaf, R., & Linscott, J. (1993). The therapeutic relationship in rational-emotive therapy: Some preliminary data. *Journal of Rational-Emotive & Cognitive-Behavior Therapy, 11*, 223–233.

Dorn, F. J. (Ed.). (1984). *The social influence process in counseling and psychotherapy*. Springfield, IL: Charles C. Thomas.

Dryden, W. (1985). Challenging, but not overwhelming: A compromise in negotiating homework assignments. *British Journal of Cognitive Psychotherapy, 3*(1), 77–80.

Dryden, W. (1990). Self-disclosure in rational-emotive therapy. In G. Stricker & M. N. Fisher (Eds.), *Self-disclosure in the therapeutic relationship* (pp. 61–74). New York: Plenum.

Dryden, W. (1997). *Therapists' dilemmas* (Revised ed.). London: Sage.

Dryden, W. (2001). *Reason to change: A rational emotive behaviour therapy (REBT) workbook*. Hove, East Sussex: Brunner-Routledge.
Dryden, W. (2011). *Counselling in a nutshell* (2nd ed.). London: Sage.
Dryden, W. (2015). *Rational emotive behaviour therapy: Distinctive features* (2nd ed.). Hove, East Sussex: Routledge.
Ellis, A. (1959). Requisite conditions for basic personality change. *Journal of Consulting Psychology, 23*, 538–540.
Ellis, A. (1977). Fun as psychotherapy. *Rational Living, 12*(1), 2–6.
Ellis, A. (2002). *Overcoming resistance: A rational emotive behavior therapy integrated approach*. New York: Springer.
Jacobs, M. (2010). *Psychodynamic counselling in action* (4th ed.). London: Sage.
Kazantzis, N., Whittington, C., & Dattilio, F. (2010). Meta-analysis of homework effects in cognitive and behavioral therapy: A replication and extension. *Clinical Psychology: Science and Practice, 17*, 144–156.
Lazarus, A. A. (1993). Tailoring the therapeutic relationship, or being an authentic chameleon. *Psychotherapy: Theory, Research & Practice, 30*, 404–407.
Lemma, A. (1999). *Humour on the couch: Exploring humour in psychotherapy and in everyday life*. London: Whurr.
Miranda, R., & Andersen, S. (2007). The therapeutic relationship: Implications from the social-cognitive process of transference. In P. Gilbert & R. L. Leahy (Eds.), *The therapeutic relationship in the cognitive behavioral psychotherapies* (pp. 63–89). Hove, East Sussex: Routledge.
Robb, H. (2010). Two REBT therapists and one client. *Journal of Rational-Emotive & Cognitive-Behavior Therapy, 28*, 141–144.
Rogers, C. R. (1957). The necessary and sufficient conditions of therapeutic personality change. *Journal of Consulting Psychology, 21*, 95–103.
Safran, J. D., & Muran, J. C. (2000). *Negotiating the therapeutic alliance: A relational treatment guide*. New York: Guilford.

Chapter 8
Rational Emotive Behavior Therapy: Assessment, Conceptualisation and Intervention

Windy Dryden

Introduction

In this chapter, I will consider how REBT therapists assess the problems that people bring to therapy, how and when they carry out a case conceptualisation and how they intervene on these problems. Throughout, my main, but not exclusive focus will be on therapists helping clients address their problems by encouraging them to change their irrational beliefs to their rational alternatives using a range of different methods. In doing so, I will not take the usual tack of considering assessment and conceptualisation separately from intervention. Rather I will consider them as REBT therapists approach them in action, as interdependent clinical activities within a developing working alliance (see Chap. 7 this volume). This focus also reflects REBT's view that cognition, emotion and behavior are interdependent processes and that these need to be considered as such throughout therapy. In this chapter, I will assume that the client and therapist have given their informed consent to proceed on the basis that REBT has the potential to be helpful to the client.

A Process View of Rational Emotive Behavior Therapy

In this chapter, I will adopt a process view of REBT. I will begin by describing, in detail, how an REBT therapist uses REBT's 'Situationally-based ABCDEFG model' (Dryden, 2018a) to deal with a specific example of a client's target problem (i.e. the problem that the client has nominated for change). I will also describe an REBT-based approach to case conceptualization which informs treatment from a broad perspective. Drawing on the skills and strategies in both of these areas, I will

W. Dryden (✉)
Goldsmiths University of London, London, UK

© Springer Nature Switzerland AG 2019

M. E. Bernard, W. Dryden (eds.), *Advances in REBT*,
https://doi.org/10.1007/978-3-319-93118-0_8

discuss how the REBT therapist helps the client to generalise learning to other examples of the target problem and other problems and in doing so encourages them to become their own REBT therapist, if they are so interested.

Using the Situationally-Based ABCDEFG Model of REBT in Clinical Practice

Understanding and dealing with clients' problems in REBT are clinical activities that are informed by the approach's theoretical framework. There are a number of similar versions of this framework in the REBT literature which include certain features and omit others. Please note that in this chapter, I will present and discuss my own version which I refer to as the 'Situationally-based ABCDEFG' model (Dryden, 2018a).

Situation

A = Adversity
B = Belief
C = Consequence of B about A
D = Disputing B
E = Effects of disputing
F = Facilitating change
G = Goals

While discussing this model, I will focus on what happens when REBT therapists help their clients deal with their emotional problems rather than their practical problems. In particular, I will begin by describing the therapy process where therapists help their clients deal with one emotional problem at a time. I will then show how therapists help clients generalise their learning to other problems, and as they do so, they help these clients become their own therapists.

In the 'Situationally-based ABCDEFG' model, clients are deemed to disturb themselves (at *'C'*) in a *situational context* about the personal inferences that they make about the situation. These are known as adversities at *'A'*. Their disturbances are underpinned by a set of rigid and extreme, irrational beliefs (at *'B'*) that they hold about the adversities. Therapists help their clients to set goals (at 'G'), and in the same way, as their problems are underpinned by (irrational) beliefs, their goals will also be underpinned by beliefs, in this case, a set of flexible and non-extreme rational beliefs also at *'B'*. The process of change is initiated by therapists helping their clients to dispute their irrational beliefs at *'D'* and to develop the alternative set of flexible and non-extreme rational beliefs. The effects of this disputing process at *'E'* are likely to represent the clients' intellectual acknowledgement that their irrational beliefs are irrational and their rational beliefs are rational, but this may not lead to emotional/behavioral change. To facilitate such change *('F')*, clients will likely need to do various things to deepen their conviction in their rational beliefs and to weaken their conviction in their irrational beliefs. When they do, then they

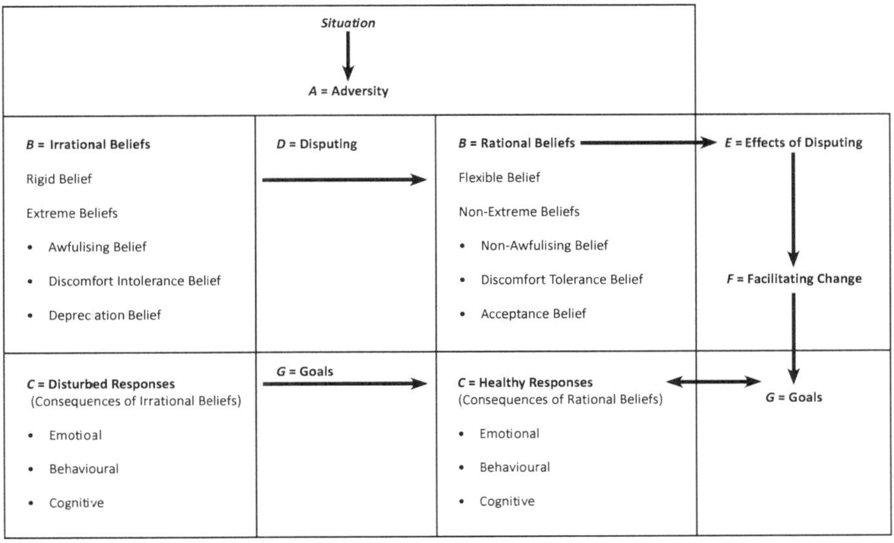

Fig. 8.1 *Situational ABCDEFG* framework

should ideally achieve their goals at '*G*'. Figure 8.1 presents a visual representation of the 'Situationally-based ABCDEFG' model.

Working with a Target Problem

REBT therapists tend to begin therapy with a focus on the problem that the client has nominated for change. This may be the first that the client has mentioned or one chosen by the client from a previously compiled problem list (Beck, 2011). Traditionally, the therapist asks the client for a specific example of this problem. This is to facilitate the gathering of clinically relevant information. A general example of this problem often yields vague generalizations that are not useful for assessment purposes. Such specific examples may be typical, recent, vivid, emotionally-laden or anticipated.

Obtaining a Brief Description of the Situation

It is useful for the therapist to gain a brief description of the specific situation in which the target problem occurred. Maultsby (1975) called this the camera check as it should indicate what a video camera with an audio-channel would record. This is useful to obtain as it facilitates the client's recall of the problem example and as such it is sometimes called the 'Situational *A*' to provide a contrast with the adversity or 'Critical *A*' which is the aspect of the situation about which the client is most disturbed.

Assessing '*C*'

When the *ABC* portion of the REBT ABCDEFG model is the target for assessment, the most common order is *CAB*, followed by *ACB*. In this chapter, I will use the *CAB* order because often the emotional part of the '*C*' best facilitates identification of '*A*'. As Fig. 8.1 shows, '*C*' stands for the *consequences* of beliefs and as we are discussing a client problem, they will tend to be disturbed consequences of irrational beliefs. There are three components of '*C*' for the therapist to assess: the emotional, the behavioral and the cognitive. When these '*Cs*' are disturbed, the person's emotions are not only very painful, they are highly disruptive for the person, their behaviors tend to maintain the problem and their cognitions are highly distorted and skewed to the negative.

When carrying out an assessment, the REBT therapist focuses not only on the client's target problem, but also on their reactions to that problem to determine whether or not they have a meta-psychological problem (i.e. a secondary problem about their primary problem). If, so, the question arises concerning which problem the therapy dyad should prioritise. While this, of course, should be jointly decided, the REBT therapist is guided by the following points which recommend beginning with the meta-psychological problem if: (i) its presence would disrupt work that the therapist and client plan to do on the primary problem in the session; (ii) its presence would disrupt work the client plans to do on the primary problem outside the session and (iii) it is clinically, the more important of the two problems (e.g. shame and, often anxiety about anxiety). In this latter case, the therapist would give the client a rationale for beginning with this secondary problem and would proceed once the client has given their agreement.

Assessing the Emotional '*C*' When the therapist is assessing the emotional '*C*', what they are looking for is the one main disturbed or dysfunctional emotion that the person experienced in the nominated example. This is sometimes referred to as an unhealthy negative emotion (UNE). The eight most common UNEs that clients seek help for from therapy are as follows: anxiety, depression, guilt, shame, hurt, unhealthy anger, jealousy and malicious envy (Dryden, 2009).

In REBT, the intensity of a negative emotion does not indicate the healthiness or unhealthiness of that emotion. While the client will most often seek help when a negative emotion is intense, it is possible, for example for a client to feel intense sadness and for this to be a healthy response to a significant loss. Thus, when assessing for the presence of a UNE, the therapist looks primarily at the consequences, both short- and long-term for the person before jointly deciding whether or not a negative response is healthy. The therapist also looks at the accompanying behaviors and cognitions while making this judgment (see below).

Sometimes, clients struggle with clearly identifying what they felt in the nominated example. Thus, they may provide a vague emotion such as 'upset' or they may give an inference and not an emotion (e.g. "I felt rejected"). The task of the therapist here is to explain the difficulties with such responses and to guide the client to provide the required information. Once, the therapist has identified a UNE, then the therapist has evidence (based on REBT theaory) of the presnec of an irrational belief.

Assessing the Behavioral '*C*' When a person experiences a disturbing emotion, they experience an urge to act (known as an action tendency) which they either act on (an overt action) or not. Since both may be problem maintenance factors, it is important for the REBT therapist to find out about them. Such behavioral factors tend to be unconstructive (i.e. self-defeating) and are either expressions of the disturbed emotion or attempts by the person to get rid of their UNEs and/or the adversity at 'A'.

Assessing the Cognitive '*C*' In the version of the 'ABC' model that I use, there are cognitive consequences of beliefs as well as emotional and behavioral consequences. In emotional problems, such cognitive consequences tend to be highly distorted and skewed to the negative. As such, it is useful to assess these as they again may serve to maintain the client's problem. Cognitive distortions that were originally identified by Burns (1980) are common examples of cognitive C's (e.g. always and never thinking). Thus when a client has been unsuccesful at a job interview and thinks, "Nobody will want to employ me ever"), this is a cognitive 'C' since is negatively skewed and highly distorted and likely to have been produced as a consequence of the client holding an irrational belief (at 'B') about the interview failiure at 'A'.

Assessing 'A'

As already noted. 'A' represents what the client was most disturbed about in the situation in which they experienced an example of their emotional problem. Assessment of 'A' may be straightforward or more complex. When the latter is the case, the therapist employs a variety of techniques such as 'inference chaining' (Neenan & Dryden, 1996). In inference chaining, the therapist takes the emotional '*C*' (e.g. anxiety) and asks the client what was most disturbing about the situation they were in until the client indicates an irrational belief (see Table 8.1 for an example). I have devised a technique for assessing 'A' that I call 'Windy's Magic Question' and an example of this technique and how to use it is presented in Table 8.2.

Once '*A*' has been assessed, it is important that the therapist encourages the client to assume temporarily that it is true even if it is clearly distorted. This is to enable both therapist and client to identify the irrational rigid and extreme beliefs that underpin the client's disturbed response to the adversity (at '*C*').

Table 8.1 An example of inference chaining

Purpose: To help the client identify the adversity in the '*ABC*' being assessed (i.e. what the client is most disturbed about at '*A*'
Therapist: So, you are anxious about giving a public presentation to a group of consultants tomorrow?
Client: Yes.
Therapist: What is anxiety-provoking to you about giving the presentation?
Client: Well, I have been over it and over it and I am not happy about it
Therapist: What is anxiety-provoking to you about you not being happy about it?
Client: I will be pre-occupied about it not being correct.
Therapist: And if that occurs, what's scary to you about such pre-occupation?
Client: On the day, I might not be fully focused.
Therapist: And if you are not fully focused on the day, what's anxiety-provoking to you?
Client: My mind may go blank during the presentation.
Therapist: And if that happens, what is scary about that for you?
Client: Oh my God! That would be terrible.
[Here, the client spontaneously mentions an irrational belief, which is a clue to the presence of the adversity. The therapist then tests this out by reviewing all the inferences that the client has mentioned and asking them to select the one about which they were most disturbed]
Therapist: So, of all the things you have mentioned: not being happy about the presentation, being pre-occupied, not being fully focused on the day and your mind going blank during the presentation what are you most anxious about?
Client: Definitely my mind going blank.

Table 8.2 Windy's Magic Question (WMQ)

Purpose: To help the client to identify the 'A' in the ABC framework as quickly as possible (i.e. what the client is most disturbed about) once 'C' has been assessed and the situation in which C has occurred has been identified and briefly described.
Step 1: Have the client focus on their disturbed 'C' (e.g. "anxiety")
Step 2: Have the client focus on the situation in which 'C' occurred (e.g. "about to give a public presentation to a group of consultants")
Step 3: Ask the client: *"Which ingredient could we give you to eliminate or significantly reduce 'C'?"* (here, anxiety)*?* (In this case the client said: "my mind not going blank"). Take care that the client does not change the situation (i.e. he does not say: "not giving the presentation")
Step 4: The opposite is probably "A" (e.g. "my mind going blank"), but check. Ask: *"So when you were about to give the presentation, were you most anxious about your mind going blank"?* If not, use the question again until the client confirms what they were most anxious about in the described situation

Setting the Goal at '*G*'

Goal-setting with clients can take place at different times in the process and with different purposes. Thus, an REBT therapist might ask the client at the outset what they would like to achieve from therapy and receive a vague or general response (e.g. "I want to overcome my anxiety"). The therapist might not want to intervene at this point unless the client's stated goal at the outset is clearly problematic.

However, at the point in the process that we have arrived at, the therapist needs to help the client to set clear, specific goals with respect to the adversity.

Thus, if the client is anxious about their mind going blank at '*A*', then the therapist asks a variant of the following question: 'Instead of being anxious about your mind going blank, what would be a constructive emotional response to the prospect of this happening that you would want to strive for? The therapist's task here is to help the client to see that given that their '*A*' is negative their choice is to experience an unhealthy negative emotion (like anxiety) or a healthy negative emotion (like un-anxious concern). Thus, if the client states that they want to strive for the absence of anxiety (absence of UNE), then the therapist points out that since '*A*' is negative i) they need to experience an emotion about '*A*', and this tends to lead to a discussion concerning what constitutes an HNE and what to call such an emotion. Alternatively, if the client nominates a goal which represents a positive statement about the situation (e.g. "I want to be confident about giving public presentations"), the therapist accepts this as a goal of a different order (i.e. something to strive for once the client has dealt constructively with their adversity at '*A*' (Dryden, 2018a) and asks the client whether their 'confidence' goal is likely to be achieved by being anxious about their mind going blank or by being concerned, but not anxious about it.

It is important to note that the therapist's goal-setting questioning at this point in the process is guided by two points a) the importance of facing adversity at '*A*' rather than bypassing it or questioning its validity (see above) and b) the distinction between an unhealthy negative emotion (UNE) and a healthy negative emotion (HNE) and the fact that it is both realistic and constructive for the client to work towards the latter rather than the former.

In my view, it is very important that the REBT therapist has a good working knowledge of the '*ABC's*' of the eight major unhealthy negative emotions (UNEs) that clients seek help for and their healthy alternatives, known, as discussed above, as healthy negative emotions (HNEs). Having an understanding of what people generally disturb themselves about at '*A*' when they experience these UNEs and what they tend to do and think while they are experiencing them serves as an important guide if clients struggle to identify this information. In addition, and relevant to our present discussion, having an understanding of what people tend to do and think while they are experiencing the healthy alternatives to UNEs serves as a guide when clients to struggle to set constructive behavioral and realistic cognitive goals that sit alongside their healthy negative emotional goals, As such, I refer the reader to the Appendix at the end of this chapter where I present the *ABCs* of the eight most common UNEs and their healthy alternatives.

Making the '*B-C*' Connections

REBT is based on a reformulation of Epictetus' famous dictum. This is as follows: "People are not disturbed by adversities. Rather, they disturb themselves by the rigid and extreme irrational beliefs that they hold about these adversities". This makes explicit what is referred to in REBT as one of two '*B*-*C*' connections. This '*B*-*C*' connection is known as 'irrational *B*-disturbed *C*' connection. In addition, the therapist needs to help the client understand the other '*B*-*C*' connection. This states that people respond healthily to adversities when they hold flexible and non-extreme rational beliefs about them. This is known as the 'rational *B*-healthy *C*' connection.

There are a number of ways of helping clients to understand these two connections. I will outline two here. I have selected them because they teach clients the two 'B-C' connections in different ways. The first such method is known as 'The Lateness Model' and is presented in Table 8.3.

As can be seen, the 'Lateness Model' first teaches the 'irrational *B*-disturbed *C*' connection first and then teaches them the 'rational *B*-healthy *C*' connection. This method also removes the client from their nominated example of their target problem and should be used when teaching the two '*B*-*C*' connections needs to be done independently from the assessment of the nominated example. The second method is what I call 'Windy's Review Assessment Procedure' (WRAP) and follows on from 'Windy's Magic Question (WMQ) – see Table 8.2. This is presented in Table 8.4.

The WRAP method employs the client' nominated example of their target problem and simultaneously teaches the two '*B*-*C*' connections while doing so. In addition, as can be seen, when this method is employed the therapist also assesses both the client's irrational and rational beliefs at '*B*'. It is, thus, a good example of the value that REBT places on therapeutic efficiency in that two tasks are achieved with one method (Dryden, 2015; Ellis, 1980a).

Assessing B

The advantage of teaching the client the two '*B*-*C*' connections before assessing '*B*' is that it makes this latter task so much easier. Thus, in the 'Lateness Model', the client is helped to see the role of a rigid belief and one extreme belief (usually awfulising) in a setting away from their problem. The therapist can now use this important point of theory to inform their questioning during the assessment of the client's irrational beliefs in their nominated example. This is an example of what DiGiuseppe (1991a) has called theory-driven questioning in the assessment phase of REBT.

Theory-Driven Questioning[1] in the Assessment of Irrational Beliefs When employing theory-driven questions, the therapist uses the 'irrational *B*-disturbed *C*' connection to assess the client's irrational beliefs. The therapist takes the 'A' and 'C' components of the nominated example of the client's target problem and asks a theory-driven question designed to discover the person's irrational belief. Here are a few examples of theory-driven questions to assess B:

[1]Also known as hypothesis-driven assessment (DiGiuseppe, 1991a)

Table 8.3 The Lateness Model

Therapist: I'd like to teach you a model which explains the factors that account for people's emotional problems. There are other explanations in the field of therapy, but this is the one I use in my work. Are you willing to hear about this explanation?
Client: Yes.
Therapist: OK. There are four parts to this model. Now here's part one. I'd like you to imagine that you are ten minutes late for an appointment and that you believe the following, 'I prefer to be on time for all my appointments but it's not essential that I am on time. It's bad to be late but it's not the end of the world'. So, if you really believed this, how do you imagine you would feel about being ten minutes late for your appointment bearing in mind that you want, but don't demand, that you arrive on time?'
Client: I guess I'd be concerned.
Therapist: That's exactly right. Now, I'd like you to take note of a very important point, in the same situation different beliefs lead to different types of feelings. Let's move on to part three of the model. This time you hold the same belief as you did in the last scenario, 'I absolutely must be on time for all my appointments, I must, must, MUST! It would be the end of the world if I was late!' This time though, you glance up at a clock in the street and realize that your watch is twenty minutes fast. So, in fact, you are actually ten minutes early for your appointment. How do you imagine you would feel about being ten minutes early when you believe that you absolutely have to be, absolutely must be on time for your appointment?
Client: Uh...I'd be relieved.
Therapist: That's right you would feel relieved. Now consider the fourth and final part of the model. Realizing that you're ten minutes early for your appointment and still holding the same belief namely 'I must be on time for all my appointments, I must, must, MUST! To be late would be the end of the world!' Despite being ten minutes early, something will occur to you that will cause you to feel panicky again. Can you think what that might be?
Client: That I'll be delayed somehow and still end up arriving late.
Therapist: Precisely. Or that the street clock was wrong or perhaps you got the appointment time wrong and you are in fact late rather than ten minutes early. Right. Now the point this model makes is that all humans- be they male or female, rich or poor, of any age or race- make themselves emotionally disturbed when they don't get what they truly believe they must get. Even when they do get or achieve what they believe they absolutely must, they are still vulnerable to further disturbance in the future. Why? Because it is always possible that they will lose it. But when humans hold non-absolute or non-dogmatic preferences and resist converting them into demands such as 'I must!', they experience healthy negative emotions like concern when they don't get or achieve what they prefer. They are also able to take constructive action when their preferences are not met and able to work toward preventing something undesirable happening in the future. So in our work together we're going to focus closely on the differences between rigid beliefs and flexible beliefs. Does that make sense to you?
Client: Yeah, it does.
Therapist: Good. Can you tell me what you've understood from the model, in your own words, so I can check that I've made the points clearly?

- "What when you were anxious ('*C*') about your mind going blank ('*A*'), what were you demanding ('*B*')"
- "When you failed the test ('*A*') and became depressed ('*C*') how much worth did you think you had as a person ('*B*')"?

Helping Clients to Construct an Alternative Rational Belief Once the therapist has identified the client's irrational belief, they have completed their ABC assessment

Table 8.4 Windy's Review Assessment Procedure (WRAP)

[This follows on from Windy's Magic Question (WMQ)]
Purpose: Once 'C' (e.g. "anxiety") and 'A' (e.g. "my mind going blank") have been assessed, this technique can be used to identify both the client's rigid and alterative flexible belief and to help the client to understand the two relevant B-C connections. This technique can also be used with any of the derivatives of the rigid and flexible belief pairing
Step 1: Say: *"Let's review what we know and what we don't know so far."*
Step 2: Say: *"We know three things. First, we know that you were anxious ('C'). Second, we know that you were anxious about your mind going blank ('A'). Third, and this is an educated guess on my part, we know that it is important to you that your mind does not go blank. Am I correct?"*
Assuming that the client confirms your hunch, note that what you have done is to identify the part of the belief that is common to both the client's rigid belief and alternative flexible belief, as we will see.
Step 3: Say: *"Now let's review what we don't know. This is where I need your help. We don't know which of two beliefs your anxiety was based on. So, when you were anxious about your mind going blank was your anxiety based on Belief 1: "It is important to me that my mind does not go blank and therefore it must not do so"* ('Rigid belief') *or Belief 2: "It is important to me that my mind does not go blank, but that does not mean that it must not do so* ('Flexible belief')?""
Step 4: If necessary, help the client to understand that their anxiety was based on their rigid belief if they are unsure.
Step 5: Once your client is clear that their anxiety was based on their rigid belief, make and emphasize the irrational belief-disturbed 'C' connection. Then ask: "*Now let's suppose instead that you had a strong conviction in belief 2, how would you feel about your mind going blank if you strongly believed that while it was important to you that your mind did not go blank, it did not follow that it must not do so?"*
Step 6: If necessary, help your client to nominate a healthy negative emotion such as concern, if not immediately volunteered, and make and emphasize the rational belief-healthy 'C' connection.
Step 7: Have the client clearly understand the differences between the two B-C connections
Step 8: Help the client set concern as the emotional goal in this situation and encourage them to see that developing conviction in their flexible belief is the best way of achieving this goal

of the client's nominated example of their target problem. At some point in the therapy process, it is important for the therapist to help the client to construct a rational alternative to their irrational belief and connect it to their goal. Some REBT therapists prefer to do so during the disputing of the client's irrational belief, using the client's responses to disputes to construct the rational belief. Other REBT therapists prefer to do so after the ABC assessment has been completed, but before the initiation of disputing. This is partly a matter of therapist preference and partly the therapist's judgment concerning which approach is likely to be effective with which client. When neophyte REBT therapists help clients to construct an alternative rational belief, they tend to skip over the disputing process (discussed below) in a bid hep their clients think rationally. This is not best practice in REBT and should be avoided.

Choice-Based, Theory-Driven Questioning Therapists new to REBT tend to have difficulties with theory-driven questioning and tend to use open-ended questioning. They do so because they think that theory-driven questioning puts words into the client's mouths. This potential problem is not encountered when the therapist encourages the client to exercise choice concerning which belief is related to their disturbed response at 'C' and which belief is related to their potential constructive response at 'G'. This is done in the WRAP method (see Table 8.4).

Here are a few other examples of 'choice-based' theory-driven questions:

- "When you thought you might fail the task you wanted to do ('*A*') and put it off ('*C*'), did you believe at the time that it would be bad, but not awful to fail or that it would be awful to fail ('*B*')?"
- "When you experienced the urge to eat that cream cake and acted on it ('*C*') to get rid of that sensation of deprivation *('A')* was your behavior based on the belief that while it would be a struggle to tolerate the deprived feeling, you could stand it, and it would be worth it to you to do so or was it based on the belief that you could not tolerate that deprived sensation?"

Open-Ended Questioning in the Assessment of Irrational Beliefs I mentioned earlier that some REBT therapists are reluctant to use theory-driven questioning of whichever type for fear of putting words into their client's mouths. Instead, they use open-ended questioning to identify the client's irrational belief. However, these therapists often get stuck or go round in circles, because they do not actively help the client to look for their irrational belief. As the therapist asks more and more open-ended questions, (e.g. "What were you telling yourself?", "What was going through your mind" or "What were you thinking?"), the client provides more and more inferences. Such questions do not help the client to look beyond their surface cognitions to discover underlying irrational beliefs. Here is an example.

Therapist: What were you telling yourself about your mind going blank that explained your anxiety?

Client: That I would not know how to continue.

Therapist: And if that were the case what would be going through your mind about that that would you to be anxious?

Client: That I'd be stuck.

Therapist: And if you were stuck, what would you think that would explain your anxiety?

Client: I would think, "What do I do?"

My suggestion is here is quite definite. It is for REBT therapists not to use open-ended questioning to identify irrational beliefs and to employ instead one of the two main theory-driven questioning methods discussed above or similar.

Using Belief Tests in Assessment

There are a number of belief tests that are employed in REBT-related research. How useful are they in clinical practice? In considering this question, I will refer to the 'Attitude and Belief Scale II' (DiGiuseppe, Leaf, Exner, & Robin, 1988) as it is the most commonly used research scale and it is included in the intake packet at the Albert Ellis Institute. The scale has 72 items and includes the four irrational beliefs and rational beliefs across three content/context areas (achievement, affiliation and comfort). Each content/context area is exemplified by three adversities each (e.g. achievement = failure; affiliation = not being liked; and comfort = frustrated by life's hassles).

As with all such scales, items are expressed in general terms and are limited to a small number of adversity ('*A*') themes (see above). As such, the ABS-II does not cover a variety of adversities (at '*A*') that are related to the eight disturbed emotions for which people seek help.

On the other hand, the completion of the ABS-II may give REBT therapists a *general* indication of in which content area a client's problems may lie and with which irrational beliefs the person is most likely to resonate.

Finally, the lack of 'C' variables in the ABS-II and similar scales make it very difficult for therapists to use them for detailed assessment of nominated examples of clients.

From this, I recommend to REBT therapists, who use the ABS-II scale (or similar scales) that they do so to obtain an overall sense of in which area(s) the clients' target problems may reside but to be mindful that these areas may not be covered in the scale. However, I recommend that therapists employ verbally-based skilful interviewing to move the therapy process forward in order to get more specific information about the client's problematic theme at 'A'. Of course, these scales can also be used to get an overall sense of which irrational beliefs to target in therapy.

Disputing '*B*' ('*D*')

So far in this chapter, I have covered the '*Situational ABCG*' components of dealing with an example of the client's target problem. The next step is disputing the client's irrational beliefs at '*D*'.

Preparing the Client for the Disputing Process Before initiating the disputing process, it is useful for the therapist to help the client understand the whys and wherefores of disputing. If the therapist begins disputing without such an explanation, they run the risk of creating resistance in the client. My own practice here is based on work alliance theory, where after explaining the process of disputing, I clarify the client's understanding and elicit their agreement to continue (see Chap. 7).

Focus in Disputing: Premise and Derivative Beliefs Traditionally, in REBT, disputing is a process in which the therapist helps the client focus on their irrational beliefs and questions them until the client sees that they are 'irrational' and that their alternative rational beliefs are 'rational'. I will say more on this point later in this section of the chapter. During intervention, the therapist generally helps the client to focus on one irrational belief at a time. This may be a 'premise' belief which is rigid and takes the form of 'demands', 'unconditional musts', etc., or it may be in the form of one of three extreme 'derivative' beliefs: awfulizing beliefs, discomfort intolerance beliefs and devaluation beliefs.

In classic REBT theory, rigid beliefs are primary (the premise), and extreme beliefs are derived from these beliefs and are regarded as primary.[2] Thus, in the classic approach to REBT, the therapist helps the client to see that their rigid belief is at the very core of their target problem and thus 'should' ideally be disputed first. When the client has been helped to see that their rigid belief is 'irrational' then the focus changes to the extreme, derivative beliefs.

The question, then, is which extreme (irrational) belief should be focused on? There are two approaches to this question. The first approach is that if the client's problem primarily concerns ego disturbance (involving unhealthy beliefs about self), then the therapist and client should focus on the latter's self-devaluation belief. However, if the client's problem primarily concerns non-ego disturbance (involving unhealthy attitudes to others, discomfort or aspects of life), then the therapist and client should focus on the latter's awfulising and/or discomfort tolerance beliefs. The second approach is client-led. Here, the therapist and client focus on whichever secondary belief the client nominates for questioning.

This client-led approach can also be employed when choosing which of the four irrational beliefs (rigid and extreme) to question first. Often the client resonates more with an extreme belief than with their rigid belief, partly because the former is more accessible in their mind than the latter.[3] In this approach, then, the therapist may not even dispute the rigid belief at all is the client does not resonate with it, a practice which is driven by pragmatism rather than by REBT theory.

My own approach to the issue of which irrational beliefs to focus on and in which sequence is that, whenever possible, I commence with disputing the rigid belief and then switch to disputing the one extreme belief that the client nominates for questioning. I do this after giving a rationale for taking this tack for which I seek and obtain my client's agreement. I find that disputing more than two irrational beliefs per problem example is unnecessary to the resolution of the problem. Other REBT therapists may employ other strategies on this issue.

Arguments in Disputing In his seminal chapter on disputing, DiGiuseppe (1991b) pointed out that when disputing a client's beliefs (both rational and irrational), the REBT therapist uses three main arguments: empirical (is this belief true or false?),

---

[2] For research on this point see Chaps. 4 & 5 in this volume.

[3] A rigid beliefs is at the very core of psychological disturbance and is thus less accessible than the extreme beliefs that are derived from it.

logical (is this belief logical or illogical?) and pragmatic (is this belief helpful or unhelpful?). The therapist uses these arguments when targeting rigid, awfulising, discomfort intolerance and devaluation beliefs and their rational alternatives as shown in Table 8.5.

Using Persuasive Arguments Table 8.5 indicates the underlying bases of irrational beliefs that the therapist needs to help the client undermine and the underlying bases of rational beliefs that the therapist needs to help the client develop. How the therapist does this is perhaps the art of therapy, and in doing so, the emphasis needs to be on the therapist using arguments that the client finds persuasive. How does the therapist discover arguments that the client might find persuasive? My approach to this issue is to use one or more of the following strategies:

- Ask the client directly (e.g. "What would help you to give up your idea that you have to do well in favour of the idea that you would like to do well, but you don't have to do so?")
- Discover a persuasive person in the person's life (e.g. "Who in your life would you believe if they told you that while you may want to do well, you don't have to do so?")
- Ask, "What would you teach your children"? (e.g. "Would you teach a child that they absolutely had to well or that it was very important for them to do so, but they don't always have to succeed?"). Once the person has answered the question, I then ask them to explain the reason for their choice.
- Pay attention in therapy to how the client responds. I often learn during the process of therapy what points clients are likely to listen to and what not. Thus, some clients are persuaded more by the therapist's use of logic than pragmatism, but for the majority, the reverse is the case. Using arguments that a particular client will find persuasive is often arrived at on a trial and error basis, but the client will often give clues along the way concerning this issue, and it is important that the therapist listens for and uses such clues.

Disputing Irrational and Rational Beliefs: Consecutively or Together One of the other points made by DiGiuseppe (1991b) is that not only does the REBT therapist need to dispute the client's irrational beliefs, they also need to help the client to construct the relevant, rational belief alternatives. For this to happen, the client needs to understand why these rational beliefs are rational and the therapist helps them to do this by questioning these rational beliefs in the same way as they questioned the client's irrational beliefs. Given that the therapist, when disputing the client's beliefs, needs to question both their irrational and rational beliefs, the following issue needs to be concerned. Is it best for the therapist to dispute the client's irrational and rational beliefs consecutively or together?

When disputing a client's beliefs consecutively, the therapist usually starts with an irrational belief (e.g. a rigid belief), disputes this belief using questions based on the three arguments discussed in the previous section and then repeats this procedure while disputing the rational alternative to this belief (e.g. a flexible belief). This

Table 8.5 Arguments Used by REBT Therapists when Disputing Irrational and Rational Beliefs

Irrational	Belief arguments	Rational belief
Rigid belief *"I want X to happen and therefore it must"*	***Empirical argument*** The preference statement, "I want X to happen", which features in both beliefs, is true, but there is no empirical law that states that having this desire guarantees that it will happen. X may happen or it may not irrespective of the person's desire. If the rigid belief were true, it would be impossible for X not to happen. But it is possible. Consequently, the rigid belief is false. The flexible belief is true because it recognises the truth of the person's desire, and allows for the possibility that it may not be met.	***Flexible belief*** *"I want X to happen, but it doesn't have to do so"*
	Logical argument In the flexible belief, the preference statement, "I want X to happen", is non-rigid. The statement, "but it doesn't have to do so" is also non-rigid. The two statements are therefore logically connected by dint of their non-rigidity. Thus, the flexible belief is logical. In the rigid belief, the preference statement, "I want X to happen" is again non-rigid and the statement, "and therefore it must" is rigid. Logically, it is not possible to derive something rigid from something non-rigid. Thus, the rigid belief is illogical.	
	Pragmatic argument Holding the rigid belief, "I want X to happen and therefore it must" leads to actual disturbed responses (emotive, behavioural and cognitive) if X does not happen. Even if X does happen holding this rigid belief renders the person vulnerable to future disturbance should it fail to continue to happen. Thus, the rigid belief is pragmatically unhelpful. Holding the flexible belief, "I want X to happen, but it doesn't have to do so" leads to actual healthy responses (emotive, behavioural and cognitive) if X does not happen and to future healthy responses if X does not happen at a later date. Thus, the flexible belief is pragmatically helpful.	

(continued)

Table 8.5 (continued)

Irrational	Belief arguments	Rational belief
Awfulising belief *"It would be bad if X does not happen and therefore it would be terrible"*	***Empirical argument*** When a person holds an awfulising belief, they mean, at the time, that if X does not happen: (a) Nothing could be worse; (b) It is worse than 100% bad; (c) No good can possibly come from this event which is wholly bad (d) The event cannot be transcended In contrast, when the person holds a non-awfulising belief, they mean, at the time, that if X does happen: (a) Things could always be worse (b) The event in question is less than 100% bad (c) Good can come from this bad event. (d) The event can be transcended. It is clear from the above that the awfulising belief is false and the non-awfulising belief is true.	***Non-Awfulising belief*** *"It would be bad if X does not happen, but it would not be terrible"*
	Logical argument In the non-awfulising belief, the evaluation of badness statement, "It would be bad if X does not happen", is non-extreme. The statement, "but it would not be terrible" is also non-extreme rigid. The two statements are therefore logically connected by dint of their non-extremity. Thus, the non-awfulising belief is logical. In the awfulising belief, the evaluation of badness statement, "It would be bad if X does not happen" is again non-extreme and the statement, "and therefore it would be terrible" is extreme. Logically, it is not possible to derive something extreme from something non-extreme. Thus, the awfulising belief is illogical.	

(continued)

Table 8.5 (continued)

Irrational	Belief arguments	Rational belief
	Pragmatic argument Holding the awfulising belief, "It would be bad if X does not happen and therefore it would be terrible" leads to actual disturbed responses (emotive, behavioural and cognitive) if X does not happen. Even if X does happen holding this awfulising belief renders the person vulnerable to future disturbance should it fail to continue to happen. Thus, the awfulising belief is pragmatically unhelpful. Holding the non-awfulising belief, "It would be bad if X does not happen, but it would not be terrible" leads to actual healthy responses (emotive, behavioural and cognitive) if X does not happen and to future healthy responses if X does not happen at a later date. Thus, the non-awfulising belief is pragmatically helpful.	
Discomfort intolerance belief *"It would be a struggle for me to tolerate it if X does not happen and therefore I could not bear it"*	***Empirical argument*** When a person holds a discomfort intolerance belief they mean, at the time, that if X does not happen: (a) They will die or disintegrate (b) They will lose the capacity to experience happiness When a person holds a discomfort tolerance belief they mean, at the time, that if X does not happen: (a) They will struggle to tolerate it, but they will neither die nor disintegrate (b) They will not lose the capacity to experience some happiness although this capacity will be temporarily diminished (c) The situation is worth tolerating, all things considered and (d) They have a choice whether to tolerate it or not It is clear from the above that the discomfort tolerance belief is false and the discomfort tolerance belief is true	***Discomfort tolerance belief*** *"It would be a struggle for me to tolerate it if X does not happen but I could bear it, it would be worth it to me to do so, I am willing to do so and I am going to do so"*

(continued)

Table 8.5 (continued)

Irrational	Belief arguments	Rational belief
	Logical argument In the discomfort tolerance belief, the 'struggle' statement, "It would be a struggle for me to tolerate it if X does not happen" is non-extreme. The statements, "but I could bear it, it would be worth it to me to do so, I am willing to do so and I am going to do so" are also non-extreme. All statements are therefore logically connected by dint of their non-extremity. Thus, the discomfort tolerance is logical. In the discomfort intolerance belief, the 'struggle statement, "It would be a struggle for me to tolerate it if X does not happen" is again non-extreme and the statement, "and therefore I could not bear it" is extreme. Logically, it is not possible to derive something extreme from something non-extreme. Thus, the awfulising belief is illogical.	
	Pragmatic argument Holding the discomfort intolerance belief, "It would be a struggle for me to tolerate it if X does not happen and therefore I could not bear it" leads to actual disturbed responses (emotive, behavioural and cognitive) if X does not happen. Even if X does happen holding this discomfort intolerance belief renders the person vulnerable to future disturbance should it fail to continue to happen. Thus, the discomfort intolerance belief is pragmatically unhelpful. Holding the discomfort tolerance belief non-awfulising belief, "It would be a struggle for me to tolerate it if X does not happen but I could bear it, it would be worth it to me to do so, I am willing to do so and I am going to do so" leads to actual healthy responses (emotive, behavioural and cognitive) if X does not happen and to future healthy responses if X does not happen at a later date. Thus, the discomfort tolerance belief is pragmatically helpful.	

(continued)

Table 8.5 (continued)

Irrational	Belief arguments	Rational belief
Devaluation belief *"If X happens, that would be bad and would prove that I am no good/ you are no good/ life is no good"*	***Empirical argument*** When a person holds a devaluation belief they mean, at the time, that if X does not happen: (a) A person (self or other) can legitimately be given a single global rating that defines their essence and the worth of a person is dependent upon the presence or absence of X (b) The world can legitimately be given a single rating that defines its essential nature and that the value of the world varies according to the presence or absence of X (c) A person can be rated on the basis of one of his or her aspects and the world can be rated on the basis of one of its aspects When a person holds an acceptance belief they mean, at the time, that if X does not happen: (a) A person (self or other) cannot legitimately be given a single global rating that defines their essence and their worth, as far as they have it, is not dependent upon the presence or absence of X (b) Life cannot legitimately be given a single rating that defines its essential nature and that the value of life does not vary according to the presence or absence of X (c) It makes sense to rate discrete aspects of a person and of the world, but it does not make sense to rate a person or the world on the basis of these discrete aspects. It is clear from the above that the acceptance belief is true and the devaluation belief is false	***Acceptance belief*** *"If X happens, that would be bad, but it would not prove that I am no good/ you are no good/life is no good. Rather, it proves that I am/you are am a fallible human being and life is a complex mixture of good, bad and neutral aspects"*

(continued)

Table 8.5 (continued)

Irrational	Belief arguments	Rational belief
	Logical argument In the acceptance belief, the evaluation of badness statement, "If X happens, that would be bad" is evaluating a part of the person's experience. The statement, "but it would not prove that I am no good/ you are no good/life is no good. Rather, it proves that I am/you are am a fallible human being and life is a complex mixture of good, bad and neutral aspects" is accepting the whole of the person, their experience and life conditions. The latter incorporates the former and as they are both non-extreme they are logically connected. As such, the acceptance belief is logical In the devaluation belief, the evaluation of badness statement, "If X happens, that would be bad" is again evaluating a part of the person's experience and is non-extreme. The statement, "and would prove that I am no good/you are no good/ life is no good" is extreme and rates the whole of the person/life logically, it is not possible to derive something extreme from something non-extreme and it is not possible to rate the whole on the basis of one of its parts. Thus, the devaluation belief is illogical.	
	Pragmatic argument Holding the devaluation belief, "If X happens, that would be bad and would prove that I am no good/you are no good/ life is no good" leads to actual disturbed responses (emotive, behavioural and cognitive) if X does not happen. Even if X does happen holding this discomfort intolerance belief renders the person vulnerable to future disturbance should it fail to continue to happen. Thus, the devaluation belief is pragmatically unhelpful. Holding the acceptance belief, "If X happens, that would be bad, but it would not prove that I am no good/ you are no good/life is no good. Rather, it proves that I am/you are am a fallible human being and life is a complex mixture of good, bad and neutral aspects" leads to actual healthy responses (emotive, behavioural and cognitive) if X does not happen and to future healthy responses if X does not happen at a later date. Thus, the acceptance tolerance belief is pragmatically helpful.	

is done until the client understands why their irrational belief is irrational and why their rational belief is rational.

When disputing a client's beliefs together, the therapist takes both the client's rational and irrational belief (e.g. rigid and flexible belief) and asks questions directed at them both at the same time (e.g. which of these beliefs is true/logical/helpful and why? and which of these beliefs is false/illogical/unhelpful and why?). The therapist then proceeds again until the client understands why their irrational belief is irrational and why their rational belief is rational.

Disputing Styles DiGiuseppe (1991b) argued that there are four basic disputing styles. Beal, Kopec, and DiGiuseppe (1996) gave examples of these styles when disputing clients' linked rigid and extreme irrational beliefs. What are these styles and when should be used?

Socratic Style When the REBT therapist employs a Socratic style of disputing irrational beliefs, they ask the client focused questions concerning the empirical, logical and pragmatic status of their irrational and rational beliefs. Depending on the client's response the therapist may ask a follow-up question or may make a corrective statement followed by a follow-question. The therapist proceeds this way guiding the client to understand the irrationality of their irrational belief(s) and the rationality of their alternative rational belief(s). Clients who tend to benefit from Socratic disputing are those who tend to think for themselves and can tolerate a period of not knowing as a route to understanding.

Didactic Style When the REBT therapist employs a didactic style of disputing irrational beliefs, they provide the client with information and explanations concerning why their irrational beliefs are irrational, and their rational beliefs are rational. This style is used with clients who cannot engage with Socratic disputing. When using a didactic approach, the therapist should provide information in easily digestible 'chunks' and ensure that the client has understood the points made and agrees with them.

Metaphorical Style When the REBT therapist employs a metaphorical style of disputing irrational beliefs, they expose the irrationality of an irrational belief by directly referring to an area which is meaningful to the client. In doing so, the therapist sheds light by identifying hidden similarities between two ideas. Beal et al. (1996: 223) provide the following example of a metaphorical dispute: 'If Martin Luther King had held the belief that 'everybody should[4] approve of me, where would we be today in the area of civil rights?' Metaphorical disputes are best employed with clients who can easily see the connection between ideas in different realms.

[4] Meaning 'must'

Humorous Style The final disputing style mentioned by DiGiuseppe (1991a, 1991b) and Beal et al. (1996) uses humour to get the client to laugh at the absurdity of their rational belief as a prelude to committing themself to the alternative rational belief. Humour was a feature of Ellis's work, particularly at his Friday Night Live workshops (Ellis & Joffe, 2002) and is currently a feature of my own demonstration work (Dryden, 2018b). As Beal et al. (1996) note, an important consideration when using humour in the disputing process is that the therapist's humorous interventions are directed at the client's irrational belief and not at the client themself and should ideally not be used with clients who find it hard to make this distinction. In addition, some clients believe that humour has no place in therapy and the therapist should preferably eschew the making of humorous disputes with such clients.

Enactive Style When using an enactive disputing style, the therapist does something in the session to expose the irrationality of an irrational belief. This approach tends to be used as a last resort as it tends to be dramatic and is high risk as a consequence. An example of this is where the therapist has failed to help the client to understand that they are not a stupid person if they do something stupid. The therapist takes a half a glass of water and pours it over themself. They then ask the client if what they did was stupid and then if they are a stupid person for doing so. Hopefully, the client is thus helped to see that when they do something stupid, this proves that they are a non-stupid, fallible person for doing so and not a stupid person.

Using a Variety of Styles It is very unlikely that a therapist will employ only one style of disputing with a given client. Rather, they will tend to use a variety of different styles at different times with that client. It is important that the therapist gets feedback from the client concerning the impact of the various disputing styles that they employ so that they can use a combination of styles that will be most effective for that client.

The Effects of Disputing at '*E*'

If disputing has been successful then the therapist has helped the client to do three things:

- To understand that their irrational beliefs are irrational (i.e. false, illogical and unhelpful) and their alternative rational beliefs are rational (i.e. true, logical and helpful) and the reasons why this is the case
- To realise that this understanding will initially be 'intellectual' in nature and will not yet impact their feelings and behavior in any meaningful way (Ellis, 1963). For this understanding to become 'emotional' and thereby produce meaningful change the person has to act and think in ways that support the development of their rational beliefs and to do this regularly over time (Ellis, 1963)

- To understand the process of facilitating change and to commit themself to it. This involves identifying and dealing with the obstacles to change that they will probably encounter as they work towards developing rational thinking and thus achieving their therapeutic goals

Facilitating Change at '*F*'

As mentioned above, interventions at '*F*' are designed to help the person increase their conviction in their developing rational beliefs so that they may achieve their therapeutic goals, namely to deal effectively (at '*C*') with their problem-related adversity (at '*A*') and thence to change '*A*' if it can be changed or to adapt constructively to '*A*' if it can't be changed. To this end, REBT therapists use a variety of interventions. While I will cover a sample of interventions in each of a number of categories, I want to make the point that the creativity of the therapist in designing tailor-made interventions to help specific clients at specific times should not be underestimated. Some of the interventions that I will discuss are implemented in the therapy session itself, but most are employed by clients as homework assignments which I discuss in my chapter on 'Rational Emotive Behavior Therapy and the Working Alliance' in Chap. 7 of this volume.

Cognitive Interventions Cognitive interventions designed to help the client increase their conviction in their develop rational beliefs (and to decrease their conviction in their existing irrational beliefs) involve the client engaging in a debate between their rational and irrational 'parts'. This debate may be done in writing, in a two-chair dialogue format, or on a recording device (see Dryden, 2001). It may also be done using role-play with the client playing the role of the therapist (advocating rationality) and the therapist playing the role of the client (advocating irrationality). In carrying out these interventions, the therapist helps the client to identify and deal with doubts, reservations and objections to rational thinking.

Another cognitive intervention that helps a client to move toward emotional insight is known as semantic disputing where the therapist helps the client to become aware of and change their language to reflect rational thinking. This helped me to overcome my own anxiety about my stammer. Thus, rather than say, "I am a stammerer", I changed my language to "I am a person who stammers some of the time, but most of the time I speak fluently".

Cognitive-Behavioral Interventions Perhaps the most powerful interventions in helping the client increase conviction in their rational beliefs are those where the person faces the adversity (at '*A*') while rehearsing their rational beliefs at '*B*'. In doing so, it is important that the person refrains from using safety-seeking strategies that prevent the person from facing '*A*' while fully processing it with their rational beliefs. The important point about these interventions is that the client employs them regularly until their conviction in their rational beliefs develops to the point where they can respond healthily (emotionally and behaviorally) to the adversity at '*A*.'

For example, consider a person who is anxious (at '*C*') about making mistakes (at '*A*') while giving presentations ('Situation') because they believe (at 'B'), "I must give a flawless performance, and if I don't, I am a failure". In order to face their adversity, they need to give regular presentations while first getting into a rational mindset, (i.e. "I don't want to make mistakes, but I don't have to be flawless and if I am not, it proves that I am human and not a failure". In doing so, the person needs to refrain from enacting safety-seeking strategies designed to eliminate the possibility of making mistakes. Thus, they neither (a) overprepare, (b) read verbatim from their previously prepared script, nor (c) face away from their audience while referring to powerpoint slides. Rather, they (a) prepare reasonably, (b) take the risk of making mistakes by only consulting bullet point notes and (c) face the audience while referring to powerpoint slides. Some REBT therapists might even encourage them to make mistakes deliberately, although others would argue that this changes the '*A*' since deliberately making a mistake is not a mistake!

Imaginal Interventions These interventions involve the client rehearsing their rational beliefs (at '*B*') while imagining themself facing the adversity (at '*A*') until they can experience a healthy negative emotion (at '*C*'). One such technique is called rational-emotive imagery (Ellis, 2000). Here is how Hickey and Doyle (2018: 123–124) describe REI. Having asked clients to focus on their problematic adversities, "the counselor asks clients to make themselves feel extremely angry, anxious, guilty, depressed and so on. Once they do so, they are asked to change the unhealthy negative emotion to a healthy negative emotion and tell the counselor how this was accomplished. The proper response is that this was done by changing the irrational beliefs to rational beliefs". Such imaginal interventions can be practised at any time, but are particularly helpful when used before the client faces the problematic adversity in reality.

Passionate Interventions Ellis (1979) argued that the therapist needs to be forceful and energetic in using interventions to facilitate emotionally insightful change and when encouraging clients to use such techniques with themselves. Given this, passionate interventions are designed to engage the client's emotions as powerfully as possible to facilitate change mediated by rationality. Such interventions include emotively enhanced use of the cognitive interventions described above, the forceful use of rational coping statements, forceful disputing, the use of humour and shame-attacking assignments. In the latter, the client acts in a way that is designed to court disapproval so that they can practise unconditional self-acceptance in the face of such disapproval. It is important that the therapist ensures that in carrying out a shame-attacking exercise that their behaviour is legal, ethical and repeated to the person's target problem.

Behavioral Interventions While REBT therapists do use behavioural interventions to bring about client change (which I will discuss later in the chapter), when these interventions are not related to overt cognitive techniques, they tend not be designed to bring about belief mediated change. Having made this point, such behavioural interventions may result in such belief change. Thus, in 'stay in there' activities, the client is encouraged to stay in situations that they think are intolerable to see what happens. Despite the fact that no deliberate attempt is made to help the person rehearse a discomfort tolerance belief, they may develop one as a result of successfully staying in such difficult-to-tolerate situations. However, without the overt and intentional focus on belief change, the person may instead come to reinterpret 'A' rather than change 'B'. Given the unpredictable outcome of non-cognitive behavioural interventions, they are used sparingly by REBT therapists where the focus is on helping clients to change their irrational beliefs to alternative rational beliefs.

Case Conceptualisation in REBT

A case conceptualisation is essentially a blueprint, which takes as its starting point a client's presenting problems and puts forward hypotheses about factors that account for these problems and explain how the client unwittingly perpetuates these problems. These factors are mainly cognitive and behavioral, but environmental and interpersonal context factors are also included.

A good case conceptualisation also considers the relationships between a client's problems and possible obstacles to progress and suggests a pragmatic order in which to tackle the person's problems. In short, it provides order to the conceptualisation and treatment of the client's problems (DiGiuseppe, Doyle, Dryden, & Backx, 2014; Dryden, 1998).

Currently, most CBT therapists carry out a formulation of a "case" before embarking on treatment unless the need is pressing to treat a client before such a formulation is undertaken. This tends to distinguish REBT therapists from other CBT therapists in that REBT therapists are more likely to initiate therapy based on problem assessment than their CBT colleagues. When case formulation is carried out in CBT, it is done so collaboratively.

As I discussed earlier, REBT therapists use a particular framework to help themselves, and their clients understand the cognitive-behavioral dynamics of the clients' target problems. As stated above, what they do not routinely do is to wait to intervene on clients' problems until we have carried out a case conceptualisation. Thus, REBT therapists tend to intervene more quickly on a client's target problem and build up a case formulation of the "case" as they go rather than structuring therapy into conceptualisation-intervention stages.

As with many other issues, the views of Albert Ellis are the driving force on the issue of assessment vs. conceptualisation. When he started his career, he became dissatisfied with an approach to therapy that saw therapeutic intervention dependent upon a thorough understanding of clients' psychopathology and personality based on the completion and analysis of a large number of questionnaires, inventories and other assessment tools. Ellis (1962) regarded this process as inefficient and noted that a significant number of clients tended to leave this process before treatment had commenced. Ellis noted the waste of therapist, client and an organisation's time when many person-hours were spent on preparing the client for an intervention based on the accumulation and analysis of much data that was subsequently not utilised because the client had left before treatment proper had commenced.

The legacy of this experience was that Ellis considered it to be the best use of everyone's time and resources if treatment was gotten underway as quickly as possible. Hence, Ellis tended to eschew a case conceptualisation approach to REBT, where a formal formulation routinely precedes treatment. Of course, Ellis was a highly skilled formulator of "cases", as anyone who had received clinical supervision from him would testify. But he tended to do this in his head rather than on paper and, as noted above, he made his formulations during therapy rather than before therapy had gotten underway. Indeed, Ellis argued that a client's response to therapy tells the therapist a great deal about the client and their problems and for this to become manifest, therapy must be initiated.

So, what have other REBT therapists had to say about the use of case formulation in REBT? I have perhaps put forward the most developed approach to the use of case conceptualisation in REBT (Dryden, 1998). I call this approach UPCP, which stands for "Understanding the Person in the Context of their Problems" because I dislike referring to a person as a "case".

'UPCP': One Approach to Case Conceptualisation (Dryden, 1998)

I argue that there are a number of factors that need to be identified when conducting a UPCP.Please bear in mind that a case conceptualisation, while formulated at the beginning of therapy, is fluid and subject to change as therapist and client proceed through the REBT treatment process.

Basic Information on the Client and Any Striking Initial Impressions In addition to collecting basic information about the client – and this will vary from therapist to therapist - it is important that the therapist obtains details of the client's past and present substance use and possible abuse. In addition, it is useful for the therapist to note any striking information about the client from their presentation and see how this may fit in with any conceptualisation that is made later.

The Client's Health and Medication Status It is important for the therapist to know about the client's physical well-being and about any medication they are taking. Such factors may play a role in the client's problems and may impact on the agreed treatment plan.

A List of Relevant Contributory Factors REBT theory posits that events past or present do not cause a client's emotional disturbance, but may contribute to it. As such, the therapist will want to know what contributes to the client's disturbance. These are specific and general factors that are properly conceptualized as factors at '*A*'.

A List of the Client's Problems It is useful for the therapist to encourage the client to develop a list of problems that they wish to address in therapy. This practice is perhaps more of a feature of therapists from the Beckian school of CBT than from REBT (Beck, 2011), but developing such a list does help the REBT therapist to see how these problems may relate to one another, to hypothesise possible connections between the problems at both an inferential level and a belief and to suggest a possible order in which these can be tackled. The REBT therapist who is mindful of working alliance issues will discuss and negotiate such an order with the client (see Chap. 7).

The Client's Goals for Change As discussed earlier, the therapist can ask for the client's goals at different points of the therapeutic process (e.g. at the outset and after specific problems have been assessed). In constructing a case conceptualisation, it is useful to know what types of goals a client has because not only do these indicate what the person is looking for across the board but again may suggest the best order in which the person's problems are addressed.

A List of the Client's Problem Emotions (UNEs) As we have seen, when working on a target problem with a client and particularly where a specific example of that problem is being addressed, it is best if the pair deal with one problem emotion at a time. By contrast, when formulating a case conceptualisation, the therapist seeks to discover the range of problematic emotions the client wants help with. When this list has been obtained, both therapist and clear look for any links among these emotions which, if discovered, would indicate how the client's problems are related to one another and may indicate that some are clustered together. Such clusters suggest that certain problems may be best dealt with in close proximity to one another.

A List of the Client's Adversities or '*A*'s Very often clients report handling similar situations and the reason for this is that struggle with one or more adversities (e.g. disapproval, uncertainty, failure, injustice). There should be consistency between the clients' listed adversities at '*A*' and their problematic emotions at '*C*' (see Appendix).

The Client's Core Irrational (Rigid and Extreme) Beliefs As therapy proceeds, the client will reveal one or more core irrational beliefs which are general in nature and underpin the range of the client's problems. These will be in the ego domain of disturbance (rigid belief + self-devaluation belief) and/or the discomfort domain of disturbance (rigid belief + awfulising belief or discomfort intolerance belief or other/life devaluation belief). In the latter domain, it is important that the therapist identifies and works with the extreme belief with which the client most resonates.

A List of the Client's Dysfunctional Behaviors and their Purpose As the tables in the appendix shows, when a person experiences an unhealthy negative emotion, they tend to act in a certain way. In constructing a case conceptualisation, the therapist and client develop a list of such behaviors together with their purpose. When these behaviors stem from irrational beliefs, it is probable that they serve to maintain the client's problem. It is also important that as therapy develops, the therapist helps the client to construct and operationalize an alternative list of constructive behaviors.

A List of the Ways in Which the Client Prevents or Cuts Short the Experience of their Problems A client may have problems because they disturb themselves about a number of adversities. They may also have problems because they may seek to avoid them or to prevent them from being experienced. These avoidance and preventative methods (which may be cognitive, behavioral or interpersonal in nature) serve only to put off the inevitable and also make it difficult for the client to deal with the adversities because they are designed to stop the person from encountering them.

A List of the Ways in Which the Client Overcompensates for Problems A client may unwittingly maintain their problems by overcompensating for them. For example, a client may be ashamed of feeling anxious and overcompensate for this by taking foolhardy risks to prove to themselves that they are not weak. Some clients use such overcompensations strategies as their major way of dealing with their problems.

A List of Meta-Psychological Problems REBT has, for many years, stressed the importance of the role of what I refer to here as 'meta-psychological problems' in explaining how clients deepen their psychological problems. These are psychological problems that clients have about their original psychological problems. Common meta-psychological problems include anxiety, depression, shame, guilt and self-anger. These problems have also been referred to as 'secondary emotional problems' and 'symptom stress' (Walen, DiGiuseppe, & Wessler, 1980) in the REBT literature.

A List of the Cognitive Consequences of Core Irrational Beliefs As I mentioned earlier, core irrational beliefs are general beliefs which underpin the range of the client's problems. Traditionally, REBT therapists are concerned with the emotional and behavioral consequences of such beliefs, but they also have cognitive consequences, and it is important to understand these in a case conceptualisation. Such consequences tend to be highly distorted and skewed to the negative and the person experiences them in a ruminative way. In the appendix, I list the cognitive consequences of irrational beliefs associated with each of the eight UNEs for which the person seeks help.

How the Client Expresses Problems and the Interpersonal Responses to these Expressions As noted in the 'Situational ABCDEFG' model, clients experience their problems in specific contexts. They also express these problems in these contexts, and it is important to understand such expressions. Thus, some clients will express their problems dramatically, while others will attempt to suppress them. Often, a client will have a particular style of problem expression and others will respond to these expressions in ways that may ameliorate the problem or serve to maintain or exacerbate it. Thus, the REBT will seek to discover the both how clients express their problems and the interpersonal responses to these expressions.

Predicting the Client's Likely Response to Therapy In developing a case conceptualisation, the therapist will gather information that will enable them to develop predictions about the client's likely response to therapy. In doing so, the therapist may be able to develop a treatment plan that helps the client to get the most out of the REBT process and minimise treatment resistance.

Conclusion

As you can see from the above, developing a UPCP takes time and this time may be better spent in helping the client to address their problems. Thus, I do not recommend that REBT therapists carry out a full UPCP with every client. But it should be conducted:

- When it is clear that the person has many complex problems.
- When resistance occurs in clients, who have, at first sight, non-complex problems and where usual ways of addressing such resistance have proven unsuccessful
- When clients have had several unsuccessful previous attempts at therapy, particularly when one or more of these previous therapies were REBT.

The Generalization Process in REBT

So far in this chapter, I have described how the REBT therapist works with a specific example of a client's target problem and, more generally, the topics the therapist covers when carrying out a case conceptualisation which guides treatment in more complex situations. Both perspectives help to inform what I call here the generalisation process where therapist and client work together to help the client use REBT across the board with their problems. You will notice from what I discuss below that the therapist is keen to help the client develop their skills at REBT assessment and intervention and this is linked to the therapist's overall goal of encouraging the client wherever possible to become their own REBT therapist. The generalisation process takes a number of forms.

Generalizing to Other Examples of the Target Problem

Once the client has dealt with one specific example of their target problem they can be prompted to deal with others. They will probably not be able to do so without such prompting at this early juncture. A number of years ago, I helped one of my clients deal with his fear of criticism. We began by focusing on his fear of being criticised by his boss, and I helped him by taking him through the 'Situational ABCDEFG' process as described earlier in this chapter. At the beginning of the next session, he wanted to talk about his fear of being criticised by his girlfriend's father. I asked if had made any use of the process he went through in the previous session. He replied, "No, was I supposed to?" So, many clients need active help generalising what they have learned from one example of their target problem to another. In helping clients to deal with examples of their problems, many REBT therapists use self-help forms which outline salient aspects of the 'Situational ABCDEFG' framework. Some of these provide instructions which outline the process of assessing and dealing with problems. One such form appears in Fig. 8.2.

As the client gets prompted to identify the ABCs of their target problem and encouraged to dispute the relevant irrational beliefs, the therapist encourages them to take greater responsibility for setting their own homework assignments.

As the client learns to deal with a range of examples of their target problem as described above, they learn to recognise the situations in which they tend to experience the problem and intervene with themself so that they prevent the problem from occurring.

Generalizing to Other Problems they May Have (at 'A' and/or 'C')

Another way in which the therapist can help the client to generalise their developing skills in using REBT is to help them use these skills with their other problems. This can be done where the focus is on a problematic emotion or behaviour at '*C*', a problematic theme at 'A' or a combination. Again the therapist encourages the client to use a self-help form to assess the problem and dispute the irrational beliefs before encouraging them to develop their own homework assignments to facilitate belief change and develop emotional insight. Again as they become more aware how they typically experience these problems and in which contexts they tend to occur they again learn to intervene with themself so that they do not experience the problems.

ABCD Blank Form with Instructions

SITUATION =

"A"=

"iB" (irrational belief) =

"rB" (rational belief) =

"C" (emotional consequence) =

(behavioural consequence) =

(thinking consequence) =

"C" (emotional goal) =

(behavioural goal) =

(thinking goal) =

1) Write down a brief, objective description of the "situation" you were in
2) Identify your "C" - your major disturbed emotion, your dysfunctional behaviour and, if relevant, your distorted subsequent thinking
3) Identify your "A" - this is what you were most disturbed about in the situation (Steps 2 and 3 are interchangeable)
4) Set emotional, behavioural and thinking goals
5) Identify your irrational beliefs ("iBs") i.e. rigid belief + awfulising belief, discomfort intolerance belief or depreciation belief
6) Identify the alternative rational beliefs ("rBs") that will enable you to achieve your goals i.e. flexible belief + non-awfulising belief, discomfort tolerance belief or acceptance belief

<u>OVERLEAF</u>

7) Develop persuasive arguments to convince yourself that your irrational beliefs are irrational and that your rational beliefs are rational - "D". These arguments will help you to achieve your emotional, behavioural and thinking goals
8) Re-examine "A" and consider how realistic it was. Given all the facts, would there have been a more realistic way of looking at "A"? - if so write it down

Fig. 8.2 ABCD Blank Form with Instructions

"D" (Disputing) =

Re-examine "A" =

Fig. 8.2 (continued)

Identifying Core Irrational Beliefs and Developing Core Rational Beliefs

Another way of helping the client to generalize their learning is to help them to identify core irrational beliefs. These are general irrational beliefs that account for a range of the client's problems across a range of situations. The therapist helps the person to dispute these core irrational beliefs in the same way as they helped them to dispute their specific irrational beliefs and as before helps them to develop alternative core rational beliefs. The latter form the substrate for a general rational philosophy of living that may serve both to prevent the development of future problems and to promote personal growth. This is what Ellis used to do a lot in therapy and is part of what REBT therapists refer to 'elegant' REBT. Also, in this area, Rational Emotive Behavior Therapy (REBT) overlaps with Rational Emotive Behavior Coaching (REBC) – see the chapter on 'REBT in Coaching' by Oana David in this volume.

What is particularly valuable is if the therapist can help the client develop the skill of using core rational beliefs to develop and use specific versions of these beliefs to deal with specific instances of their problems.

Identifying and Dealing with Obstacles to Change

During the process of REBT, the client is likely to experience a variety of obstacles to change. The task of the therapist is to work with the client to identify and deal with these obstacles as efficiently as possible. Space precludes a comprehensive discussion of this issue (see Dryden & Neenan, 2011; Ellis, 2002), but common obstacles include failing to take responsibility for change, a need to feel familiar, avoiding discomfort and harboring a variety of doubts, reservations and objections about REBT concepts and salient aspects of the REBT process.

Unless these obstacles are identified and dealt with, then clients will struggle to get the most out of what REBT has to offer. In my view, in particular, the therapist needs to help the client to identify and deal with specific vulnerability factors (factors to which the client is particularly vulnerable) which if not dealt with could lead to lapses (brief returns to a problem state) and even relapse (a more profound and enduring return to a problem state).

General Versus Specific REBT

In this chapter, I have focused on the prime directive of REBT therapists which is to promote psychological change through the development and implementation of rational beliefs. This is what Ellis (1980b) called 'specific REBT'. However, REBT therapists can and often do help their clients in ways other than the promotion of rational thinking. When REBT therapists do this, they are practising what Ellis (1980b) called 'general REBT' which he argued, at the time, was indistinguishable from CBT. I will briefly review general REBT here.

Questioning and Changing Distorted Inferences

As I have previously discussed in this chapter, once the REBT therapist has accurately assessed the client's adversity at '*A*' (i.e. what the client was most disturbed about in the problem-related situation), they encourage the client to assume temporarily that 'A' was true. The therapist does this because it is the best way of helping the client to identify the irrational beliefs that they held about the adversity which best explains their disturbed reaction to 'A'. If the therapist were to encourage the client to question 'A' at this point, if it clearly appears to be distorted, then the therapist would help the person change their feelings but would do so by encouraging inference change rather than belief change.

There are two occasions when REBT therapist are advised to encourage clients to question or reconsider 'A' and thus effect inference change. The first is after belief change has been facilitated. This might be termed, 'inference change after belief change'. The second is when the person is not interested in or resists interventions aimed at belief change. This may be termed, 'inference change instead of belief change'. This latter fits in with the focus of this part of the chapter. The strategies and techniques that the therapist employs in effecting inference change are the same in both the above situations.

As an example of 'inference change instead of belief change, I cite one that Richard Wessler, a former Director of Training at what is now the Albert Ellis Institute, used to give in his training workshops. He was working with a woman who was unhealthily angry (at '*C*') at what she saw was her father's intrusiveness (at '*A*'). She inferred that he was intrusive whenever he asked her, "Noo, what's doing?" Initially, Wessler tried to teach the woman the B-C connection that her unhealthy anger was based on her demand that her father absolutely should not be intrusive and was not directly caused by his intrusiveness. However, no matter how Wessler put it, the client steadfastly resisted the B-C explanation of her problematic anger. At this point, Wessler moved from a belief change strategy to an inference change strategy which resulted in the client seeing that, 'Noo, what's doing?' was her father's standard way of beginning a conversation and was not intrusiveness on his part.

What to Ask When Questioning Inferences?

The purpose of questioning a client's inference at '*A*' is to encourage them to make the 'best bet' when settling on an interpretation about what happened in the situation under consideration. Here is a sample of such questions:

- How likely is it that *A* happened (or might happen)?
- Would an objective jury agree that *A* actually happened or might happen? If not, what would the jury's verdict be?
- Did I view (am I viewing) the situation realistically? If not, how could I have viewed (can I view) it more realistically?
- If I asked someone whom I could trust to give me an objective opinion about the truth or falsity of my inference about the situation at hand, what would the person say to me and why? How would this person encourage me to view the situation instead?
- If a friend had told me that they had faced (were facing or were about to face) the same situation as I faced and had made the same inference, what would I say to him/her about the validity of their inference and why? How would I encourage the person to view the situation instead?

Changing Behaviour

When REBT therapists focus on helping clients to change their behaviour without targeting their irrational beliefs for change, this is based on the idea that the person will profit from such behavioural change. Here are a few examples.

Changing Interpersonal Behaviour

Quite often, people disturb themselves about what they see as the aversive behaviour of others. When it is not possible for the therapist to first help the client to undisturb themself about another person's behaviour before helping them to influence the other, the therapist focuses on helping that person to change their own behaviour as a way of eliciting a more positive response from the other person.

Skills Training

Often people suffer because they lack important skills in an area of life that is important to them. When this is the case, the REBT therapist can help them by teaching them the requisite skills. Common skills training includes the development of assertion skills, social skills, parent skills and study skills. Learning and refining such skills will encourage clients to achieve their goals even though they may potentially disturb themselves when they encounter adversities because they still hold irrational beliefs which were not targeted for change with their therapist. When a client sees that improved skills development has not led to problem solution they may be more open to working with the therapist on changing their irrational thinking.

Changing the Situation

There are times in therapy when it is important for the person to change the situation they are in rather than to work towards un-disturbing themself about the situation before deciding to change it. A good example is when a female client is being abused by their partner. While other scenarios are not so clear-cut, sometimes the best thing is for the client to leave an aversive situation, particularly if they cannot or will not un-disturb themself first.

Utilising Strategies and Techniques from Other CBT

REBT theory promotes flexibility not only for clients' belief systems but also for its own hypotheses about how to understand clients' problems and how to best help them with these problems. This flexibility means considering in an open-minded way what other approaches to CBT have to offer the practice of REBT. This topic is considered by Matweychuk et al., in Chap. 3 of this volume so I will only raise a few issues that REBT therapists need to consider. This is best done together with their clients, rather than alone:

- When is it best to target clients' irrational beliefs for change and when not?
- When is it best to encourage clients to accept mindfully how they think and feel without attempting to change these processes and when is it best to target such cognitions and emotions for change?
- When should therapists encourage clients to act in ways that are consistent with their values without first targeting their irrational beliefs for change and when should belief change precede the promotion of value-based action?

REBT does not exist in its own therapeutic bubble, and it is healthy for its practitioners

to learn from their CBT colleagues as well as showing these colleagues what REBT has to offer. In this way, REBT will maintain its position as a significant contributor to the ongoing development of CBT tradition.

Appendix

Appendix: A Guide to the Eight Emotional Problems and their Healthy Alternatives with Adversities, Beliefs and Associated Behaviour and Thinking

Anxiety Versus Concern

A = Adversity	You are facing a threat to your personal domain	
B = Belief	**Irrational (rigid and extreme)**	**Rational (flexible and non-extreme)**
C = Emotion	**Anxiety**	**Concern**
C = Behaviour	You avoid the threat	You face up to the threat without using any safety-seeking measures
	You withdraw physically from the threat	
	You ward off the threat (e.g. by rituals or superstitious behaviour)	You take constructive action to deal with the threat
	You try to neutralise the threat (e.g. by being nice to people of whom you are afraid)	You seek support from others to help you face up to the threat and then take constructive action by yourself rather than rely on them to handle it for you or to be there to rescue you
	You distract yourself from the threat by engaging in other activity	
	You keep checking on the current status of the threat hoping to find that it has disappeared or become benign	You prepare to meet the threat but do not over-prepare
	You seek reassurance from others that the threat is benign	
	You seek support from others so that if the threat happens they will handle it or be there to rescue you	
	You over-prepare in order to minimise the threat happening or so that you are prepared to meet it (NB it is the over-preparation that is the problem here)	
	You tranquillise your feelings so that you don't think about the threat	
	You overcompensate for feeling vulnerable by seeking out an even greater threat to prove to yourself that you can cope	

C = Subsequent thinking	*Threat-exaggerated thinking*	
	You overestimate the probability of the threat occurring	You are realistic about the probability of the threat occurring
	You underestimate your ability to cope with the threat	You view the threat realistically
	You ruminate about the threat	You realistically appraise your ability to cope with the threat
	You create an even more negative threat in your mind	You think about what to do concerning dealing with threat constructively rather than ruminate about the threat
	You magnify the negative consequences of the threat and minimise its positive consequences	
	You have more task-irrelevant thoughts than in concern	You have more task-relevant thoughts than in anxiety
		You picture yourself dealing with the threat in a realistic way
	Safety-seeking thinking	
	You withdraw mentally from the threat	
	You try to persuade yourself that the threat is not imminent and that you are 'imagining' it	
	You think in ways designed to reassure yourself that the threat is benign or if not, that its consequences will be insignificant	
	You distract yourself from the threat e.g. by focusing on mental scenes of safety and well-being	
	You over-prepare mentally in order to minimise the threat happening or so that you are prepared to meet it (NB once again it is the over-preparation that is the problem here)	
	You picture yourself dealing with the threat in a masterful way	
	You overcompensate for your feeling of vulnerability by picturing yourself dealing effectively with an even bigger threat.	

Depression Versus Sadness

A = Adversity	You have experienced a loss from the sociotropic and/or autonomous realms of your personal domain	
	You have experienced failure within the sociotropic and/or autonomous realms of your personal domain	
	You or others have experienced an undeserved plight	
B = Belief	**Irrational (rigid and extreme)**	**Rational (flexible and non-extreme)**
C = Emotion	**Depression**	**Sadness**
C = Behaviour	You become overly dependent on and seek to cling to others (particularly in sociotropic depression)	You seek out reinforcements after a period of mourning (particularly when your inferential theme is loss)
	You bemoan your fate or that of others to anyone who will listen (particularly in pity-based depression)	You create an environment inconsistent with depressed feelings
	You create an environment consistent with your depressed feelings You attempt to terminate feelings of depression in self-destructive ways You either push away attempts to comfort you (in autonomous depression) or use such comfort to reinforce your dependency (in sociotropic depression) or your self- or other-pity (in pity-based depression)	You express your feelings about the loss, failure or undeserved plight and talk in a non-complaining way about these feelings to significant others You allow yourself to be comforted in a way that helps you to express your feelings of sadness and mourn your loss
C = Subsequent thinking	You see only negative aspects of the loss, failure or undeserved plight	You are able to recognise both negative and positive aspects of the loss or failure
	You think of other losses, failures and undeserved plights that you (and in the case of the latter, others) have experienced	You think you are able to help yourself
	You think you are unable to help yourself (helplessness)	You look to the future with hope
	You only see pain and blackness in the future (hopelessness)	
	You see yourself being totally dependent on others (in autonomous depression)	
	You see yourself as being disconnected from others (in sociotropic depression)	
	You see the world as full of undeservedness and unfairness (in plight-based depression)	
	You tend to ruminate concerning the source of your depression and its consequences	

Guilt Versus Remorse

A = Adversity	You have broken your moral code	
	You have failed to live up to your moral code	
	You have hurt someone's feelings	
B = Belief	**Irrational (rigid and extreme)**	**Rational (flexible and non-extreme)**
C = Emotion	**Guilt**	**Remorse**
C = Behaviour	You escape from the unhealthy pain of guilt in self-defeating ways	You face up to the healthy pain that accompanies the realisation that you have sinned
	You beg forgiveness from the person you have wronged	You ask, but do not beg, for forgiveness
	You promise unrealistically that you will not 'sin' again	You understand the reasons for your wrongdoing and act on your understanding
	You punish yourself physically or by deprivation	You atone for the sin by taking a penalty
	You defensively disclaim responsibility for wrongdoing You make excuses for your behaviour You reject offers of forgiveness	You make appropriate amends You do not make excuses for your behaviour or enact other defensive behaviour You accept offers for forgiveness
C = Subsequent thinking	You conclude that you have definitely committed the sin	You take into account all relevant data when judging whether or not you have 'sinned'
	You assume more personal responsibility than the situation warrants	You assume an appropriate level of personal responsibility
	You assign far less responsibility to others than is warranted	You assign an appropriate level of responsibility to others
	You dismiss possible mitigating factors for your behaviour	You take into account mitigating factors
	You only see your behaviour in a guilt-related context and fail to put it into an overall context	You put your behaviour into overall context
	You think that you will receive retribution	You think you may be penalised rather than receive retribution

Shame Versus Disappointment

A = Adversity	Something highly negative has been revealed about you (or about a group with whom you identify) by yourself or by others	
	You have acted in a way that falls very short of your ideal	
	Others look down on or shun you (or a group with whom you identify) or think that they do	
B = Belief	**Irrational (rigid and extreme)**	**Rational (flexible and non-extreme)**
C = Emotion	**Shame**	**Disappointment**
C = Behaviour	You remove yourself from the 'gaze' of others	You continue to participate actively in social interaction
	You isolate yourself from others	You respond positively to attempts of others to restore social equilibrium
	You save face by attacking other(s) who have 'shamed' you	
	You defend your threatened self-esteem in self-defeating ways	
	You ignore attempts by others to restore social equilibrium	
C = Subsequent thinking	You overestimate the negativity of the information revealed	You see the information revealed in a compassionate self-accepting context
	You overestimate the likelihood that the judging group will notice or be interested in the information	You are realistic about the likelihood that the judging group will notice or be interested in the information revealed
	You overestimate the degree of disapproval you (or your reference group) will receive	You are realistic about the degree of disapproval self (or reference group) will receive
	You overestimate how long any disapproval will last	You are realistic about how long any disapproval will last

Hurt Versus Sorrow

A = Adversity	Others treat you badly (and you think you do not deserve such treatment)	
	You think that the other person has devalued your relationship (i.e. someone indicates that their relationship with you is less important to them than the relationship is to you)	
B = Belief	**Irrational (rigid and extreme)**	**Rational (flexible and non-extreme)**
C = Emotion	**Hurt**	**Sorrow**
C = Behaviour	You stop communicating with the other person	You communicate your feelings to the other directly
	You sulk and make obvious you feel hurt without disclosing details of the matter You indirectly criticise or punish the other person for their offence You tell others how badly you have been treated, but don't take any responsibility for any contribution you may have made to this	You request that the other person acts in a fairer manner towards you You discuss the situation with others in a balanced way, focusing on the way you have been treated and taking responsibility for any contribution you may have made to this
C = Subsequent thinking	You overestimate the unfairness of the other person's behaviour	You are realistic about the degree of unfairness in the other person's behaviour
	You think that the other person does not care for you or is indifferent to you	You think that the other person has acted badly rather than as demonstrating lack of caring or indifference
	You see yourself as alone, uncared for or misunderstood	You see yourself as being in a poor situation, but still connected to, cared for by and understood by others not directly involved in the situation
	You tend to think of past 'hurts' You think that the other person has to make the first move to you and you dismiss the possibility of making the first move towards that person	If you think of past hurts you do so with less frequency and less intensity than when you feel hurt
		You are open to the idea of making the first move towards the other person

Unhealthy Anger Versus Healthy Anger

A = Adversity	You think that you have been frustrated in some way or your movement towards an important goal has been obstructed in some way	
	Someone has treated you badly	
	Someone has transgressed one of your personal rules	
	You have transgressed one of your own personal rules	
	Someone or something has threatened your self-esteem or disrespected you	
B = Belief	**Irrational (rigid and extreme)**	**Rational (flexible and non-extreme)**
C = Emotion	**Unhealthy anger**	**Healthy anger**
C = Behaviour	You attack the other(s) physically You attack the other(s) verbally	You assert yourself with the other(s) You request, but do not demand, behavioural change from the other(s)
	You attack the other(s) passive-aggressively	You leave an unsatisfactory situation non-aggressively after taking steps to deal with it
	You displace the attack on to another person, animal or object	
	You withdraw aggressively	
	You recruit allies against the other(s)	
C = Subsequent thinking	You overestimate the extent to which the other(s) acted deliberately	You think that the other(s) may have acted deliberately, but you also recognise that this may not have been the case
	You see malicious intent in the motives of the other(s)	You are able to see the point of view of the other(s)
	You see yourself as definitely right and the other(s) as definitely wrong	You have fleeting, rather than sustained thoughts to exact revenge
	You are unable to see the point of view of the other(s)	You think that other(s) may have had malicious intent in their motives, but you also recognise that this may not have been the case
	You plot to exact revenge	You think that you are probably rather than definitely right and the other(s) as probably rather than definitely wrong
	You ruminate about the other's behaviour and imagine coming out on top	

Jealousy Versus Concern for Your Relationship

A = Adversity	A threat is posed to your relationship with your partner from a third person.	
	A threat is posed by uncertainty you face concerning your partner's whereabouts, behaviour or thinking in the context of the first threat	
B = Belief	**Irrational (rigid and extreme)**	**Rational (flexible and non-extreme)**
C = Emotion	**Jealousy**	**Concern for your relationship**
C = Behaviour	You seek constant reassurance that you are loved	You allow your partner to initiate expressing love for you without prompting her or seeking reassurance once she has done so
	You monitor the actions and feelings of your partner	You allow your partner freedom without monitoring his/her feelings, actions and whereabouts
	You search for evidence that your partner is involved with someone else You attempt to restrict the movements or activities of your partner You set tests which your partner has to pass You retaliate for your partner's presumed infidelity You sulk	You allow your partner to show natural interest in members of the opposite sex without setting tests You communicate your concern for your relationship in an open and non-blaming manner
C = Subsequent thinking	You exaggerate any threat to your relationship that does exist	You tend not to exaggerate any threat to your relationship that does exist
	You think the loss of your relationship is imminent	You do not misconstrue ordinary conversations between your partner and another men/women
	You misconstrue your partner's ordinary conversations with relevant others as having romantic or sexual connotations	You do not construct visual images of your partner's infidelity
	You construct visual images of your partner's infidelity	You accept that your partner will find others attractive but you do not see this as a threat
	If your partner admits to finding another person attractive, you think that s/he finds that person more attractive than you and that s/he will leave you for this other person	

Malicious Envy Versus Non-malicious Envy

A = Adversity	Another person possesses and enjoys something desirable that you do not have	
B = Belief	**Irrational (rigid and extreme)**	**Rational (flexible and non-extreme)**
C = Emotion	**Malicious envy**	**Non-malicious envy**
C = Behaviour	You disparage verbally the person who has the desired possession to others	You strive to obtain the desired possession if it is truly what you want
	You disparage verbally the desired possession to others	
	If you had the chance you would take away the desired possession from the other (either so that you will have it or that the other is deprived of it)	
	If you had the chance you would spoil or destroy the desired possession so that the other person does not have it	
C = Subsequent thinking	You tend to denigrate in your mind the value of the desired possession and/or the person who possesses it	You honestly admit to yourself that you desire the desired possession
	You try to convince yourself that you are happy with your possessions (although you are not)	You are honest with yourself if you are not happy with your possessions, rather than defensively trying to convince yourself that you are happy with them when you are not
	You think about how to acquire the desired possession regardless of its usefulness	You think about how to obtain the desired possession because you desire it for healthy reasons
	You think about how to deprive the other person of the desired possession	You can allow the other person to have and enjoy the desired possession without denigrating that person or the possession You think about what the other has and lacks and what you have and lack
	You think about how to spoil or destroy the other's desired possession You think about all the other things the other has that you don't have	

References

Beal, D., Kopec, A. M., & DiGiuseppe, R. (1996). Disputing clients' irrational beliefs. *Journal of Rational-Emotive & Cognitive-Behavior Therapy, 14*, 215–229.

Beck, J. S. (2011). *Cognitive therapy: Basics and beyond* (2nd ed.). New York, NY: Guilford.

Burns, D. D. (1980). *Feeling good: The new mood therapy*. New York, NY: Morrow.

DiGiuseppe, R. (1991a). A rational–emotive model of assessment. In M. E. Bernard (Ed.), *Using rational–emotive therapy effectively* (pp. 151–172). New York, NY: Plenum.

DiGiuseppe, R. (1991b). Comprehensive cognitive disputing in rational-emotive therapy. In M. E. Bernard (Ed.), *Using rational-emotive therapy effectively* (pp. 173–195). New York, NY: Plenum.

DiGiuseppe, R., Leaf, R., Exner, T., & Robin, M.V. (1988). *The development of a measure of rational/irrational thinking*. Paper presented at the World Congress of Behavior Therapy, Edinburg, Scotland.

DiGiuseppe, R. A., Doyle, K. A., Dryden, W., & Backx, W. (2014). *A practitioner's guide to rational emotive behavior therapy* (3rd ed.). New York, NY: Oxford University Press.

Dryden, W. (1998). Understanding persons in the context of their problems: A rational emotive behavior therapy perspective. In M. Bruch & F. W. Bond (Eds.), *Beyond diagnosis: Case formulation approaches in CBT* (pp. 43–64). Chichester, UK: Wiley.

Dryden, W. (2001). *Reason to change: A rational emotive behaviour therapy (REBT) workbook*. Hove, UK: Brunner-Routledge.

Dryden, W. (2009). *Understanding emotional problems: The REBT perspective*. Hove, UK: Routledge.

Dryden, W. (2015). *Rational emotive behavior therapy: Distinctive features* (2nd ed.). Hove, UK: Routledge.

Dryden, W. (2018a). *Cognitive-emotive-behavioural coaching: A flexible and pluralistic approach*. Abingdon, UK: Routledge.

Dryden, W. (2018b). *Very brief therapeutic conversations*. Abingdon, UK: Routledge.

Dryden, W., & Neenan, M. (2011). *Working with resistance in rational emotive behaviour therapy*. Hove, UK: Routledge.

Ellis, A. (1963). Toward a more precise definition of "emotional" and "intellectual" insight. *Psychological Reports, 13*, 125–126.

Ellis, A. (1979). The issue of force and energy in behavioral change. *Journal of Contemporary Psychotherapy, 10*(2), 83–97.

Ellis, A. (1980a). The value of efficiency in psychotherapy. *Psychotherapy: Theory, Research and Practice, 17*, 414–418.

Ellis, A. (1980b). Rational-emotive therapy and cognitive behavior therapy: Similarities and differences. *Cognitive Therapy and Research, 4*, 325–340.

Ellis, A. (2000). Rational-emotive imagery. In M. E. Bernard & J. L. Wolfe (Eds.), *The REBT resource book for practitioners* (2nd ed., pp. II-8–II-10). New York, NY: Albert Ellis Institute.

Ellis, A. (2002). *Overcoming resistance: A rational emotive behavior therapy integrated approach*. New York, NY: Springer.

Ellis, A., & Joffe, D. (2002). A study of volunteer clients who experienced live sessions of rational emotive behavior therapy in front of a public audience. *Journal of Rational-Emotive & Cognitive-Behavior Therapy, 20*, 151–158.

Ellis, A. (1962). Reason and emotion in psychotherapy. New York: Lyle Stuart.

Hickey, M., & Doyle, K. A. (2018). Rational emotive behavior therapy. In A. Vernon & K. A. Doyle (Eds.), *Cognitive behavior therapies: A guidebook for practitioners* (pp. 109–141). Alexandria, VA: American Counseling Association.

Maultsby, M. C., Jr. (1975). *Help yourself to happiness: Through rational self-counseling*. New York, NY: Institute for Rational Living.

Neenan, M., & Dryden, W. (1996). The intricacies of inference chaining. *Journal of Rational-Emotive and Cognitive-Behavior Therapy, 14*, 231–243.

Walen, S. R., DiGiuseppe, R., & Wessler, R. L. (1980). *A practitioner's guide to rational emotive therapy*. New York, NY: Oxford University Press.

Chapter 9
Brief Interventions in Rational Emotive Behavior Therapy

Windy Dryden

Introduction

In this chapter, I will consider the role of brief interventions in Rational Emotive Behavior Therapy. With its initial emphasis on problem assessment rather than on case formulation, REBT lends itself quite well to brief work. In this chapter by 'brief', I mean between 1 and 11 sessions and I will focus on REBT that is brief by design rather than by default. Although often when clients end therapy quickly, and the end is not planned, it should not be necessarily assumed that they have terminated the process 'prematurely' as their decision is often 'mature' and they are pleased with what they have achieved (Talmon, 1990). In this chapter, I focus on three different formats when discussing brief interventions in REBT (see below).

What Are Brief Interventions in REBT?

While at first glance, the term 'brief' when describing therapy, in general and REBT, in particular, is straightforward, i.e. it refers to therapeutic help that does not last a long time, the reality is far more complex. For example, REBT is described on the Albert Ellis Institute website as 'short-term therapy, long-term results'. If we take such an approach then it is meaningless to consider brief interventions in REBT as a special topic because, by definition, REBT is intrinsically brief. However, as any REBT practitioner will tell you for a number of clients, therapy involves long-term work. This may be due to the fact that the client has several problems that are difficult to deal and, additionally, they may encounter several obstacles when dealing with these problems. Alternatively, a client may seek longer-term REBT because

W. Dryden (✉)
Goldsmiths University of London, London, UK

© Springer Nature Switzerland AG 2019

M. E. Bernard, W. Dryden (eds.), *Advances in REBT*,
https://doi.org/10.1007/978-3-319-93118-0_9

they first want to address their emotional problems and then want to work towards greater self-development which Mahrer (1967) argued, a number of years ago, were the two major goals of psychotherapy.

There is also the issue of time versus number of sessions. Thus, if a client has a small number of sessions (e.g. 5), but these are spread over a long period of time, (e.g. a year) then should we refer to this as 'brief' therapy? Alternatively, if a person has a large number of sessions (e.g. 30) over a short period of time (e.g. 6 weeks) would this be considered 'brief'? Intensive, surely, but 'brief'?

As you can see there is no consensus in the field concerning what constitutes 'brief' therapy and thus, in this chapter, I will make it quite clear that I will be taking a 'session number' focus, not a 'time' focus. Thus, for me, brief therapy is 11 sessions or less and I will discuss an 11-session protocol for brief REBT that I have published (Dryden, 1995). I refer to this approach as 'brief REBT' as it contains, as will be seen, the major components of REBT, albeit in truncated form. I contrast this with the other two formats which I will refer to as 'single session therapy using REBT principles and practice' (Dryden, 2017) and 'very brief therapeutic conversations using REBT principles and practice' (Huber & Backlund, 1991). Such conversations, for example, occur at the Albert Ellis Institute's 'Friday Night Live'[1] evenings where two volunteers discuss their problems of living with an REB therapist in front of an audience (Ellis & Joffe, 2002).

Brief REBT: An 11 Session Protocol

I developed a protocol for brief REBT that lasts 11 sessions. I selected this number of sessions after trialing ten, eleven and twelve sessions and found that eleven sessions gave me and other REB therapists sufficient time to cover what needed to be covered.

Suitability Criteria

The following are good indicators for brief REBT:

1. The person is able and willing to present their problems in specific form and set goals that are concrete and achievable
2. The person's problems can be addressed within brief REBT. In my experience, these problems tend to be:

[1]When Albert Ellis was alive and running these sessions, they were called 'Friday Night Workshops'. I run a similar event in England at monthly UKCBT Meetup groups where I give a lecture on a theme and then interview two volunteers who have problems with that theme and are seeking help.

- Acute rather than chronic
- Disruptive to the person's life in one or two particular life areas but not to the person's entire life
- Distressing to the person, but the person's distress lies within a mild to moderate range of distress. If the person's level of distress is severe the problem may still be amenable to brief REBT as long as the other criteria listed here are met.
- In addition, the person is not defensive with respect to the problem(s) and is open to address and change the problem(s)

3. The person is able and willing to target, at the most, two problems that they particularly want to work on during therapy.
4. The person has understood the 'Situational ABCDEFG' framework used in REBT (Dryden, 2018) - or salient parts of that framework- and has indicated that this way of conceptualising and dealing with their problems makes sense and is potentially helpful to them.
5. The person has understood the therapist's tasks and their own tasks in brief REBT, has indicated that these seem potentially useful to them and is willing to carry out their tasks.
6. The person's level of functioning in their everyday life is sufficiently high to enable them to carry out their tasks both inside and outside therapy sessions.
7. There is evidence that a good working bond can be quickly developed between the therapist and the person seeking help.

Getting Brief REBT Off on the Right Foot

It is very important that the brief REB therapist gets therapy off to a good start and they do this by completing the following tasks. The therapist:

1. Begins by suggesting an agenda for the session. This should outline the following items and incorporate what the person wants to put on the agenda.
2. Encourages the person to talk about their problem(s) in their own way, but briefly. In doing so, the therapist shows the person empathic understanding of their problem(s). but does so without reinforcing the client's idea that 'A' causes 'C'.
3. Helps the person to specify their problems and suggests that they work with two of these problems for brief REBT, if they specify more than two. If two are selected, the therapist asks the person to nominate one of these problems that they would like to focus on first. This becomes the person's 'target' problem.
4. Helps the person to set a goal in line with the target problem as it has been *specified*. As the person does so, the therapist ensures that this goal are within the person's control, stated positively, observable (or have a referent that is observable), achievable and health promoting.[2]

[2] The therapist helps the client set a goal in line with their second problem at the appropriate time later in the process.

5. Teaches the person the 'Situational ABCDEFG' model of REBT (Dryden, 2018) either using one of the person's problems as content or a generalised problem example.
6. Explains their tasks as a brief REB therapist and suggests what the person's tasks would be if they become a client in brief REBT.
7. Decides with the person whether or not they are a good candidate for brief REBT. If so, the two contract for brief REBT and the person becomes a 'brief REBT' client. If not, the two may contract for longer term REBT or the therapist may refer the person to a practitioner of a therapeutic approach better suited to what the person is looking for.
8. Negotiate the first homework assignment with the client with the target problem in mind.

Assessment and Goal Setting

The next task that the therapist has in brief REBT is to help themself and the client understand the target problem using the 'Situational ABC' part of the 'Situational ABCDEFG' framework used in REBT. At the same time, the therapist also helps the client to learn how to assess their problems themself, if they are interested in doing so. In doing this, they may use one of a number of REBT self-help forms that are freely available in the professional domain (e.g. Dryden & David, 2009). As is typical in REBT, the therapist encourages the client to select a specific example of the target problem to facilitate assessment. Assessment involves the therapist first identifying the client's unhealthy negative response, unconstructive behavioural response and highly and negatively distorted thinking response (at 'C') to the adversity (at 'A'). Then and most importantly, the therapist helps the client to identify the irrational beliefs that they hold (at 'B') about the adversity that accounts for these problematic responses. Once the client has seen this, they can be said to understand the 'irrational belief-disturbed C' connection.

An important part of assessment is to determine whether the client has a meta-emotional problem (an emotional problem about their target problem). If so, the therapist and client need to deal with this first, if the client agrees and if its presence interferes (a) with the two of them working on the target problem in the therapy room and (b) with the client working on the target problem outside the therapy room.

Once assessment has been completed the therapist helps the client to set a goal in line with the problem as *assessed* ('G' in the 'Situational ABCDEFG' framework). What is important here is that the client's goal represents a healthy response to the adversity identified at assessment. In particular, the client is helped to nominate a healthy negative emotional response, a constructive behavioural response and a realistic and balanced cognitive response to the adversity and to identify the rational beliefs that they would need to hold about the adversity that would enable them to experience these healthy responses. Once they have seen this they can be said to understand the 'rational belief-healthy C' connection.

Disputing and Understanding

Once the client's target problem has been assessed and they have understood the role that their irrational and rational alternative beliefs play in their problem and in achieving their goal, the therapist can help them to stand back and dispute these beliefs (at 'D') and to commit themself to developing their rational beliefs. Disputing involves the therapist encouraging the client to examine their irrational and rational beliefs from an empirical standpoint, a logical standpoint and a pragmatic standpoint. The goal of disputing is to help the client understand (at 'E') that their irrational beliefs are false, illogical and lead to predominantly unhealthy results and that their alternative rational beliefs are true, logical and lead to predominantly healthy results. Where appropriate, the client is also taught how to question their irrational and rational beliefs for themself and the therapist suggests appropriate self-help material to facilitate the client doing this (Dryden, 2001).

The client is helped to see that this understanding is likely to be 'intellectual' rather than 'emotional' in nature. Ellis (1963) distinguished between intellectual insight and emotional insight. He argued that intellectual insight involves a cognitive understanding of why an irrational belief is irrational and why the alternative rational belief is rational without this impacting on the person's feelings and behaviour. By contrast, he argued that emotional insight involves a deeper felt conviction into the same point which does impact on the person's feelings and behaviour. While a minority of clients do experience an immediate change in feelings, behavior and related thinking once they have recognised and changed their irrational belief to a rational belief for such change to last, all clients need to internalise their rational beliefs which is the subject of the next section.

Engaging Emotions in the Disputing Process

As I will discuss below, perhaps the best way of promoting belief change *outside* the session is for the client to act repeatedly in ways that support their developing rational beliefs while facing the adversity at *'A'*. However, the best way of promoting such change inside the session is for the client to be helped to argue in favour of these beliefs in a forceful manner while their healthy emotions are engaged. This is particularly important in brief therapy where time is at a premium. REBT has a number of techniques that can be grouped under this heading. The following techniques are a few examples of those that can be used in brief therapy to encourage belief cahnge in this respect.

Rational-emotive imagery Here, the client is asked to imagine disturbing themself in response to the adversity at *'A'* and then to develop a healthy emotional response to the same *'A'* with the therapist ensuring that this was achieved by a belief change from irrational to rational.

Forceful recorded disputing Here the client is encouraged to record themself disputing beliefs and to ensure that the rational part of themself is more forceful and more persuasive than the irrational part.

Chairwork (Kellogg, 2015) The use of chairs in REBT where the client can play both their rational belief and their irrational belief having a dialogue is a particularly vivid and emotional way of engaging the client in the belief change process. The therapist searches for ways of encouraging the client in the rational belief chair to respond persuasively to their irrational belief in the other chair. This method is also useful in helping both therapist and client to discover irrational arguments to which the client struggles to respond. This can then be discussed outside of chairwork before it is resumed once the client has developed a persuasive argument to their irrational voice. A variety of emotive techniques can be negotiated for use as homework assignments to ensure that the client retains their focus on belief change between sessions.

Repeated Integrated Action and Thinking to Promote Change

In REBT, in general, it is thought that the best way for the client to facilitate change (at 'F') is for them to (i) face adversity while rehearsing their developing rational beliefs and (ii) act and think in ways that are consistent with these beliefs and that will support their development and (iii) do such practice repeatedly. I refer to this practice as 'integrated action and thinking' because it brings together, in integrated form, rational beliefs, constructive behavior and realistic thinking. In brief REBT, in particular, the client is called upon to do more of this practice to benefit from its limited number of sessions than in ongoing REBT. Consequently, it is important that the client commits sufficient time to do this practice. Negotiating and reviewing homework tasks are key for both therapist and client here. Emotional change is deemed to occur as a result of this repeated, integrated action and thinking.

While change is best promoted between sessions, brief REB therapist often use techniques within sessions which also aid this change process and which can be taught to the client for their later use (Dryden, 1995). Common techniques which are designed to do this include those which (i) encourage the client to develop and use persuasive arguments in support of their rational beliefs; (ii) promote a variety of rational and irrational dialogues where the client accesses both rational and irrational beliefs and engages in a debate designed to help them to develop conviction in the former and to let go of the latter; (iii) enable the person to use imagery to rehearse the integration of rational beliefs with constructive action and realistic thinking while imagining facing adversity. This is often done before the client faces adversity in reality.

Dealing with Obstacles to Change

Obstacles to change probably occur in all types of psychotherapy and REBT is no exception. In brief REBT, the more such obstacles can be anticipated and dealt with in advance the better. However, if such obstacles are encountered in reality, these often take the form of (a) adversities unrelated to the target problem or (b) discomfort-related adversities. The therapist and client use the 'Situational ABCDEFG' framework with the therapist encouraging the client to take the lead to deal effectively with these adversities. Obstacles to change may also take the form of one or more doubts, reservations and objections (DROs) to some aspect of brief REBT. Here, the therapist helps the client to identify the misconception that usually is at the heart of the DRO and to correct it.

Most of the time, the therapist can help the client deal with such obstacles within the paradigm of brief REBT. When this is not the case then the therapeutic contract needs to be renegotiated.

Generalization and Ending

When the client has achieved their goal with respect to their first target problem, then the therapist encourages them to generalize their learning to deal with their second target problem (when they have selected such a problem). Here, the client is invited to take the lead and use the REBT emotional problem-solving process that they learned in dealing with their first target problem with the therapist prompting the client when needed. In addition, the therapist encourages the client to generate rational beliefs and to use specific variants of these general beliefs in other problem areas beyond the two problems targeted for change in brief REBT.

It is at the generalization stage that therapist and client are likely to agree to increase the interval between therapy sessions and while brief REBT formally ends at the 11th session, a follow-up session can be carried-out at a suitable future date to enable both to evaluate the client's progress.

Single Session Therapy Using REBT Principles and Practice

Single session therapy (SST) has been defined as "one face-to-face meeting between therapist and a patient with no previous or subsequent sessions within one year" (Talmon, 1990: xv). In my view, the main feature of REBT-inspired SST is to offer the client one thing that the person can take away from the experience that would make a difference to their problem and which they can maintain after SST has been concluded. This, ideally, should be a rational belief with which the client resonates and which the person can implement in a relevant part of their life (Keller & Papasan, 2012).

In the REBT-inspired approach to SST that I have developed (Dryden, 2017) there are four points of contact: (i) When the person contacts the therapist for the very first time; (ii) the pre-session telephone contact; (iii) the face-to-face session; (iv) the follow-up telephone session after 3 months. As you can see, as only one of these four points of contact takes place face-to-face within the 1 year period stipulated by Talmon, my approach is an example of single session therapy. Before I discuss each point of contact in more depth, let me say a little about the indications and contra-indications of REBT-inspired SST.

Indications and Contra-Indications for REBT-Inspired SST

I will first outline some of the indications for this approach to SST.

Indications In my experience, the following are indications for REBT-inspired SST;

- A person who experiences an everyday, non-clinical emotional problem of living (anxiety, non-clinical depression, guilt, shame, anger, hurt, jealousy and envy)
- A person who has a relationship issue at home and at work or who is seeking advice and help with dealing with others
- A person who experiences an everyday problem of self-discipline
- A client who is in ongoing therapy but who wants brief help with a problem with which their therapist can't or won't help them. It is important that the other therapist agrees to you seeing them for SST
- A therapy trainee who wants to find out what it is like to have therapy from a different perspective
- A person who is ready to 'take care of business now' and whose problem is 'non-clinical', but amenable to a single session approach. This problem may become 'clinical' if not dealt with
- A person who is ready to take care of business now and whose problem is 'clinical', but amenable to a single session approach (e.g. simple phobias – Davis, Ollendick, & Öst, 2012 and panic disorder – Reinecke, Waldenmaier, Cooper, & Harmer, 2013).

- A person who is stuck and needs some help to get unstuck and move on
- A person who views therapy as providing intermittent help across the life cycle
- A person who has a self-development or coaching goal
- A person with a clinical problem, but who is ready to tackle a 'non-clinical' problem
- A person who is open to therapy, but wants to try it first before committing themself
- A person who wants some prophylactic assistance
- A person who has a meta-emotional problem
- A person who requires prompt and focused crisis management
- A person who has a life dilemma
- A person who is required to make an important, imminent decision
- A person who is finding it difficult to adjust to life in some way
- A person who is seeking advice on how REBT would tackle their problem

Contra-indications The following are some contra-indications for REBT-inspired SST

- A person who does not want REBT or CBT of any description
- A person who requests ongoing therapy
- A person who needs ongoing therapy
- A client who has many vague complaints and can't be specific
- A client who is likely to feel abandoned by the therapist at the end of the process

The Process of REBT-Inspired SST

As I mentioned above there are four points of contact in REBT-inspired SST. In outlining these I will refer to my own experience as a single session therapist using REBT principles and practice (Dryden, 2017).

Point of contact 1: The very first contact. When a person first contacts an REB therapist they are either making an enquiry about the therapist's services or applying for that person's help. At that contact, I outline my services including single session therapy. If they show an interest in SST, I then have a brief conversation with them to determine whether they are suitable for and may benefit from SST and agree with its practicalities (format, timing and fees). If the signs are promising, then I schedule a 30-min telephone schedule to confirm the person's suitability for SST and to help them get the most out of the process. This telephone call should be arranged as soon as possible to create a momentum.

Point of contact 2: The pre-session telephone contact. The tasks of the SS therapist in this contact are to:

Confirm that the person is suitable for SST. If the person is suitable then they have a clear and realistic idea what they want to gain from the process and are ready to take immediate steps to achieve their goal.

Elicit the client's view of the therapist's role in helping them to achieve their goal. Here, the client often says that the therapist's role is to "help me to put things into a different perspective" or "help me to approach the problem differently". The therapist uses such statements to show that they are consistent with REBT-inspired SST.

Ask the client to outline what they already have they done to address the problem. In doing so, the therapist discovers what has been helpful and unhelpful about doing so. The therapist aims to build on the latter and distance their approach from the latter.

Discover the client's strengths and resources. The purpose of SST is to build on the client's pre-existing strengths and help them draw upon extant resources rather than to start from scratch in each area. One discovered, the therapist's role is to remind the client to use these strengths and resources in the face-to-face session.

Encourage the client to do any relevant homework task before the face-to-face session. Depending upon what emerges in the pre-session telephone contact, the therapist will want to suggest something that the client can do before the face-to-face session to initiate the process. Once again this session should be arranged as soon as possible after the phone call.

Point of contact 3: The face-to-face session. The face-to-face session usually lasts for approximately 50 min (unless there is good reason to extend it as in a single extended session when working with simple phobias, Davis et al., 2012).

Build a bridge between the phone-call and the session. The first thing that the therapist should do is to pick up on any preparatory work that the client has done between the end of the phone contact and this session. In addition, the therapist should enquire about any changes that the client may have noticed since they had the phone call and build on any such changes.

Create a focus. The therapist's next task is to help the client to create a focus for the session and then to identify the person's target problem (i.e. the problem they want to be helped with) and the goal with respect to that problem. Problem and goal assessment follow, based on a selected example of the problem. There is some value in the client selecting an anticipated example of the problem to help the person apply their learning in the session to that situation.

Identify the central mechanism. By the central mechanism I mean the major irrational belief (s) and associated behavior and thinking that are responsible for the existence and maintenance of the problem.

Dispute the irrational belief(s). The next stage is for the therapist to help the client to examine at least the one major irrational belief that is deemed largely responsible for the problem and to modify this and plan on acting on the new rational belief. Throughout this process the therapist looks for ways to help the client to generalize learning.

Rehearse the rational belief in the session. It is very useful if the therapist can find a way to make an emotional impact on the client which may encourage learning and later application. This is best done when the therapist gives the client an opportunity to rehearse their new belief in the session. Some variant of two chair work (see Kellogg, 2015) or rational-emotive imagery (Dryden, 2001) are often useful in this context.

Implementation. After such rehearsal, the therapist should initiate discussion concerning how the client is going to implement their learning in their everyday life as soon as possible after the session. Any potential obstacle should be identified and addressed. At the end of the session a final summary should be made preferably by the client and augmented by the therapist and any loose ends tied up. A definite appointment should be made for the follow-up session 2–3 months in the future.

One of the features of my approach to REBT-inspired SST (Dryden, 2017) is that I record the session and offer my client the digital voice recording (DVR) of the session and/or a typed transcript of the session. I find that doing so aids client reflection and gives the client something to review after the final session and provides a useful bridge between the face-to-face session and the follow-up session.

Point of contact 4: The follow-up session. Some clients say that knowing that they were going to have further contact with the therapist is a motivation to help them maintain the gains that they made from the session. Others welcome the chance to reflect on the process and it also serves as a reminder of what was achieved since the face-to face session and what can yet be achieved.

Follow-up also enables the therapist to discover what was helpful and not so helpful about their contribution to the process and thus, it aids their development as an REBT-inspired SS therapist. Finally, if the therapist works in a service that collects data on intervention effectiveness, follow-up is crucial in finding out just how effective REBT-inspired SST is with certain groups and populations. It also yields data on differential effectiveness among therapists.

Very Brief Therapeutic Conversations (VBTCs) Using REBT Principles and Practice

The final brief intervention in REBT that I will discuss in this chapter is what I refer to as 'very brief therapeutic conversations using REBT principles and practice'. This form of brief intervention was developed initially by Albert Ellis in his 'Friday Night Workshops' in 1965. At these workshops, Ellis publicly interviewed two volunteers from the audience on so-called 'problems of living' which were normally emotional and/or behavioral in nature, These sessions lasted for about 30 min and were followed by a question and answer session involving audience members. Research has shown that such short interviews are frequently rated as 'helpful' or 'very helpful' by the volunteers themselves and seem also to benefit audience members (Ellis & Joffe, 2002). After Ellis's death in 2007, the Albert Ellis Institute has continued this tradition of 'very brief therapeutic conversations' at its 'Friday Night Live' event. In Britain, I have done over 300 of such public demonstration sessions of REBT which are generally 20–30 min in length and sometimes considerably less (see the session transcript below). Before the sessions, I usually give a lecture on a particular theme (e.g. shame) and invite volunteers who wish to be helped with their particular problem of the evening's focused theme. The purpose of these demonstrations are twofold. First, they have a therapeutic purpose: to provide the volunteers with some help for their problems. Second, they have an educational purpose: to give people an idea of REBT in action.

When calling for volunteers, it is important that the therapist asks that the person volunteering brings a genuine, current problem or issue for which they are sincerely seeking help. Role-played problems are neither helpful to the person playing the role, to the therapist providing the 'help' and showing how REBT works, nor to the watching audience who may want to learn more about the practice of REBT or may want to apply what they see to their own, similar problems.

One of the features of VBTCs that take place in a public setting is that the therapist knows nothing about the client[3] or about the issue they are going to raise. Consequently, there are no indications or contra-indications for this type of help other than the aforementioned point about the importance of the client seeking help for a genuine problem or issue.

Let me outline some of the features of 'VBTCs using REBT principles and practice' as I see them. These principles apply mainly where the conversation takes place in a public setting, but also apply whn it is taking place in private.

'Primum non nocere'

The principle of 'first, do no harm' is enshrined in the helping professions, but is particularly important in public VBTCs where the therapist knows nothing about the person that they are meeting for the first time, but knows that the time that they have together is very limited. While the therapist may wish to show REBT in action to those present, their first duty is the client's welfare and when the two clash, the latter is prioritized. Having said that, in the 300 public VBTCs that I have conducted, I have never felt that the client's well-being was being compromised. Even when the client felt and displayed distress, they never opted to stop the interview when asked if they wanted to do so. Nevertheless, the therapist does need to be prepared to offer extra help if needed and I am happy to do so directly after the event finishes or soon after,

Therapeutic Style

In public VBTCs, the most effective REB therapists display a therapeutic style comprising the following three elements.

[3] I refer to the volunteer as a 'client' throughout this section.

Creating and maintaining a focus REBT is a form of active-directive therapy (Ellis, 1994). This is certainly true of REBT-inspired VBTCs. Perhaps what is even more important is the ability of the therapist to create and maintain a focus throughout the conversation.

Demonstrating empathy It is important that the client experiences the therapist as empathic, but it is also important that the therapist does not reinforce a causal 'A-C' connection while doing so even if the client makes this connection themself.

Using appropriate humor I pointed out above that VBTCs have therapeutic and educational value. While the entertainment value of VBTCs should always be secondary to its other values, it should be noted that humor, which is an important feature of VBTCs, is both entertaining, therapeutic and educational. Indeed, therapist humor often helps the client to keep an open mind about the therapist's message, particularly where this may be otherwise unpalatable. Ellis (1977) has written on the role of humor in REBT, but cautioned against the use of humor that can be construed as 'ad hominem' (directed at the person) rather than 'ad opinionem' (directed at the person's belief).

Just One Thing

The therapist's goal in a VBTC is to provide the client with one meaningful point that they can take away with them that will make a difference to the way they deal with their problem or issue (Keller & Papasan, 2012). While the REB therapist may hope that this point may refer to the therapeutic value of a rational belief, this may not necessarily be the case (unlike in REBT-inspired SST where it is more likely to be the case). The important factor is that this one thing is meaningful to the client and can potentially lead to some kind of therapeutic change.

One Problem/Issue

Due to the very limited time available in the VBTC, it is important that the therapist ensures that they work with only one client problem or issue. When the client brings up more than one at the outset, then the therapist urges them to select the one problem which they would like to focus on. This may be the problem that the person thinks can be most easily solved or it may be one about which they are most troubled. The most important point here is that once a particular problem has been selected then both therapist and client keep to this problem unless there is a good reason not to do so.

One Example

While therapist and client can deal with a problem or issue in general terms, it is preferable for them to work with a specific example of the problem or issue as selected by the client, if this is at all possible. Indeed, I usually suggest to the client that they choose a specific example of their problem/issue that is imminent. I do so to facilitate them putting into practice whenever they learn from the VBTC. This is a more direct way of proceeding than using a past example of their target problem, working that through and then applying learning to a nominated future example. A specific example of the target problem should be located in a specific setting, with specific people present and occurring a specific time. A specific example may be actual or imaginal.

Accurate Assessment Is Important and Worth Spending Time Over

In my experience conducting VBTCs, it is important to devote sufficient time to assessing accurately the specific example of the client's target problem using the ABC assessment framework of REBT. In particular, pinpointing the 'A', with accuracy, is perhaps the most important part of the assessment. In addition, when identifying the client's irrational beliefs, it is useful to help them to identify their rational alternative beliefs at the same time. Helping the client to understand the 'irrational belief-disturbed C' connection and the related 'rational belief-healthy C connection' both within the context of the adversity at 'A' is particularly important.

Goal Setting

Helping the client to select a goal can be done at any point in the VBTC process, but in my view, it is best done just after the assessment and where the client indicates that they understand the relationship between their beliefs and their responses to the adversity, both disturbed and healthy. Such understanding encourages the client to set a healthy response to the adversity at 'A' before the work proceeds.

Disputing and Choice

The reason that I recommend that the therapist helps the client to identify both irrational and rational beliefs at the same time during the assessment process, is to help them to dispute these beliefs at the same time during the disputing process. In doing so I recommend that the therapist helps the client to see clearly that they can either choose to hold an irrational belief or choose to hold a rational belief about the same adversity and that the consequences are very different. It can also be useful during the disputing process to ask the client that they have a choice of teaching the same irrational or rational belief to their children or other relevant group and to enquire what they would choose to teach and why.

Practice rB in the Session If Possible

Once the client has been helped to formulate a rational belief, then if possible, the therapist suggests that the client gains some practice at holding this rational belief during the session. This may be done within and imagery context or with some kind of rational-irrational dialogue e.g. rational role reversal (Dryden, 1995) or two chair dialogue (see Kellogg, 2015). If possible, this in-session practice should have an emotional impact on the client.

Practice rB outside the Session

While in-session rehearsal of a rational belief is desirable, what is more important is that the client commits themself to practising their rational belief in a context where they are likely to encounter their adversity at 'A'. In doing so, they should be encouraged to act in ways that strengthen their rational belief. This context may have already been selected if the therapist was able to encourage the client to use an anticipated example of their problem. The therapist should suggest that the client rehearses this in their mind's eye before they carry it out in reality and if there is time they should give the client an opportunity to do such rehearsal in the session. Unlike in ongoing therapy, the therapist will not get to learn the outcome of the work that they have done with the client, unless they invite the client to report back.

Generalization, If Relevant

While the REB therapist has the time in brief REBT to help the client to generalize the learning to other problems and they may have some time to do this in REBT-inspired SST, there is little if any time to do this kind of work in REBT inspired the VBTC. However, when I can I make a few closing remarks referring to generalization and suggest that the client consults these remarks either in the recording of the session or in the transcript that I routinely provide for my VBTC clients (see Dryden, 2017).

A Transcript of a VBCT Session

In what follows, I provide a verbatim transcript of an REBT-inspired VBTC held at a meeting of the United Kingdom CBT Meetup group. The conversation lasted for 10 min. I present this transcript with the full written consent of the client whose name has been changed. It gives an idea of what can be achieved in a very brief period of time.

Windy: OK, Tony, what problem can I help you with this evening?

Tony: I think that I suffer from chronic shame.

Windy: Chronic shame, OK. Can you tell us a little bit about that in more detail, please?

Tony: Sure. I was born in the mid-50s when gay activity between men was illegal. I came out to myself at the age of 12, just as the law was changing, and really kept that very much to myself as much as I could, right the way through until I was 28. So I didn't come out until I was 28, properly. In the meantime, at university, I had a crisis, so severe depression, and was referred, initially, to the psychiatrist, who tried to convert me, unsuccessfully.

Windy: To convert you?

Tony: To convert me to heterosexuality.

Windy: Right. He'd be struck off today.

Tony: Yeah, indeed. Then a hypnotherapist had a go, and that didn't work either. I can still remember the opening line of every hypnotherapy session was, 'Hey Tony, are you still a homo?' which was very affirming.

Windy: Happy days!

Tony: Indeed. So I seemed to achieve more equilibrium over time, but I wasn't really noticing the amount of alcohol I was consuming. I hit rock bottom in 2000, so 17 years ago, and really was in a situation there of total crisis, and it was when I decided that sobriety was the only way forward for me, that I also realised that the only circumstances under which I could countenance a physical relationship was under the influence of alcohol.

Windy: Which blocked what out?

Tony: Disinhibition, really. I mean there are sexual acts – I will spare everybody's blushes – that would make me feel uncomfortable, for example. So that disinhibiting effect, the alcohol did the trick, up to a point. Of course, it was a very negative way of coping. So the dilemma I've faced since then is really whether or not I'm going to come to terms, at the age of 62 now, with living my life on my own and work on my own resilience, or whether I…

Windy: Resilience for being on your own?

Tony: For being on my own, yes; for solitude. I don't mean isolation, but I mean solitude in terms of a relationship that's romantic or sexual. Or whether, in fact, this is something I should still work on. So that's the dilemma. I've tried various ways, which have been partly helpful, to disinhibit myself, such as regular mindfulness practice, and so on.

Windy: And that disinhibits you by what?

Tony: It doesn't disinhibit to the point where I'm actually having any sexual relationships, and I still find the whole concept, actually, quite scary. So, in some ways, I feel as if I'm 62 intellectually, but, probably, emotionally, about 15, and that's difficult to come to terms…

Windy: And, if we were successful this evening, what would we have achieved?

Tony: I would feel, whatever decision I made, whether it was to work towards being more resilient in a solitary life or whether it was better to be in a relationship, I feel that I was making a free choice. At the moment, I don't think I have the freedom to make that choice.

Windy: Because your choice is being influenced by what?

Tony: I think my fears are too great for me to accept the second option at the moment.

Windy: And the chronic shame, how does that fit in?

Tony: It's kind of paradoxical because I do a lot of active work within and beyond the LGBT community for gay rights and so forth, and equality, and, on the one hand, I'm able to give a lot of other people, I think, a lot of support around this, but, paradoxically, I find it very hard to turn the same trick on myself, if you like.

Windy: So is the chronic shame pushing you in the direction of one fork in the road?

Tony: Yes.

Windy: And which road is it?

Tony: That's the solitary one.

Windy: That's the solitary one. So the solitary fork is being driven by fear and chronic shame.

Tony: It is, plus the fact there's familiarity there, because now, having spent more than a quarter of my life in a solitary existence and survived so far, I know I could. I'm pretty sure I could.

Windy: Could what?

Tony: I could survive down that path. I'm not sure what the risks are, for example, of relapse if I go down the other route.

Windy: Right, OK. So, if I helped you with your chronic shame, that would help you how?

Tony: Well, I think it would unlock a lot of the processes that are going on in my mind at the moment of running against brick walls.

Windy: So what do you feel most shamed about?

Tony: I'm not shamed about my identity as a gay man and I feel quite comfortable to come into an environment like this, which is mixed, and share my sexual orientation. So it's not that. I do feel shame around sexual activity, and that was also true when I had a one-off relationship with a girl; I also felt guilty about that.

Windy: OK. So I'm going to invite you to be as honest and free as you can, and they can take care of their own blushes, alright?

Tony: OK.

Windy: So what sexual acts do you feel most ashamed about, if I could help you deal with the shame, that might be something you could really take forward?

Tony: OK, well, for me, I've never been a receptive partner in anal sex, for example. I've been the active partner, again with a large amount of alcohol inside me. I wouldn't say it was something I was totally thrilled about. I think, even with the level of inebriation, I was still conscious that it didn't feel right. So I think there are issues around that. In terms of, if you like, activities that are probably more common to heterosexual and homosexual people, such as oral sex and other…

Windy: OK, so what do you want to focus on: the anal or oral?

Tony: Let's go for anal.

Windy: So let's suppose that you are going to try anal sex as the penetrator. What, for you, is shameful about doing that?

Tony: I suppose it's a very basic notion of what the organs of the body are designed for and the notion that the anus is not designed, primarily, as a sex organ. So unnatural, I suppose, the idea of unnatural.

Windy: Alright, so let's suppose the act is unnatural. So you would be engaging in an unnatural act, let's suppose. Then what do you think you'd have to tell yourself about you, Tony, to create shame about engaging in that unnatural act?

Tony: Well, bluntly, 'You must not commit an unnatural act.'

Windy: Because, if you do, what kind of person are you?

Tony: I'm not particularly religious, but sinful, I suppose, is the word I'd use.

Windy: OK, so that's guilt.

Tony: Guilt, yeah.

Windy: Let's suppose it is a sin, it's unnatural and sinful to act in that way, how does that make you a sinful person?

Tony: In a global sense?

Windy: Yeah, because that's where guilt comes from.

Tony: Yeah, I don't think it does affect me in a global way.

Windy: So why don't you practise that, try it and see how you go in reality, because you might like it, you might not, but, if you really practise that from saying, 'I am not a sinful person, even though some people think this is sinful and some people think it's unnatural.' Presumably other people don't, right?

Tony: Sure.

Windy: So why couldn't you do that, without alcohol?

Tony: I think the way you unpicked it actually made it seem far smaller an obstacle, because you've kind of fragmented it: it's not something like this, it's now a series of…

Windy: Because I'm saying to you and asking you to invite yourself to see that the act doesn't identify you; you incorporate the act. How many other acts do you have to incorporate in this complex, fallible, very human organism called Tony? How many other acts do we have to include?

Tony: Well, quite a range, if you're talking about sexual activity, for example.

Windy: Yeah. So, you can practise anal sex, it doesn't define you unless you choose to allow it to define you.

Tony: So it's my choice?

Windy: Yeah.

Tony: I take your point.

Windy: A choice that's been…

Tony: It's been heavily conditioned by external factors.

Windy: But, you see, you, as a human being, can recondition yourself. You don't have to be a slave to that conditioning, even though you still might like it, you might not.

Tony: But it puts me in a position of choice then, as well, doesn't it?

Windy: That's right.

Tony: So that's a question of more freedom. That makes total sense, actually. That's very helpful.

Windy: So when can you put this into practice?

Tony: I can't give you a precise date.

Windy: In REBT, we want specific times and dates.

Tony: It doesn't just involve me.

Windy: Do you have somebody in mind?

Tony: Not at this moment, but I think, if I work on the concept and I think, also, if I bring some of this into my mindfulness practice, that would actually be a useful thing to do.

Windy: Yeah. How would you do that?

Tony: Well, particularly focusing during a body scan, for example. During a full body scan you include the anus and you include the genitals, and so forth. I think, maybe, in my head, having more of a connection between the genitals and the anus would be a way of breaking down my own, if you like, internalised prejudice.

Windy: Yeah, and to recognise that the totality of you, Tony, is not marked by your sexual activity.

Tony: Yeah, sure.

REBT lends itself to brief therapy and in this chapter, I have outlined three different ways that REBT can be practiced when time is at a premium. With the development of online and social media platforms together with the increasing use of smartphone applications for therapeutic purposes, in my view the future is bright with respect to how REBT therapists can bring the power of REBT to increasing numbers of people – briefly!

References

Davis, T. E., III, Ollendick, T. H., & Öst, L.-G. (Eds.). (2012). *Intensive one-session treatment of specific phobias*. New York, NY: Springer.

Dryden, W. (1995). *Brief rational emotive behaviour therapy*. Chichester, UK: John Wiley & Sons.

Dryden, W. (2001). *Reason to change: A rational emotive behaviour therapy (REBT) workbook*. Hove, UK: Brunner-Routledge.

Dryden, W., & David, D. (2009). *REBT self-help form*. New York: Albert Ellis Institute.

Dryden, W. (2017). *Single-session integrated CBT (SSI-CBT): Distinctive features*. Abingdon, UK: Routledge.

Dryden, W. (2018). *Cognitive-emotive-behavioral coaching: A flexible and pluralistic approach*. Abingdon, UK: Routledge.

Ellis, A. (1963). Toward a more precise definition of 'emotional' and 'intellectual' insight. *Psychological Reports, 23*, 538–540.

Ellis, A. (1977). Fun as psychotherapy. Rational Living, 12(1), 2–6.

Ellis, A. (1994) Reason and emotion in psychotherapy. Revised and updated edition. New York: Birch Lane Press.

Ellis, A., & Joffe, D. (2002). A study of volunteer clients who experienced live sessions of rational emotive behavior therapy in front of a public audience. *Journal of Rational-Emotive & Cognitive-Behavior Therapy, 20*, 151–158.

Huber, C. H., & Backlund, B. A. (1991). *The twenty minute counselor: Transforming brief conversations into effective helping experiences*. New York, NY: Continuum.

Keller, G., & Papasan, J. (2012). *The one thing: The surprisingly simple truth behind extraordinary results*. Austin, TX: Bard Press.

Kellogg, S. (2015). *Transformational chairwork: Using psychotherapeutic dialogues in clinical practice*. Lanham, MD: Rowman & Littlefield.

Mahrer, A. (Ed.). (1967). *The goals of psychotherapy*. New York, NY: Appleton-Century.

Reinecke, A., Waldenmaier, L., Cooper, M. J., & Harmer, C. J. (2013). Changes in automatic threat processing precede and predict clinical changes with exposure-based cognitive-behavior therapy for panic disorder. *Biological Psychiatry, 73*, 1064–1070.

Talmon, M. (1990). *Single session therapy: Maximising the effect of the first (and often only) therapeutic encounter*. San Francisco, CA: Jossey-Bass.

Chapter 10
REBT in Group Therapy

Kimberly A. Alexander and Kristene A. Doyle

History: How Ellis Defined and Practiced REB Group Therapy

Albert Ellis began practicing group therapy with deviant adolescents utilizing a psychoanalytic approach in the early year of 1949 at the New Jersey State Diagnostic Center. For many of the same reasons he criticized individual therapy using psychoanalysis, he had similar views about conducting group therapy with psychoanalysis.

REBT group therapy was born in 1959, when Ellis decided that the progress his individual clients were making with REBT could in fact be applied to group therapy as well using the ABCDE model (Yankura & Dryden, 1997). Although this model is the established core of REBT, the process by which the therapist identifies the client's ABCDE's often varies in technique whether it be in an individual or group setting and is driven by theory and emerging research.

Arguably, the therapist's decision to treat clients in a group versus individual setting can serve as a unique contribution to the success of treatment. Albert Ellis found that in his practice of group therapy using REBT, clients were actively participating in disputing other group members' irrational beliefs thereby strengthening the disputation (Yankura & Dryden, 1997). Members also benefited from being exposed to other's irrational beliefs and its disputation, which may have been similarly held. It should be noted that in more recent years, there has been a

K. A. Alexander (✉) · K. A. Doyle
Albert Ellis Institute, New York, NY, USA
e-mail: kimberly.alexander@albertellis.org; krisdoyle@albertellis.org

© Springer Nature Switzerland AG 2019

M. E. Bernard, W. Dryden (eds.), *Advances in REBT*,
https://doi.org/10.1007/978-3-319-93118-0_10

movement among many REBT practitioners to replace the word "dispute" with that of "debate," or "restructure" to partially address the criticism of REBT that it is confrontational and argumentative (DiGiuseppe, Doyle, Dryden, & Backx, 2013).

When Albert Ellis conducted group therapy, he viewed it as individual therapy within a group setting, with individuals talking to one member, debating their irrational belief(s), and encouraging problem-solving. Each member received an equal amount of time to discuss a particular problem, with a follow-up on their week's homework assignment as a starting point (the exception being in cases of clinical emergencies in which a member required more time to discuss their problem). Ellis typically had two trainees serve as co-leaders who assisted the 2 h session, and for the last 30 min the group continued in a different room without Ellis. During that time, further discussion of members' problems continued, as well as collaborating with members on homework assignments. Ellis' groups were typically referred to as "General Group," which were heterogeneous groups consisting of both men and women experiencing a range of emotional and behavioral problems including, but not limited to, anger, eating problems, relationship difficulties, procrastination, mood disorders, and anxiety. Therapy is also conducted with homogenous groups such as anger disorders, women's group, social anxiety, and emotional eating, to name a few. REB groups are conducted with various age groups, including children and adolescents (often in the school setting), and adults. Therapy can be offered as an open or closed group, depending on the goals of the leader as well as the goals of the group. Ellis' groups, the women's group led for many years by Dr. Janet Wolfe, and then carried on by Dr. Kristene Doyle, and the long-running Anger Group led by Dr. Raymond DiGiuseppe, all followed a similar model of an open group (members joining and terminating at various stages) of individual therapy within a group format. However, this is not to suggest that REB group therapy cannot be and is not done as more of a process group, with members addressing their relationships with one another. Therapy is also offered via a closed group model in which the membership is consistent, with no new members joining after the start of group and all members terminate at the same time at the end of the predetermined number of sessions.

The number of group members depends on several factors, including, the experience of the group leader, the problems being addressed in group, and the age and developmental level of the members. Adult groups typically have between 7 and 9 members over the course of a 2-h session. This range takes into account fatigue on the part of the members (and leaders), and ensures that each member will receive an adequate amount of time to discuss their particular problem. When there are fewer members, there is the risk of several members missing the same particular week and group therapy becomes more like individual therapy with 3 group leaders for two to three members. Having a size between 7 and 9 allows for member absences while still offering a group experience. However, if one is leading a group for adolescents with ADHD, the group size as well as the time length for sessions may need to be adjusted given some of the obstacles such a diagnosis has.

Distinctive Features and Benefits of REB Group Therapy

REBT group therapy, compared to individual therapy, offers several benefits, including:

1. Better learning on the part of members to dispute their own and other members' irrational beliefs;
2. Yalom's Universality Therapeutic Factor, in which group member's feeling of being unique in their problems is disconfirmed by hearing other members discuss similar issues (Yalom, 1995);
3. There tends to be not only more feedback provided, but group members tend to give more critical feedback to one another than individual and group therapists may give;
4. Group members tend to learn REBT better compared to individual therapy as there are more opportunities to teach the concepts given the number of clients in the room;
5. Problem-solving aspects are also benefited from the group experience, again, largely the result of more people coming together with various experiences and backgrounds;
6. Furthermore, group therapy affords the opportunity for enhanced vocational knowledge;
7. In mixed gender groups, members learn and are educated about the opposite gender;
8. In individual REBT therapy, modeling occurs by the practitioner; however, in group settings, there is the added component of other members (hopefully) modeling healthier beliefs, emotions;
9. A specific benefit of REBT group therapy is the opportunity for many members to model Unconditional Other-Acceptance (UOA) to one another, as well as Unconditional Self-Acceptance (USA) for themselves. Perhaps there is a dose effect that occurs in group regarding this issue. Does the presence of more individuals modeling UOA and USA have a stronger positive impact for clients than just an individual REBT therapist modeling these concepts?;
10. Group has a positive effect on members such that when one member opens up about a particular problem, irrational belief s/he is holding, or some dysfunctional negative emotion or maladaptive behavior being experienced, other group members tend to share their experiences, again, speaking to the principle of Universality;
11. Another added benefit seen in REBT group therapy is the mild competition that can take place amongst group members. For example, oftentimes there is a group member who is diligent about doing homework assignments, and consequently, experiences progress towards stated goals. When other, less committed, group members observe this progress being made, it is not uncommon for them to begin pushing themselves to achieve similar progress. Finally, groups have the unique ability to allow therapist to observe members in action and in the moment with one another and can therefore report on any

similarities and/or discrepancies between verbal and nonverbal behaviors or between what the member reports happening outside of group and what is occurring within the group (this intervention is referred to as confrontation in REBT). This in-the-moment observation can serve as an opportunity for members to correct themselves immediately rather than have to wait until the next time it occurs;

12. While not specific to REBT groups, we do think it is important to point out that the promotion of positive mental health is also carried out by the support system that often is engendered in groups. For many REBT groups, support is not only evidenced in the group setting, but it is also encouraged to continue outside of the group in between sessions. For example, if it becomes evident that one member is currently experiencing an abnormally big stressor, group members may volunteer to take turns checking in on that particular member in between group sessions and help challenge any irrational thinking that may be perpetuating emotional and/or behavioral disturbance. Naturally, there is the need to have an endorsement of this philosophy by the group leader(s) as well as an agreement amongst group members for this to occur.

Disadvantages of REB Group Therapy

While group therapy has multiple benefits for the conceptualization, assessment and treatment of many clinical conditions, there are aspects of group that do not carry such benefits.

1. Ideally, REBT groups conduct a screening session(s) to determine a goodness of fit between the potential member and the group. During the screening, it is important to ascertain whether the potential member's goals align with the group's stated goals. However, in some settings, including, but not limited to, schools, prisons, inpatient settings, and court-referred outpatient groups, individuals are mandated and a screening session is not always feasible, and there may be little if any goal alignment between the member and the group. When this is the case, we have observed REBT having more disadvantages;
2. The issue of confidentiality is not as straightforward in group therapy as it is in individual therapy, and is especially challenging for school, prison, and hospital settings, where there is access to patient information for many different individuals operating in various roles in their setting (i.e., teachers, social workers, psychiatrists, inpatient unit coordinators, etc.). In individual therapy, there is a "guarantee" that one's confidentiality will be protected by the therapist, with the obvious exceptions of harm or abuse. However, in group therapy, such a clear guarantee cannot be made to members. Of course, group leaders can assure members that they will hold what is discussed in confidence. What group leaders *cannot* do is promise members that their discussions will be kept confidential by other group members. In our experience, we have found that this

limitation has impacted some group members from being forthright about their challenges and disturbances. As a result, it can be difficult for therapists to fully conceptualize and effectively treat a group member's difficulties. We have found that one way to address the issue of confidentiality and to assuage members' concerns is to, throughout the course of the group, periodically discuss the importance of respecting members' confidentiality. Furthermore, we encourage members who wish to share with significant others insights they have learned in a particular group session about their beliefs, emotions, and behaviors by discussing *what* they learned, as opposed to *how* they learned it. Doing so helps to circumvent sharing specific details that may inadvertently disclose another member's identity;

3. REBT group therapy is also inefficient regarding the amount of time allocated for each member to speak. Most adult groups have between 6 and 8 members for a 2 h time span. This allows for approximately 15 min per group member to discuss a particular problem. As a result, group therapy requires members to be acutely aware that they have more limited time than they would in individual therapy and therefore be more focused. This poses a problem for some members who are experiencing an acute stressor or crisis, or simply require more time to discuss their problem. The time constraints also present challenges to the group leader. It is often more difficult to conceptualize members' problems, do a thorough assessment and finally provide treatment if one has only approximately 15 min per week. This is not to say that one cannot provide help or facilitate progress for members, but the time limitation is a consideration and needs to be factored into expectations on the part of both leader and member;
4. While one advantage of group therapy is that it tends to be cost effective compared to individual therapy, we have discovered that this has embedded within it a disadvantage for some members. In the more recent years, in the face of economic hardship, coupled with the lack of participation in insurance carriers, we have encountered an increasing number of individuals attending group therapy because it is more affordable, when in fact, their clinical conditions suggest they require individual therapy (e.g., clinically depressed individuals with active suicidal ideation). As a result, REBT is not as effective as it could be due to the need for more of a crisis intervention approach. The majority of the time spent in group is conducting a suicide/risk assessment, and not necessarily debating irrational beliefs, strengthening the conviction of rational beliefs, or collaborating on homework assignments that reinforce relevant REBT concepts;
5. In as much as REBT group therapy has the benefit of supporting members, there are circumstances in which a group has compulsive talkers and/or interrupters that can disrupt a member's discussion of a particular problem. Without a proper screening to determine goodness of fit, it is virtually impossible for a group leader to prevent this from occurring. To address this issue, the leader can utilize REBT to ascertain what irrational beliefs are driving the maladaptive behavior of interrupting group members or talking compulsively. However, we have found that while this is an important task for leaders, it has the unintended consequence of taking time away from other group members;

6. From an REBT perspective, therapy has not worked very well for individuals who join a group for the sole purpose of socialization. While this is a benefit of groups in general, our experience has shown us that group participation for *just* this purpose does not allow for the application of REBT interventions. We cannot discount the importance social support has for individuals; however, when members come to group merely for support in the absence of specific emotional and behavioral goals, and rely on the group for meeting all of his/her social needs, we have not found group to be as effective;
7. Having led groups for many years, we have found that many individuals who could benefit a great deal from an experience in group therapy often are intimidated by the idea of it and therefore do not take the opportunity to give it a try. For example, individuals with social anxiety, whose common irrational beliefs include "If I get rejected that would be awful," or "I couldn't tolerate being thought of negatively," or "If I am rejected by others that would prove I am worthless." It is not a leap to see the many advantages of group therapy for such individuals, as attending sessions is an exposure exercise in and of itself. Furthermore, endorsing these irrational beliefs leads to a vicious cycle of avoidance of group therapy, which in turn further reinforces the irrational thinking, leading to further avoidance. These individuals therefore do not seize the opportunity to prove to themselves, that while highly uncomfortable, REBT group therapy is tolerable and can be beneficial. In addition, such individuals do not experience many of Yalom's therapeutic factors, including Universality and Instillation of hope, known to influence change and facilitate healing (Yalom, 1995). As a result, treating social anxiety and promoting positive mental health in a group therapy setting is often not the first avenue individuals pursue. It is not uncommon to begin with individual therapy to work on the irrational beliefs preventing these individuals from attending group therapy, and eventually "graduating" to a group format;
8. Group therapy also has not worked well at times regarding the treatment of clinical conditions when there are members who are highly suggestible, coupled with members who have a penchant for giving practical solutions that are not necessarily the most helpful, or even worse, are harmful. From an REBT perspective, we are referring to members who have a belief such as, "I *need* other people to tell me what to do because I cannot figure it out for myself," (e.g., dependent personality types) as well as those who are interested in the *practical solution* of changing or escaping the Activating Event, rather than working on the *emotional solution* of changing one's irrational beliefs to change one's dysfunctional negative emotions and/or maladaptive behavior(s). This scenario speaks to the aforementioned importance of a thorough group screening to determine whether the goals of the potential group member are in synch with the goals set forth by the group leader(s). When a screening is not done, or not done thoroughly, it is not uncommon for the group to never reach the working stage, and never to experience cohesion. In other words, rather than the group members taking ownership of their group and doing the majority of the work themselves by actively challenging each others' irrational beliefs, group leaders find

themselves having to intervene to stop an unhelpful suggestion by a group member, as well as ensure that each member is taking emotional and behavioral responsibility for his/her stated goals, and coming to conclusions on their own, thereby becoming their own therapists, two fundamental goals of REBT.

Case Example

A women's group was run at the Albert Ellis Institute for many years, started by Dr. Janet Wolfe, and co-led by an intern or post-doctoral fellow. When Dr. Wolfe retired, the tradition of this group continued. The group, despite the fact that it was an open group with changing membership, was very cohesive. Members challenged one another to achieve their goals, as well as support each other when necessary. The membership demographics were diverse in age, race, and ethnicity. Given that it was an open group, members were pre-screened for eligibility and goodness of fit, and entered the group as other members terminated, to avoid a break in cohesion. This approach has an embedded benefit of new members having the opportunity to see first-hand how other members have made progress towards their goals through hard work.

At one point in the life of this group, there was one member, who we will call Jane for confidentiality purposes, who was particularly goal-driven and hard working. She accepted challenging homework assignments from other members, she pushed herself to do the work needed to make change (i.e., she was *committed*), and week after week she came in and reported her successes as well as her obstacles. Overall, this group member was making the most progress in group. This is not to say that REBT group leaders create an environment of competition amongst their members; that is not necessary. Mild competition occurs organically in many groups that are in the working stage and cohesive. This is precisely what occurred in the women's group. There was one member, who we will call Melissa, who appeared motivated, as she attended group regularly, had stated goals although they kept changing from week to week, and actively participated in helping other group members. However, what Melissa was lacking was the *commitment* that Jane demonstrated. When it came to homework, there were always reasons for non-compliance that typically boiled down to frustration intolerance. During one session, Melissa confronted Jane about her progress and how she managed to achieve so much success. It was a great opportunity to have Jane specify what particular cognitions she held to push through the discomfort and make progress. This also afforded the chance for Melissa, as well as the other members, see that progress usually does not "just happen." It is up to each member to assume responsibility for their goals and work in therapy. Following this encounter, in the weeks thereafter, the group members pushed themselves harder than they had been, and experienced success and progress towards their goals.

Case Example Demonstrating the Application of Interpersonal Processing in REB Group Therapy

Jennifer, an African American woman in an interracial marriage, sought to participate in an REBT group focusing on individuals with anger as the primary emotional problem. Over the course of group therapy, Jennifer began to explore triggers for her anger and determined that they were related to experiences with prejudice and racism. Utilizing the traditional REBT model, the emotional goal would be to move from a place of unhealthy anger to healthy anger through the debating of irrational beliefs that precede the unhealthy anger. However, the challenge in Jennifer's case is that the demands that Jennifer placed on others to not speak or behave in prejudicial and racist ways became identified as the irrational belief, which, safe to say is quite difficult to help a client "accept", because on a surface level, a rational alternative may be perceived as "accepting" the prejudicial and racist statements others have made. As a result, Jennifer demonstrated an intensely overt anger response within the group session and discontinued attendance thereafter. Of course, it was not the intention of the therapists and group members to help Jennifer identify a rational alternative that involved acceptance of prejudicial and racist statements made by others. However, a rational statement might look like, "While I prefer people to be non-racists, there is no law that they must be non-racists. I can disapprove/dislike racist behaviors and statements, but work toward accepting that these beliefs unfortunately exist while also not condemning the offender's overall worth and value as a person." This rational statement would serve to help Jennifer acknowledge the difficult reality that racist ideologies and behaviors exist but she cannot place a demand that it must not, nor that global worth and value is based on a person's ideology.

An additional point to make note of regarding Jennifer's case is that the activating event that she presented was complex, as it not only had political and historical implications for Jennifer's present state, but also involved a multi-layered emotional experience for this client that likely included sadness and beliefs about her own worth. With this in mind, in retrospect, a few group variables are also worth noting.

Jennifer happened to be the only identified female in the group aside from a co-facilitator in the group, and furthermore, she was the only individual who identified as African American. In addition, much of her activating events that she would describe involved racial and prejudicial interactions with individuals perceived to be White or Hispanic men and women. Drawing from interpersonal theory, there can sometimes be a recapitulation of the client's problem in session between client and therapist or in this case, amongst group members (Teyber, 2000). That is, session after session, Jennifer discussed various activating events that involved her anger towards individuals who were responding to her in racist and prejudicial ways that left her feeling threatened by the invalidation of her experience as an African American woman. When she perceived herself to be invalidated by her therapists and group members because of their attempt to challenge Jennifer's demand (that others behave in non-prejudicial/racist ways) as these beliefs were making her unhealthily angry, Jennifer reenacted the same intensely overt anger responses within session.

Research in REB Group Therapy

An extensive review of the literature on REB group therapy indicated that there are different terms used to refer to REB group therapy, including, REBT group therapy, RE/CBT group therapy, and RE & CBT group therapy. Although there is variation in the terms used, this is not to suggest that there is variation in the techniques used in group therapy that warrants one term over another. Additionally, the studies in this review do not place an emphasis defining or describing the rationale for the use of one term over another. Instead the focus is placed on the effects of REB group therapy on different populations and within different contexts.

Although Ellis provided the theoretical rationale for REBT group therapy, empirically-supported data is lacking. While intervention is informed by theory and emerging research, multiple researchers have identified that there is a deficiency in the literature to support the efficacy of REB group therapy. Recently, David, Cotet, Matu, Mogoase, and Stefan (2017) conducted a systematic review and meta-analysis to examine the empirical evidence for the efficacy of REBT interventions, its effect on the change from irrational to rational beliefs, and the relationship between this change and intervention outcomes. David et al. (2017) found medium and significant effect sizes of REBT on outcomes (including emotional, behavioral, cognitive, health, quality of life, and school performance) and change from irrational beliefs to rational beliefs for both between and within group at post-intervention and follow-up. David et al. (2017) demonstrated that these findings transcend clinical status, age or sample, and delivery format, that being individual versus group. Although determining the efficacy of REBT in a group versus individual setting was not the primary focus of this study, it can be deduced from the inclusion of both individual and groups interventions that there might be some supporting for the efficacy of REBT in a group setting.

In addition, a 2015 randomized clinical trial conducted by Iftene, Predescu, Stefan, and David examined the efficacy of group RE/CBT, pharmacotherapy, and their combination for depression in youth. Iftene, Predescu, Stefan, and David (2015) found that group RE/CBT, pharmacotherapy, and their combination were equally effective in treating youth depression. Although it may not be surprising that this outcome suggests the utility of the combined treatment of pharmacotherapy and group therapy, the conclusions that can be drawn about the specific use of REBT group therapy is of great value given the deficit in literature identifying the efficacy of REBT group therapy. Iftene et al. (2015) added to the body of literature reporting that there is a deficiency in the research demonstrating the efficacy of REBT group therapy. Often research primarily focuses on individually-delivered CBT, although there is evidence to support similar efficacy of group CBT as well (Weisz, Mccarty, & Valeri, 2006). However, Iftene et al.'s (2015) research is likely the first randomized clinical trial comparing RE/CBT group therapy, pharmacotherapy, and their combination. Furthermore, the focus on youth participants managing depression also supports the use of RE/CBT with a variety of populations including youth with depression. When the treatment is described as RE/CBT reader not clear on whether this is orthodox REBT or hybrid RE/CBT.

Research has also identified the efficacy of REBT group therapy when compared to relaxation training when treating aggressive youth. Research conducted by Barekatain, Taghavi, Salehi, and Hasanzadeh (2006) examined the effectiveness of REBT group therapy and Relaxation therapy in reducing aggressive behaviors of male adolescents whose fathers have war related PTSD. Results suggested that group size may be an interesting caveat to the effectiveness of group therapy and can vary depending on the type of therapy used. Ellis (1997) suggested in his practice that up to ten members would be sufficient to run an REBT group. He explained that it is acceptable to have more members than typical psychotherapy groups of six to eight participants due to the structured nature of the REBT group session.

In Barekatain et al.'s (2006) study, participants in both treatment groups, REBT group therapy and Relaxation Group Therapy, demonstrated improvements in the reduction of aggressive behaviors. However, their research indicated a statistically significant positive relation between the reduction in reported aggressive behaviors in REBT group therapy and the number of patients' participation in each group session. Whereas, for the Relaxation Therapy group, the reduction in reported aggressive behaviors was negatively related to the number of patients' participation in group sessions. Their research revealed that when the number of participants in treatment sessions increased, in the Relaxation Therapy group, the efficacy decreased. Whereas, in the REBT group, the more participation in the group sessions for each patient resulted in a greater reduction in reported aggressive behaviors. Barekatain et al. (2006) suggested that their findings on the difference in self-report of aggression may be explained by the difference in therapeutic focus. That is, for the Relaxation Therapy group, participants are guided through relaxation exercises and follow up discussion post exercise. Though relaxation exercises are an important behavioral component to therapy, it is possible that as group size increases, there are increased demands of the group facilitator to offer feedback on participants' proper execution of the exercise. In addition, participants are unable to learn vicariously through other participants. Instead, members will rely on the anecdotal experiences and feedback that each participant offers. However, as REBT group therapy focuses on deficits and distortions in maladaptive cognitive processes, that being irrational beliefs, increasing the number of participants likely adds to the generalizability of cognitive restructuring because members may learn how to dispute their own beliefs if they likely hold similar irrational beliefs that are challenged by the group facilitator.

The efficacy of REBT group therapy also encompasses treatment for anxiety disorders and by incorporating both cognitive and behavioral approaches. Typically, a key feature of treatment for anxiety disorders is the exposure exercises that are often implemented. Thus, it should not be assumed that there is no room for behavioral interventions when implementing group REBT therapy. In fact, Ellis highlighted multiple behavioral techniques that he used in addition to the cognitive work (Yankura & Dryden, 1997). For example, the in vivo desensitization technique encourages group members to engage in active-experimental behaviors to address neurotic fears of social avoidance, public speaking, etc. (Yankura & Dryden, 1997).

Cowan and Brunero (1997) found in their research examining the efficacy of REBT group therapy on clients with anxiety disorders, that mean scores on the Beck Anxiety Inventory (BAI) and Beck Depression Inventory (BDI) significantly decreased post REBT group therapy intervention suggesting that REBT group therapy is an effective treatment approach. Clients were better able to identify when they were responding to events based on the irrational beliefs they may be holding and relate these beliefs to emotional disturbance they may be experiencing. Cowan and Brunero (1997) state that therapists in this study adopted an active-directive approach, using "dynamic and interactive" techniques. Some techniques referenced included visual illustration, role plays, and in-session behavioral disputes. Although detailed descriptions on what these techniques looked like in session were not provided, this study highlights the importance of using a dynamic and interactive approach that can not be standardized apart from complying with REBT theory, as different techniques, whether cognitive or behavioral, are applied depending on the needs of the group members.

When taking a look at treatment studies applying a more traditional model of REBT group therapy, statistically significant changes in irrational beliefs have been identified in women during pregnancy and the immediate period after giving birth. Anton and David (2015) conducted a randomized clinical trial in which participants were assigned to either 9 weeks of an REBT preventive program conducted mostly in a group format or community care (control). For the treatment condition, each session lasted 90 min. The first session was conducted as an individual session to develop a more accurate list of problems for the entire group and allow for the client to become comfortable with self-disclosure. The eight sessions that followed were conducted in a group format that used restructuring techniques focused on irrational beliefs related to participants physical health, the moment of giving birth, fears related to the baby and baby's health, the marital relationship, and participants body image. Anton and David (2015) found that REBT was more efficient at post-treatment (prepartum) than community care on depression symptoms, negative emotionality, and anxiety. However, at 3-month postpartum the effects were only maintained for negative emotionality and anxiety, but with a non-statistically significant decrease in symptoms of depression. Due to the significant improvements seen in the areas of negative emotionality and anxiety, Anton and David suggest that REBT-based psychological intervention can work as a preventive intervention for anxiety and negative emotionality in pregnant women.

When examining the extant literature on REBT group therapy it is important to consider that because there is not a great deal of comparison studies examining the effectiveness of REBT group therapy to individual therapy, this does not necessarily mean that REBT group therapy is not an effective form of treatment. That is, there is not a great deal of evidence to support that REBT group therapy is a better form of treatment than individual therapy, but there is evidence to support that REBT group therapy is an effective form of treatment for clinical populations. The research that has been highlighted in this chapter provides some support for this notion that REBT group therapy is an effective form of treatment for variety of emotional problems within different contexts.

Implication of Recent Findings of REBT Research to the Practice of REB Group Therapy

The research previously discussed in this chapter serves to demonstrate some of the advances in REBT theory, research, and practice by highlighting the developments in our understanding of what treatment modalities and interventions are efficacious. While there is need for added empirical support of REBT group therapy, there is outcome data to support the efficacy of REBT group therapy with a variety of clinical problems and diagnoses. However, as the research community continues to demonstrate the efficacy of REBT group therapy, a critical look must be taken to also consider questions about treatment process that have been left unanswered and how identifying these questions may inform the future direction of REBT.

There is a common understanding of what the typical structure of REBT group sessions might look like. As previously described, traditional REBT groups look to offer each participant a brief amount of time within the group session to present an emotional and/or behavioral problem for analysis and restructuring the relevant irrational beliefs. Other participants are encouraged to support the process by reflecting on similar experiences, providing validation when appropriate, offering insight when identifying the ABCDEs, and helping one another debate their irrational beliefs. This traditional model to REBT group therapy has received research support insofar as when compared to treatment as usual (TAU) groups or in pretest/posttest outcome studies, as demonstrated earlier in this chapter. However, the question that remains, structurally, is this the only way to conduct REBT group sessions?

Research has recently begun to examine the effects of conducting REBT group therapy using a more didactic approach. What may be best described as REBT educational workshops, participants are generally educated on the basic theoretical ideas of REBT, the ABCDE framework, the relationship between beliefs and emotions and behaviors, and the debating of irrational beliefs and development and promotion of rational beliefs (Vertopoulos & Turner, 2017).

Vertopoulos and Turner (2017) examined the effects of this modified form of REBT group therapy on a non-clinical sample of adolescent athletes that had participated in REBT educational workshops. After completion of the REBT educational workshops, a group of athletes participated in an extension of treatment termed Personal-Disclosure Mutual-Sharing (PDMS). Originally, PDMS was an applied sport psychology approach to team building in which athletes disclose facts and stories about themselves to their teammates (Dunn & Holt, 2004; Holt & Dunn, 2006; Mohammed & Dumville, 2001). Vertopoulos and Turner (2017) thought to modify the application of PDMS to fit REBT resulting in Rational Emotive PDMS (REPDMS). REPDMS requires that athletes share their experiences of using the ABCDE model using real issues in which they specify their irrational and rational beliefs and how they operationalized their disputation. In addition, whereas PDMS is typically use to develop group cohesion, the REPDMS' purpose is to increase individual benefits of strengthening disputation, reducing emotional problems and developing rational beliefs. When the treatment group (receiving REBT education and REPDMS) was compared with the REBT education-only group, both groups demonstrated a decrease in irrational beliefs and increase in rational beliefs from pre- to post-REBT education. However, for the REPDMS intervention there was a further reduction in irrational beliefs and a stable elevation in rational beliefs. Additionally, although differences in irrational beliefs between groups were not statistically significant, the REBT education-only group did depict an increase in irrational beliefs and a decrease in rational beliefs. Therefore, REPDMS seems to have a boosting effect on REBT education.

Vertopoulos and Turner's (2017) work examined this difference in approach insofar as their between group comparisons were with an REBT educational workshop group compared to an REBT workshop with the added REPDMS sessions group. As previously described, the REPDMS sessions incorporated personal disclosure which served to provide vicarious learning experiences typical to traditional REBT group therapy. However, a notable difference worth considering is the preparation for personal disclosure that is required before session. That is, Vertopoulos and Turner (2017) specify that the positive effects of the REPDMS may be explained by the group members preparing a speech about personal experiences using the REBT ABCDE framework. Therefore, while their research suggests the importance of the conscious participation and personal disclosure components of group therapy when taking a more didactic approach, this still raises an important question. Is there something particular about the out-of-session preparation that increases efficacy as opposed to the more traditional model of REBT group therapy in which participants present an emotional or behavioral problem that has not necessarily been "worked through" prior to group session? Furthermore, perhaps the effort that is required by REPDMS functions to, structurally, hold each member accountable for their personal application of REBT in a different way than the traditional way of assigning homework. Moreover, REPDMS may serve to be an important component, in addition to the traditional way of assigning homework to members.

This discussion about the structure of REBT group sessions relates to another question about "interpersonal process" or the way in which information is communicated between group members and group facilitators. That is, to what extent can discussing the interpersonal interactions occurring between group members and therapist enhance the effectiveness of the REBT group session? Although when managing problematic interactions within the group, it is essential to conduct group screenings to determine goals and fit, as well as, to address problematic behaviors that sometimes occur during sessions. However, in addition to that, it is safe to say that interpersonal interactions are occurring in real time by the fact that members are participating in interpersonal communication. Obviously, this holds true for both individual and group settings. As such, borrowing from interpersonal theory and literature on the interpersonal process approach to psychotherapy, the relational process of how members and therapist are interacting may be a means for further exploration within the REBT group therapy framework.

What We Have Learned About REB Group Therapy

From its inception in 1959 by Dr. Albert Ellis, REB group therapy continues to show it is an effective approach to treating a variety of clinical problems with many populations. One of the many benefits of REB group therapy includes the flexibility of the model as it can be applied to a variety of contexts and modified to meet the varying needs of group members. REB group therapy offers a cost-effective treatment for individuals and lends itself to more rigorous debating of irrational beliefs and restructuring to rational alternatives. However, while there is some research to support its effectiveness, the REBT community preferably should acknowledge the need for additional research to continue to explore the idiosyncratic considerations of REB group therapy.

References

Anton, R., & David, D. (2015). A randomized clinical trial of a new preventive rational emotive and behavioral therapeutical program of prepartum and postpartum emotional distress. *The Journal of Evidence-Based Psychotherapies, 15*(1), 3–15.

Barekatain, M., Taghavi, T., Salehi, M., & Hasanzadeh, A. (2006). The efficacy of rational-emotive-behavioral versus relaxation group therapies in treatment of aggression of offspring of veterans with post traumatic stress disorder. *Journal of Research in Medical Sciences, 11*(1), 34–40.

Cowan, D., & Brunero, S. (1997). Group therapy for anxiety disorders using rational emotive behaviour therapy. *Australian and New Zealand Journal of Mental Health Nursing, 6*, 164–168.

David, D., Cotet, C., Matu, S., Mogoase, C., & Stefan, S. (2017). 50 years of rational-emotive and cognitive-behavioral therapy: A systematic review and meta-analysis. *Journal of Clinical Psychology*. https://doi.org/10.1002/jclp.22514

DiGiuseppe, R. A., Doyle, K. A., Dryden, W., & Backx, W. (2013). *A practitioner's guide to rational-emotive therapy* (3rd ed.). New York, NY: Oxford University Press.

Dunn, J. G., & Holt, N. L. (2004). A qualitative investigation of a personal-disclosure mutual-sharing team building activity. *The Sport Psychologist, 18*(4), 363–380. https://doi.org/10.1123/tsp.18.4.363

Ellis, A. (1997). REBT and its application to group therapy. In J. Yankura & W. Dryden (Eds.), *Special applications of REBT: a therapist's casebook.* (pp. 131–161). New York, NY: Springer.

Holt, N. L., & Dunn, J. G. (2006). Guidelines for delivering personal-disclosure mutual-sharing team building interventions. *The Sport Psychologist, 20*(3), 348–367. https://doi.org/10.1123/tsp.20.3.348

Iftene, F., Predescu, E., Stefan, S., & David, D. (2015). Rational-emotive and cognitive-behavior therapy (REBT/CBT) versus pharmacotherapy versus REBT/CBT plus pharmacotherapy in the treatment of major depressive disorder in youth; a randomized clinical trial. *Psychiatry Research, 225*(3), 687–694. https://doi.org/10.1016/j.psychres.2014.11.021

Mohammed, S., & Dumville, B. C. (2001). Team mental models in a team knowledge framework: Expanding theory and measurement across disciplinary boundaries. *Journal of Organizational Behavior, 22*(2), 89–106. https://doi.org/10.1002/job.86

Teyber, E. (2000). *Interpersonal process in psychotherapy: A relational approach* (4th ed.). Belmont, CA: Brooks/Cole.

Vertopoulos, E., & Turner, M. J. (2017). Examining the effectiveness of a Rational Emotive Personal-Disclosure Mutual-Sharing (REPDMS) intervention on the irrational beliefs and rational beliefs of Greek adolescent athletes. *The Sport Psychologist, 31*(3), 264–274. https://doi.org/10.1123/tsp.2016-0071

Weisz, J. R., Mccarty, C. A., & Valeri, S. M. (2006). Effects of psychotherapy for depression in children and adolescents: A meta-analysis. *Psychological Bulletin, 132*(1), 132–149. https://doi.org/10.1037/0033-2909.132.1.132

Yankura, J., & Dryden, W. (1997). *Special applications of REBT: A therapist's casebook.* New York, NY: Springer.

Yalom, I. D. (1995). *The theory and practice of group psychotherapy.* New York, NY: BasicBooks.

Chapter 11
REBT and Positive Psychology

Aurora Szentagotai-Tătar, Diana-Mirela Cândea, and Daniel O. David

The Modern Study of Well-Being: Positive Psychology

The nature of happiness and the good life have preoccupied people for millennia and the idea that what matters is not just to live, but to live well has been central to both Eastern and Western philosophical thought (Kesebir & Diener, 2008). In psychology, interest in this topic can be traced back to the origins of the field itself, in William James' writings about "healthy mindedness "(James, 1902; Linley, Joseph, Harrington, & Wood, 2006). Human flourishing was also a fundamental issue for the humanistic movement (Huta, 2013). However, the systematic empirical study of the conditions and processes that lead to flourishing and well-being is related to the emergence positive psychology, at the end of the 1990s (Gable & Haidt, 2005).

Proponents of positive psychology argued that, after World War II, research in psychology had mainly focused on understanding and treating psychopathology and, as a result, little was known about thriving and about how to encourage it (Seligman & Csikszentmihalyi, 2000; Sheldon & King, 2001). In the attempt to remedy this problem, positive psychology turned its attention to three major issues (Seligman & Csikszentmihalyi, 2000): (1) positive subjective experiences (e.g., well-being and contentment regarding the past, happiness and flow in the

A. Szentagotai-Tătar (✉) · D.-M. Cândea
Department of Clinical Psychology and Psychotherapy,
Babeş-Bolyai University, Cluj-Napoca, Romania
e-mail: auraszentagotai@psychology.ro; dianacandea@psychology.ro

D. O. David
Department of Clinical Psychology and Psychotherapy,
Babeş-Bolyai University, Cluj-Napoca, Romania

Department of Oncological Sciences, Icahn School of Medicine at Mount Sinai,
New York, NY, USA
e-mail: danieldavid@psychology.ro

© Springer Nature Switzerland AG 2019
M. E. Bernard, W. Dryden (eds.), *Advances in REBT*,
https://doi.org/10.1007/978-3-319-93118-0_11

present, hope and optimism for the future); (2) positive individual traits (e.g., wisdom, courage, kindness, leadership, curiosity, creativity, open mindedness); and (3) institutions that foster positive subjective experiences and adaptive individual traits.

While there is no clear definition about what makes people feel happy and fulfilled, investigations tend to cluster around two related but distinct perspectives, stemming from different philosophies: the *hedonic* view and the *eudaimonic* view (Keyes, Shmotkin, & Ryff, 2002; Ryan & Deci, 2001; Waterman, 1993). The hedonic approach equates happiness with pleasure, enjoyment and comfort, resulting from fulfilling one's desires and valued outcomes in a variety of realms (Huta & Ryan, 2010; Ryan & Deci, 2001). Research in this paradigm has mainly used *subjective well-being* (Diener, 1984) as an index of happiness (Kesebir & Diener, 2008; Ryan & Deci, 2001). Subjective well-being reflects a general evaluation of a person's life (Diener, Napa Scollon, & Lucas, 2003), and involves the following components: life satisfaction (global and domain-related), positive affect (i.e., the prevalence of positive emotions and moods) and negative affect (i.e., low levels of negative emotions and moods) (Kesebir & Diener, 2008). The eudaimonic perspective rejects the idea of reducing well-being to enjoyment. It rather views it as a life of purpose, of cultivating personal strengths, of living in accordance with individual potentialities, which ultimately lead to flourishing and fulfillment (Ryff & Singer, 2006; Waterman, 1993).

One of the most influential theories of well-being in positive psychology was developed by Martin Seligman (2002), and it is a combination of the two approaches, with a heavier accent on the eudaimonic perspective. The *Authentic happiness theory* describes three types of happiness: *the pleasant life*, *the good life* and *the meaningful life* (Seligman, 2002), which are not exclusive, but stem from one another. A pleasant life is about positive emotions regarding the past, present and future, a good life is about developing positive traits and practicing strengths, while a meaningful life involves anchoring these traits and strengths into goals that transcend the individual and serve a higher purpose (Seligman, 2002). A more recent development of the theory, the *PERMA model* (Seligman, 2011), conceptualizes well-being as characterized by five core elements: (1) positive emotions - P; (2) engagement - E; (3) positive relationships - R, (4) meaning - M and (5) accomplishment - A. The model builds on the *Authentic happiness theory* by retaining positive emotions, engagement and meaning, and acknowledges that accomplishment and healthy relationships also play an important role in determining well-being (Seligman, 2011).

Interest in Well-Being Before Positive Psychology: Rational Emotive Behavior Therapy

Positive psychology as a field was established at the end of the 1990s. However, an examination of the literature makes it clear that interest in happiness and well-being has existed much longer in psychology (Linley et al., 2006). Human flourishing and self-realization were fundamental issues not only for humanistic psychology (see Maslow, 1950/1973; Rogers, 1961), but also for an influential approach to mental health and disturbance that has evolved over the past 60 years: Rational emotive behavior therapy (REBT) (Bernard, Froh, DiGiuseppe, Joyce, & Dryden, 2010).

REBT was founded in the 1950s by Albert Ellis (Dryden, David, & Ellis, 2010). In addition to its focus on reducing psychological disturbance and suffering, REBT has always had a distinct interest in well-being, in that it aims to help people: (1) develop their individuality and increase their freedom, self-interest and self-control, and (2) live involved and committed lives, facilitating individual and social interest (Dryden et al., 2010; Ellis, 1984). The aims of REBT thus anticipate the ones expressed later by positive psychology, which is also *"concerned with understanding what makes life worth living, with helping people become more self-organized, and self-directed, and with recognizing that people and experiences are embedded in a social context"* (Maddux, 2002, pp. 21–22). The "ingredients" of well-being proposed by REBT also anticipate the ones later found in positive psychology models. Specifically, REBT holds that humans are purposeful or goal-seeking creatures (Ellis, 1973), and that their main goals are to stay alive and to have a happy existence (Bernard et al., 2010; Ellis, 1976). According to Ellis, these goals are met when: (1) people experience a minimum of pain and misery and a maximum of comfort and pleasure; (2) they develop healthy, satisfying relationships with others, and (3) they fully realize their potential, both professionally and in recreational activities (e.g., hobbies) (Bernard et al., 2010; Ellis, 1976).

The REBT Perspective on Mental Health and Well-Being

REBT sees people as complex, biosocial organisms with a strong tendency to establish and pursue a wide range of goals and purposes (Dryden et al., 2010). As there is no universal road to well-being, each individual must establish his/her goals in accordance with his/her preferences and talents. However, in Ellis' view, long-term happiness is very likely to be related to the pursuit and achievement of goals that reduce emotional pain and maximize comfort and pleasure, and that lead to profound and satisfying relationships and excellence at work and in other activities (Bernard, 2011). More important than the content of goals, however, is whether they are formulated in rational or irrational terms. The emphasis on the relevance of *how* we wish for something, in addition to *what* we wish for is a major, often neglected, contribution of REBT to the understanding of well-being (Szentágotai & David, 2013).

According to REBT, cognitions, emotions and behaviors are tightly interconnected, with cognitions (more specifically, evaluative cognitions) playing a major role in the generation of our feelings and actions (Ellis, 1995; Ellis & Dryden, 1997). A distinction is made in REBT between two types of thinking patterns: *rational and irrational*. Ellis maintains that both these thinking patterns, the self-enhancing (i.e., rationality) and self-defeating (i.e., irrationality), are biologically based, not just the result of interacting with a particular environment (Ellis, 1995; Ellis & Dryden, 1997). Thus, in addition to a self-actualizing tendency, human beings are also characterized by a natural self-defeating tendency, one that, however, they can learn to control (Ellis, 1995).

The core of irrationality is the rigid formulation of goals and desires, expressed in the dogmatic insistence that certain conditions must or must not exist. These rigid requirements are reflected in the form of "musts", "shoulds" and "oughts". Embracing a philosophy of demands leads to three other irrational cognitions that are hypothesized to be the derivatives of demands (Dryden et al., 2010). *Awfulizing* beliefs refer to the extreme dichotomous evaluation of a negative event as worse than it absolutely should be. They exaggerate the consequences of past, present, or future events, conceptualizing them as terrible, horrible, or the worst thing that could happen (MacInnes, 2004). *Low frustration tolerance* beliefs assert the fact that one cannot tolerate or bear an event or set of circumstances, thereby making a situation appear to be intolerable. Finally, *global evaluation* reflects the tendency of people to rate a specific trait, behavior or action according to a standard of desirability or worth, and then apply this evaluation to their entire being (MacInnes, 2004). Global evaluation can also be applied to others or to life conditions. Irrational thinking is an obstacle to happiness and well-being by generating problematic emotions and behaviors, and by sabotaging the person's goals and purposes (for reviews see David, Szentágotai, Kállay, & Macavei, 2005; Szentágotai & Jones, 2010).

At the heart of mental health and well-being lie flexible, non-dogmatic formulations of personal goals and desires (Dryden et al., 2010). These are assertions of what the person wants, coupled with the acceptance of the fact that we cannot insist that we absolutely get what we want. The hypothesized rational derivatives of non-dogmatic preferences are *anti-awfulizing*, *high frustration tolerance*, and *unconditional acceptance*. Anti-awfulizing beliefs occur when people's preferences are not met, and they conclude that the circumstances may be "bad", but not "awful". This approach allows for the fact that worse outcomes are possible (Dryden, 2002), and relies on a continuum of badness, rather than a dichotomous judgment of either awful or not bad at all. High frustration tolerance beliefs assert that events may be difficult to tolerate, but they are not intolerable (Dryden, 2002). Acceptance occurs when a person understands that although people do bad things they cannot be globally rated as bad, and when he/she accepts himself/herself and others as fallible human beings. In addition, life conditions are accepted as they exist (Dryden et al., 2010). While irrational thinking is an obstacle to well-being, rationality promotes happiness by helping people reach their goals or formulate new ones when old ones cannot be reached (Dryden et al., 2010).

The relation between irrationality and psychological distress is well-documented in the literature. Reviewing this evidence is beyond the scope of the chapter. We will only note that a recent meta-analysis of 83 studies, including 100 independent samples, indicated a positive association between irrational beliefs and general distress, and irrational beliefs and negative emotions such as anxiety, depression, anger and guilt (Vîslă, Flückiger, grosse Holtforth, & David, 2015). There is also evidence supporting the association between rationality, or less irrationality, and fewer self-reported life stressors, and better stress management in various life areas, ranging from general response to negative life events, to job stress, relational problems, bereavement and health-related issues (for a review see Caserta, Dowd, David, & Ellis, 2010).

Significantly fewer studies have examined the relationship between low levels of irrational beliefs or high levels of rational beliefs and positive outcomes, such as positive emotions or well-being, but existing evidence does support this association. For example, a study by Ciarrochi (2004) that involved over 450 student participants, showed that self-downing, need for approval and demanding perfection were negative predictors of joviality, self-assurance and life satisfaction. A few studies have specifically focused on unconditional self-acceptance and well-being. Thus, Chamberlain and Haaga (2001) reported a positive association between unconditional self-acceptance on the one hand, and happiness and satisfaction with life on the other hand. These results were confirmed by MacInnes (2006), who found a positive correlation between unconditional self-acceptance and psychological well-being, and by Davies (2006), who showed that unconditional self-acceptance was significantly negatively related with neuroticism, one of the most important personality predictors of subjective well-being (Davies, 2006).

The REBT Perspective on Positive and Negative Emotions

Healthy and Unhealthy Positive Emotions

In positive psychology, happiness is seen as reflecting the balance of the frequency of positive and negative emotions, with the former outnumbering the latter in happy individuals (Diener, Sandvik, & Pavot, 1991), and playing an important role in mental and physical health (Fredrickson, 1998; Fredrickson & Joiner, 2002; Seligman, 2011). REBT also recognizes the importance of positive emotions, and advocates teaching the client to achieve both pleasure of the moment and of the future (Ellis & Dryden, 1997). However REBT also proposes that not all positive emotions are created equal, and that positive emotions can be *functional* or *dysfunctional,* depending on the beliefs they result from (Dryden et al., 2010). Positive emotions that stem from irrational thinking (e.g., elation after being praised, related to the belief that "people MUST appreciate my work") are seen as dysfunctional, as they reinforce the underlying irrational beliefs, and focus people on short-term rather than long-term benefits (David et al., 2005). On the other hand, positive emotions that result from rational beliefs (joy after being praised, related to the belief that "I would like people to appreciate my work, and this time they did, but I accept that it might not always happen") are seen as helpful or functional.

Unfortunately, to date, there is almost no research exploring this distinction. Understanding dysfunctional positive emotions could have implications both for the way we conceptualize happiness from a hedonic perspective, as well as for clarifying their role in emotional disorders. For example, pride is an important emotion that plays a critical role in several domains of psychological functioning, particularly in prosocial behavior and achievement-related behavior (Tracy & Robins, 2007). However, pride can be also profoundly dysfunctional, and associated with aggression, interpersonal problems, and a variety of self-destructive behaviors, as in the case of narcissism (Tracy & Robins, 2004). It has already been proposed that the difference between healthy and unhealthy (i.e., hubristic) pride lies in the appraisals each involves (Tracy & Robins, 2004); focusing on rational/irrational beliefs as antecedents of pride could definitely contribute to a better understanding of the adaptive and maladaptive facets of this emotion.

Although the distinction between functional and dysfunctional positive emotions as proposed by Ellis has not been theoretically and practically explored and exploited, evidence has accumulated over the last years confirming some of the characteristics proposed by REBT for maladaptive positive emotions (see Gruber, Mauss, & Tamir, 2011 for a review). For example, studies have shown that very high levels of positive emotions may not be associated with benefits, or may even lead to negative outcomes (e.g., Davis, 2009; Johnson, 2005); that people who overvalue happiness and pursue it excessively report less well-being, more loneliness, and higher depressive symptoms (e.g., Ford, Shallcross, Mauss, Floerke, & Gruber, 2014; Mauss, Tamir, Anderson, & Savino, 2011; Mauss et al., 2012; Schooler, Ariely, & Loewenstein, 2003); and that positive emotions based on dysfunctional evaluations, such as hubristic pride, can have negative effects on social processes such as liking, connectedness, and the development of long-term satisfying relationships (Tracy, Cheng, Robins, & Trzesniewski, 2009).

Healthy and Unhealthy Negative Emotions

Positive psychology studies show that, across cultures, the experience of positive emotions is related to happiness judgments more strongly that the experience of negative emotions, leading to the conclusion that positive experience is an important route to greater happiness and life satisfaction (Kuppens, Realo, & Diener, 2008). However, it is also recognized that, under certain conditions, having negative emotions is more reflective of healthy functioning than not having them or avoiding them (Ryan & Deci, 2001). The REBT perspective on the relation between negative emotions on the one hand, and mental health and happiness on the other, is more refined. In this case too, a distinction is made between *functional* negative emotions, resulting from rational beliefs regarding negative situations, and *dysfunctional* negative emotions, generated by irrational beliefs regarding negative life events. As they are the product of qualitatively different ways of thinking, functional and dysfunctional negative emotions are also conceptualized as qualitatively, rather than only quantitatively, different (David, 2003; Ellis & DiGiuseppe, 1993). Thus, while dysfunctional negative emotions are associated with psychological disturbance, and incompatible with happiness, functional negative emotions are considered reflective of mental health under conditions of adversity, and even compatible with happiness (Bernard et al., 2010).

The relation between irrational beliefs and psychological distress and disturbance has been confirmed by numerous studies (see Vîslă et al., 2015 for a meta-analysis). Moreover, a recent meta-analysis of 26 studies, that included a total number of 5247 participants, reported a moderate negative association between rational beliefs and distress (Oltean & David, 2018). The authors of the meta-analysis conclude that their results confirm the protective role of rational beliefs against emotional suffering, as hypothesized by REBT (Oltean & David, 2018).

Two Types of Happiness: Short-Term Satisfaction and Long-Term Fulfillment

Over the last years, positive psychology has been among the most important advocates of the need to study human happiness, conditions that lead to it, and ways in which it can be developed and maintained (Seligman & Csikszentmihalyi, 2000). As we have indicated, positive psychology conceptualizes happiness as involving both hedonic elements (i.e., pleasure and positive emotions), and eudaimonic ones (i.e., pursuing virtue and meaning, seeking to use and develop the best in oneself, reaching excellence).

From the beginning of his work, Albert Ellis was also deeply interested in what made people happy and in how happiness could be achieved (Bernard, 2011). Titles of some of his most popular books are a reflection of this interest: *A Guide to Personal Happiness; How to Make Yourself Happy and Remarkably Less Disturbed; How to Stubbornly Refuse to Make Yourself Miserable About Anything – Yes, Anything; A Guide to Successful Marriage; How to Raise an Emotionally Healthy, Happy Child.* An overview of his approach also reflects the twofold goal of helping people attain happiness both from hedonic and eudaimonic point of view:

> [REBT] primarily deals with disturbed human evaluations, emotions and behaviors. It is rational and scientific but uses rationality and science to enable humans to live and be happy. It is hedonistic, but it espouses long-range instead of short-term hedonism so that people may achieve the pleasure of the moment and of the future, and may arrive at maximum freedom and discipline (Ellis & Dryden, 1997, p. 5).

A distinction is thus made between two types of happiness – both of which people are encouraged to pursue – short-term satisfaction, and long-term fulfillment (see Bernard, 2011; Ellis & Harper, 1975). Short-term happiness is defined in terms of feelings of pleasure, which can be achieved through active involvement in a wide range of activities (Bernard, 2011; Ellis & Becker, 1982). Long-term happiness is also conceptualized as positive emotions, resulting from the realization of individual potential, striving towards excellence and self-actualization (Bernard, 2011; Ellis, 1995). It involves a choice, an active quest, and it is intimately related to goals (Ellis & Dryden, 1997). As there is no universal road to well-being, each person must establish his/her goals in accordance with his/her preferences and talents. However, in Ellis' view, long-term happiness is very likely to be related to the pursuit and achievement of goals that reduce emotional pain and maximize comfort and pleasure, and that lead to profound and satisfying relationships and excellence at work and other activities (Bernard, 2011).

The contribution of hedonic and eudaimonic motives to well-being continues to be debated in the literature (Huta & Ryan, 2010). The few studies that have actually compared them, to determine how each relates to happiness, confirm Ellis' perspective that both short-term satisfaction and long-term fulfillment are important contributors to a life worth living. For example, a series of four studies conducted by Huta and Ryan (2010) showed that hedonic motives related more to positive affect and carefreeness, and more negatively to negative affect, and that hedonia was more frequently linked to life satisfaction than eudaimonia. On the other hand, eudaimonic motives related more to meaning and experiences such as awe, inspiration and the sense of being connected to a greater whole (Huta & Ryan, 2010). People high in both hedonic and eudaimonic motives had higher well-being that people low in both, higher positive affect and carefreeness than predominantly hedonic individuals, and higher meaning, elevating experiences and vitality than predominantly hedonic individuals (Huta & Ryan, 2010). Moreover, Huta and Ryan (2010) also found that an intervention focused on hedonia produced more well-being on the short run, while an intervention focused on eudaimonia resulted in more well-being on the longer run, confirming the importance of both types of pursuits.

Rational Principles for a Happy Life

REBT outlines several principles that should guide people in their pursuit of emotional health and happiness. These principles have also been discussed elsewhere (see Bernard et al., 2010; Ellis & Bernard, 1985; Ellis & Dryden, 1997), but we revisit them in light of new research findings regarding well-being.

Self-Interest and Social Interest

REBT hypothesizes that emotionally healthy people tend to put their own interest at least slightly above the interest of others. They do sacrifice themselves to a certain extent for those whom they love, but not completely (Ellis & Bernard, 1985). The importance of following self-interest is illustrated by data on happiness and goal attainment. A series of studies by Sheldon and collaborators show that high levels of goal progress and attainment predict increased well-being, which persists in time and sustains future goal attainment (Sheldon & Elliot, 1999; Sheldon & Houser-Marko, 2001). The effect is dependent, however, on goal type (i.e., intrinsic vs. extrinsic motives) and reasons for pursuing the goal (i.e., autonomous vs. controlled motives). Specifically, while intrinsic and autonomous motives are positively related to well-being, extrinsic and controlled motives are significant negative predictors of well-being (Sheldon, Ryan, Deci, & Kasser, 2004). Experimental methods used to test the self-interest assumption usually involve directly choosing between helping oneself or helping others (Berman & Small, 2012). Research shows that under such conditions, if possible, people often avoid making trade-offs between self and others (Dana, Weber, & Xi Kuang, 2005). However, when the tension generated by this trade-off is removed from the situation, people's happiness increases by pursuing self-interest (Berman & Small, 2012).

Studies thus confirm the REBT assumption that establishing relevant goals in life and actively pursuing them makes people happy. At the same time, REBT argues that, when setting goals and following them, people must keep in mind that they live among other people, and that social interest must come at close second to self-interest (Ellis & Dryden, 1997). The benefits of focusing on others' well-being is well documented in the literature, and research shows that altruistic behavior is associated with significant and lasting benefits in terms of emotional and physical health (e.g., Brown, Consedine, & Magai, 2005; Brown, Nesse, Vinokur, & Smith, 2003; Schwartz, Meisenhelder, Ma, & Reed, 2003).

Self-Direction and Frustration Tolerance

Self-direction involves people assuming responsibility for their own happiness, rather than placing it on others or relying on others for it (Bernard et al., 2010; Ellis & Dryden, 1997). In this context, Ellis talks about having the *will*, and having the *willpower* to pursue happiness (Ellis, 1999). Having the will refers to making the choice, expressing the decision of working towards being happy; having the willpower is harder, and it involves persisting in trying to reach a goal, taking the appropriate actions doing them again and again, until the goal is reached (Ellis, 1999). This requires frustration tolerance, which Ellis defines as preferring, but not demanding that life provides you with what you want easily, and understanding that in order to achieve pleasant results on the long term, you sometimes have to tolerate discomfort on the short run (Bernard et al., 2010). According to REBT, low frustration tolerance discourages people from contending with unpleasant circumstances, and short-circuits their ability to confront obstacles to goal attainment. Alternatively, high frustration tolerance promotes active efforts to confront or eliminate obstacles to happiness and achievement (Dryden, 2002).

Indeed, studies in positive psychology confirm the importance of intentional activity as one of the most promising ways of increasing well-being (Lyubomirsky, 2008). Moreover, as Ellis hypothesized, it seems that *will* and *willpower* are both necessary to attain happiness. More specifically, data on the effect of happiness boosting activities indicate that these are most beneficial in the case of people who explicitly express a desire to become happier (Lyubomirsky, Dickerhoof, Boehm, &

Sheldon, 2011), and that long-term gains are to be expected only when individuals invest energy into reaching their goals, and then, continuous and sustained effort into maintaining gains (Sheldon et al., 2010).

Self-Acceptance and Acceptance of Others

The essence of the REBT idea of unconditional acceptance is the affirmation of human worth above and beyond human behavior. In this view, a person cannot be given a single global rating that defines him/her and his/her worth. Personal value is not to be defined by conditions that change (Dryden & Neenan, 2004). Unconditional self- and other-acceptance involve acknowledging that we are complex beings, subject to constant change, that defy rating by ourselves or others, while at the same time accepting that we are essentially fallible (Ellis & Dryden, 1997). However, this does not mean that individual behaviors cannot be subject to evaluation. Unconditional acceptance allows people to rate their (and others') actions and traits, and encourages such ratings as a means of personal change and improvement, but not their (or others') self or essence (Bernard, 2011).

Acceptance in this form is considered "crucial to solid emotional and behavioral health" (Ellis & Robb, 1994, p. 91). By eliminating self-rating, people become liberated of anxiety, feelings of inadequacy and fear of criticism and rejection, and are free to explore and pursue the things that really make them happy (Bernard, 2011). Being happy and enjoying life is, in Ellis' view, far more important than proving oneself (Bernard, 2011). Self-rating and other-rating, although not responsible for all human emotional problems, "very possibly create most of them" (Ellis, 2005, p. 157).

As mentioned above, studies indicate a positive relation of self-acceptance with life satisfaction, happiness (Chamberlain & Haaga, 2001), and psychological well-being (MacInnes, 2006), and a negative one with neuroticism, one of the most important [negative] personality predictors of well-being (Davies, 2006), anxiety and depression. Conversely, global self-rating has a negative effect on most components of well-being, and is associated with dysfunctional negative emotions (e.g., DiGiuseppe & Tafrate, 2007), relationship and marital problems (Addis & Bernard, 2002; Möller & De Beer, 1998; Möller, Rabe, & Nortje, 2001), and poor goal setting and pursuit (Flett, Besser, Davis, & Hewitt, 2003; Wicker, Brown, Hagen, Boring, & Wiehe, 1990).

Just as people can chose to accept themselves, they can choose to accept others, despite occasional problematic thoughts, emotions and behaviors. They may evaluate these thoughts, emotions and behaviors as "bad" and decide not to accept them, but they will not rate the person as a whole. Although, to our knowledge, research has not specifically examined the relation between unconditional other acceptance, as defined by REBT, and well-being, studies focused on *blaming others* as an emotion regulation strategy support the REBT perspective. For example, Martin and Dahlen (2005) found that blaming others was positively related with anxiety, depression and stress in a sample of college students, while Stuewig and collaborators (2010) showed that it was associated with higher levels of aggression. A study that examined the predictors of negative self-referential emotions in adolescence (N = 706) found that lower levels of blaming others significantly predicted lower guilt-proneness (Szentágotai-Tătar & Miu, 2016). Moreover, a study comparing emotion regulation strategies in a clinical sample and a matched non-clinical control group reported that both self-blame and other-blame significantly differentiated between the two groups (Garnefski et al., 2002).

Acceptance of Uncertainty

Acknowledging and accepting the idea that we live in a world of probabilities, where absolute certainties are unlikely to ever exist is, according to REBT, another condition for mental health and happiness (Ellis & Dryden, 1997). Individuals who are intolerant of uncertainty view ambiguity as stressful and believe uncertain situations must be avoided (Yook, Kim, Suh, & Lee, 2010); as a result, they experience problematic cognitions and emotions. A recent meta-analysis (Şoflău & David, 2017) found that irrational beliefs related to certainty are significant predictors of dysfunctional automatic thoughts. Intolerance of uncertainty also predicts high levels of worry, and is considered an important vulnerability factor for generalized anxiety disorder (Koerner & Dugas, 2008). It is related to a host of other psychological problems such as social phobia, panic disorder, obsessive compulsive disorder and depression (Gentes & Meron Ruscio, 2011; McEvoy & Mahoney, 2012), and to reduced well-being in the context of life changes (Bardi, Guerra, & Ramdeny, 2009). These findings support the legitimacy of the REBT recommendation that people learn to see uncertainty as a challenge, not as a threat, and learn to live with it if they want to reach important goals in life (Bernard, 2011; Ellis & Dryden, 1997).

Psychological Flexibility and Scientific Thinking

REBT maintains that healthy individuals tend to be flexible in their thinking, open to change, and pluralistic in their views of others (Ellis & Dryden, 1997). When people adopt a flexible perspective, they will not become disturbed, even when confronted with unpleasant conditions or negative life events (Dryden et al., 2010). On the other hand, psychological inflexibility (i.e., the tendency to hold on to rigid, dogmatic beliefs in the form of demands) is considered a central element of emotional and behavioral disturbance (Dryden et al., 2010). According to Ellis (1997, 2003), there are three main types of demands that create problems for people: (1) demands that they should perform well, (2) demands that others must treat them nicely, and (3) demands that living conditions must be free of hassles and that life should be fair.

The role of psychological inflexibility, expressed as dogmatic demands, in creating a range of dysfunctional negative emotions and behaviors is well-established empirically (see David, Schnur, & Belloiu, 2002; David et al., 2005; Szentágotai & Jones, 2010), and so is its negative association with indices of well-being such as life satisfaction, joviality and self-assurance (Ciarrochi, 2004). To our knowledge, the relation between flexibility and well-being has not yet been examined by REBT scholars, but has been given some attention in positive psychology (Kashdan, 2010), which defines flexibility as the way a person: (1) adapts to fluctuating situational demands; (2) reconfigures mental resources, (3) shifts perspectives and (4) balances competing desires, needs and life domains (Kashdan, 2010). There is evidence that flexibility, expressed this way, is associated with higher well-being (see Kashdan, 2010 for a review).

Scientific thinking is seen by Ellis as one of the best prevention methods and one of the most efficient antidotes against the psychological misery resulting from inflexibility (Ellis, 1995). Unlike irrational thinking, scientific thinking is flexible and non-dogmatic, and involves the testing of our beliefs against evidence from reality (Ellis, 1995). If a belief proofs to be wrong, it should be replaced with a valid idea, as unrealistic thinking is one of the main sources of psychological distress (Ellis, 1995). An ongoing scientific approach to desires and preferences precludes their escalation into irrational "musts" and prevents emotional problems. Moreover, scientific thinking is also the way to eliminate emotional problems in individuals who, for various reasons, have endorsed dogmatic demands. Ellis suggests that scientific thinking entails passing our beliefs through the following filters (Ellis, 1995): establishing if they are realistic or factual; establishing if they are logical; determining if they are flexible and unrigid; establishing if they can be falsified; determining if they prove deservingness; and evaluating if they will lead to good and happy outcomes for ourselves and the others.

Commitment to Creative and Absorbing Activities and Risk Taking

From the beginning, REBT emphasized the role of action as a fundamental element of therapeutic change ("Rational emotive therapy is one of the relatively few techniques which include large amounts of actions, work and homework assignments of so called nonverbal nature"; Ellis, 1962, p. 334), but also as an essential vehicle to happiness (Bernard et al., 2010). Getting involved in creative and absorbing activities was seen by Ellis as a way of gaining both short-term happiness and long-term fulfillment, and he recommended that people discover and pursue those activities that can lead to both (Ellis & Harper, 1975). He also identified three main forms of such pursuits: (1) loving or feeling absorbed in other people,

(2) creating or getting absorbed in things, and (3) philosophizing or getting absorbed in ideas (see Bernard et al., 2010).

Research in positive psychology confirms the benefits of these recommendations. Indeed, it seems that intentional activity, more specifically, discrete actions and practices in which people can chose to get involved, is one of the most efficient ways of enduringly influencing happiness levels (Lyubomirsky, Sheldon, & Schkade, 2005). Also, activity can be both a source of short-term and of long-term happiness. A series of studies comparing the endorsement of three different ways to be happy: through pleasure (i.e., getting involved in activities that lead to enjoyable experiences), through engagement (i.e., engaging in activities that are fully immersive) and through meaning (i.e., undertaking activities that contribute to the greater good) found that all three individually predicted happiness. However, orientation towards pleasure was a less strong predictor of happiness than orientation towards engagement and meaning (Peterson, Park, & Seligman, 2005; Vella-Brodrick, Park, & Peterson, 2008). Moreover, Peterson, Ruch, Beernann, Park, and Seligman (2007) showed that character strengths most associated with happiness (i.e., humor, zest, curiosity, perseverance and religiousness) were also most highly associated with engagement and meaning.

In addition to emphasizing the importance of engagement for long-term happiness, REBT also encourages people to take risks and get involved into activities that entail a high likelihood of failure (Bernard et al., 2010; Ellis, 1962). This helps fight fear of failure and performance anxiety, and, at the same time, can lead to the discovery of new sources of well-being (Bernard et al., 2010). In support of these recommendations, there is evidence showing that people who plan their daily goals so as to avoid their worst fears report significantly lower levels of happiness than those who plan their daily goals so as to help them reach their broader life objectives (King, Richards, & Stemmerich, 1998). Also, studies looking at the relations between personality traits and happiness found that while openness to experience is not a very robust predictor of the hedonic aspects of well-being (i.e., pleasure), it is a robust predictor of eudaimonic aspects, such as self-actualization (Keyes et al., 2002).

REBT as a Tool for Promoting Well-Being and Preventing Emotional Disturbance

As frequently pointed out by Ellis (e.g., 1973, 1994), REBT is not only intended to alleviate psychological disturbance and suffering, but also, due to its humanistic-existential outlook, to promote psychological health and well-being (Ziegler, 2003). However, similar to research in Psychology in general, which has primarily focused on understanding and "repairing" the negative, rather than on the positive (Seligman & Csikszentmihalyi, 2000; Sheldon & King, 2001), research in REBT has mainly concentrated on assessing REBT efficacy in reducing emotional disturbance, rather than in increasing well-being. The advantage of this approach is the fairly solid evidence confirming the efficacy of REBT in managing a variety of disorders and problems. For example, a recent meta-analysis by David and collaborators (2017) reports significant effect sizes in favour of REBT compared to control groups in reducing distress, depression, anger, anxiety and irrational thinking, and in increasing school performance and health-related outcomes.

The downside is that less is known about the benefits of REBT in terms of preventing psychological problems and promoting happiness. Of course, it can be argued that reducing dysfunctional emotions and behaviors is automatically related to increases in well-being. However, considering that positive and negative affect seem to be independent in daily life (Diener & Emmons, 1984), and that flourishing mental health is characterized by a ratio of positive to negative affect of about 2.9 (Fredrickson & Losada, 2005), more studies that focus specifically on the impact of REBT on positive outcomes are needed. Existing evidence does support the promises of REBT in this direction. For instance, in their meta-analysis, David, Coteț, Matu, Mogoaşe, and Ştefan (2017) report a significant effect of REBT on increasing quality of life in a variety of clinical and non-clinical populations. Also, data indicate that REBT school interventions for children and adolescents lead to increases in well-being, social-emotional competences and academic achievement (Ashdown & Berbard, 2012; Bernard & Walton, 2011; Shannon & Allen, 1998). These results support the recommendations of Ellis who, for many years, argued for the importance of introducing REBT principles in the school curriculum and the home as way of preventing psychopathology and increasing well-being (Weinrach et al., 2006).

Conclusions

Happiness and well-being have preoccupied people for millennia, and the idea that what matters is not just to live, but to live well has been central to both Eastern and Western philosophical thought (Kesebir & Diener, 2008). More recently, well-being has also become the subject of scientific scrutiny, as behavioral and social sciences have begun to devote increased attention to this topic (Kesebir & Diener, 2008; Ryan & Deci, 2001). Understanding well-being, through the study of positive emotions, positive individual traits and the institutions that foster them, is one of the main goals of positive psychology, established as a field at the end of the 1990s. However, interest in well-being has existed much longer in psychology, as illustrated by REBT, the influential approach to mental health and disturbance developed by Albert Ellis in the 1950s (Bernard et al., 2010). Indeed, in addition to his preoccupation with emotional problems, Ellis was deeply interested in what made people happy and in how happiness could be achieved (Bernard, 2011), and some of his most popular works are witness to this interest. His contribution to the understanding of well-being was acknowledged by Martin Seligman, founder of positive psychology, who has called Ellis an "unsung hero of positive psychology".

Rational thinking is central to the REBT theory of happiness, whereas irrational thinking is central to the theory of unhappiness and psychopathology. While rational thinking is hypothesized to lead to functional positive and negative emotions, both characteristic of well-being. REBT thus advances the idea of what can be called *rational/irrational* happiness (Szentágotai & David, 2013), maintaining that the way our goals and desires are formulated is equally important as their content and their attainment. It also proposes several principles that should guide people in their pursuit of short-term satisfaction and long-term fulfillment. Thus, in addition to being an influential approach to psychopathology and its treatment, REBT also offers valuable insight and a fertile ground for research on well-being, and on how it can be attained and maintained. In light of the analysis in this chapter, important topics for future research include: (1) exploring the nature and correlates of functional and dysfunctional positive emotions; (2) describing the relation between rational/irrational thinking and indicators of well-being; (3) empirically evaluating the principles of a happy life as proposed by REBT; (4) conducting longitudinal studies to assess the efficacy of REBT in preventing psychopathology and maintaining mental health; and (5) evaluating the impact of REBT programs on increasing happiness.

References

Addis, J., & Bernard, M. E. (2002). Marital adjustment and irrational beliefs. *Journal of Rational-Emotive & Cognitive-Behavior Therapy, 2*(1), 3–13.

Ashdown, D. M., & Berbard, M. E. (2012). Can explicit instruction in social and emotional learning skills benefit the social-emotional development, well-being and academic achievement of young children? *Early Childhood Education Journal, 39*(6), 397–405.

Bardi, A., Guerra, V. M., & Ramdeny, G. S. D. (2009). Openness and ambiguity intolerance: Their differential relations to well-being in the context of academic life transition. *Personality and Individual Differences, 47*(3), 219–223.

Berman, J. Z., & Small, D. A. (2012). Self-interest without selfishness: The hedonic benefit of imposed self-interest. *Psychological Science, 23*(10), 1193–1999.

Bernard, M. E. (2011). *Rationality and the pursuit of happiness. The legacy of Albert Ellis*. Chichester, UK: Wiley-Blackwell.

Bernard, M. E., Froh, J. J., DiGiuseppe, R., Joyce, M. R., & Dryden, W. (2010). Albert Ellis: Unsung hero of positive psychology. *The Journal of Positive Psychology, 5*(4), 302–310.

Bernard, M. E., & Walton, K. (2011). The effect of you can do it! Education in six schools on student perceptions of wellbeing, teaching, learning, and relationships. *Journal of Student Wellbeing, 5*(1), 22–37.

Brown, S. L., Nesse, R. M., Vinokur, A. D., & Smith, D. M. (2003). Providing social support may be more beneficial than receiving it: Results from a prospective study of mortality. *Psychological Science, 14*(4), 320–327.

Brown, W. M., Consedine, N. S., & Magai, C. (2005). Altruism relates to health in an ethnically diverse sample of older adults. *The Journals of Gerontology Series B: Psychological Sciences and Social Sciences, 60*(3), 143–152.

Caserta, D. A., Dowd, E. T., David, D., & Ellis, A. (2010). Rational and irrational beliefs in primary prevention and mental health. In D. David, S. J. Lynn, & A. Ellis (Eds.), *Rational and irrational beliefs. Research, theory and clinical practice* (pp. 173–194). New York, NY: Oxford University Press.

Chamberlain, J. M., & Haaga, D. A. F. (2001). Unconditional self-acceptance and psychological health. *Journal of Rational-Emotive and Cognitive-Behavior Therapy, 19*(3), 163–176.

Ciarrochi, J. (2004). Relationship between dysfunctional beliefs and positive and negative indices of well-being: A critical evaluation of the common beliefs survey-III. *Journal of Rational-Emotive & Cognitive-Behavior Therapy, 22*(3), 171–188.

Dana, J., Weber, R. A., & Xi Kuang, J. (2005). Exploiting moral wiggle room: Experiments demonstrating and illusory preference for fairness. *Economic Theory, 33*(1), 67–80.

David, D. (2003). Rational emotive behavior therapy (REBT): The view of a cognitive psychologist. In W. Dryden (Ed.), *Rational emotive behaviour therapy: Theoretical developments* (pp. 130–159). London, UK: Brunner-Routledge.

David, D., Coteţ, C., Matu, S., Mogoaşe, C., & Ştefan, S. (2017). 50 years of rational-emotive and cognitive-behavioral therapy: A systematic review and meta-analysis. *Journal of Clinical Psychology*. https://doi.org/10.1002/jclp.22514

David, D., Schnur, J., & Belloiu, A. (2002). Another search for "hot" cognitions: Appraisal, irrational beliefs, attributions, and their relation to emotion. *Journal of Rational Emotive & Cognitive Behavior Therapy, 20*(2), 93–131.

David, D., Szentágotai, A., Kállay, E., & Macavei, B. (2005). A synopsis of Rational-Emotive Behavior Therapy (REBT); fundamental and applied research. *Journal of Rational-Emotive & Cognitive-Behavior Therapy, 23*(3), 175–221.

Davies, M. F. (2006). Irrational beliefs and unconditional self-acceptance. I. Correlational evidence linking the key features of REBT. *Journal of Rational-Emotive & Cognitive-Behavior Therapy, 24*(2), 113–124.

Davis, M. A. (2009). Understanding the relationship between mood and creativity. *Organizational Behavior and Human Decision Processes, 108*, 25–38.

Diener, E. (1984). Subjective well-being. *Psychological Bulletin, 95*(3), 542–575.

Diener, E., & Emmons, R. A. (1984). The independence of positive and negative affect. *Journal of Personality and Social Psychology, 47*(5), 1105–1117.

Diener, E., Napa Scollon, C., & Lucas, R. E. (2003). The evolving concept of subjective well-being: The multifaceted nature of happiness. *Advances in Cell Aging and Gerontology, 15*, 187–291.

Diener, E., Sandvik, E., & Pavot, W. (1991). Happiness is the frequency, not the intensity, of positive versus negative affect. In F. Strack, M. Argyle, & N. Schwarz (Eds.), *Subjective well-being: An interdisciplinary perspective. International series in experimental social psychology* (pp. 119–139). Oxford, UK: Pergamon Press.

DiGiuseppe, R., & Tafrate, R. C. (2007). *Understanding anger disorder*. New York, NY: Oxford University Press.

Dryden, W. (2002). *Fundamentals of rational emotive behaviour therapy*. London, UK: Whurr Publishers Ltd.

Dryden, W., David, D., & Ellis, A. (2010). Rational emotive behavior therapy. In K. S. Dobson (Ed.), *Handbook of cognitive-behavioral therapies* (pp. 226–276). New York, NY: The Guilford Press.

Dryden, W., & Neenan, M. (2004). *The rational emotive behavioural approach to therapeutic change*. London, UK: Sage Publications Ltd.

Ellis, A. (1962). *Reason and emotion in psychotherapy*. New York, NY: L. Stuart.

Ellis, A. (1973). *Humanistic psychotherapy: The rational emotive approach*. New York, NY: Crown & McGraw-Hill.

Ellis, A. (1976). RET abolishes most of the human ego. *Psychotherapy: Theory, Research and Practice, 13*(4), 343–348.

Ellis, A. (1984). The essence of RET. *Journal of Rational-Emotive Therapy, 2*(1), 19–25.

Ellis, A. (1994). *Reason and emotion in psychotherapy* (2nd ed.). New York, NY: Birch Lane Press.

Ellis, A. (1995). *How to stubbornly refuse to make yourself miserable about anything – yes, anything*. Secaucus, NJ: Lyle Stuart.

Ellis, A. (1997). Extending the goals of behavior therapy and cognitive behavior therapy. *Behavior Therapy, 28*(3), 333–339.

Ellis, A. (1999). *How to make yourself happy and remarkably less disturbable*. Atascadero, CA: Impact Publishers.

Ellis, A. (2003). Differentiating preferential from exaggerated and musturbatory beliefs in rational emotive behavior therapy. In W. Dryden (Ed.), *Rational emotive behaviour therapy: Theoretical developments* (pp. 22–34). New York, NY: Brunner Routledge.

Ellis, A. (2005). Can rational-emotive behavior therapy (REBT) and acceptance and commitment therapy (ACT) resolve their differences and be integrated? *Journal of Rational-Emotive & Cognitive-Behavior Therapy, 23*(2), 153–168.

Ellis, A., & Becker, I. (1982). *A guide to personal happiness*. North Hollywood, CA: Wilshire Books.

Ellis, A., & Bernard, M. E. (1985). What is rational-emotive therapy (RET)? In A. Ellis & M. E. Bernard (Eds.), *Clinical applications of rational-emotive therapy* (pp. 1–30). New York, NY: Plenum Press.

Ellis, A., & DiGiuseppe, R. (1993). Are inappropriate or dysfunctional feelings in rational-emotive therapy qualitative or quantitative? *Cognitive Therapy & Research, 17*(5), 471–477.

Ellis, A., & Dryden, W. (1997). *The practice of rational emotive behavior therapy* (2nd ed.). New York, NY: Springer Publishing Company.

Ellis, A., & Harper, R. A. (1975). *A new guide to rational living*. North Hollywood, CA: Wilshire Books.

Ellis, A., & Robb, H. (1994). Acceptance in rational-emotive therapy. In S. C. Hayes, N. S. Jacobson, V. M. Folette, & M. J. Dougher (Eds.), *Acceptance and change: Content and context in psychotherapy* (pp. 13–32). Reno, NV: Context Press.

Flett, G. L., Besser, A., Davis, R. A., & Hewitt, P. (2003). Dimensions of perfectionism, unconditional self-acceptance, and depression. *Journal of Rational-Emotive & Cognitive-Behavior Therapy, 21*(2), 119–138.

Ford, B. Q., Shallcross, A. J., Mauss, I. B., Floerke, V. A., & Gruber, J. (2014). Desperately seeking happiness: Valuing happiness is associated with symptoms and diagnosis of depression. *Journal of Social and Clinical Psychology, 33*(10), 890–905.

Fredrickson, B. L. (1998). What good are positive emotions? *Review of General Psychology, 2*(3), 300–319.

Fredrickson, B. L., & Joiner, T. (2002). Positive emotions trigger upward spirals toward emotional well-being. *Psychological Science, 13*(2), 172–175.

Fredrickson, B. L., & Losada, M. F. (2005). Positive affect and the complex dynamics of human flourishing. *American Psychologist, 60*(7), 678–686.

Gable, S. L., & Haidt, J. (2005). What (and why) is positive psychology? *Review of General Psychology, 9*(2), 103–110.

Garnefski, N., Van Den Kommer, T., Kraaij, V., Teerds, J., Legerstee, J., & Onstein, E. (2002). The relationship between cognitive emotion strategies and emotional problems: Comparison between a clinical and a non-clinical sample. *European Journal of Personality, 16*(5), 403–420.

Gentes, E. L., & Meron Ruscio, A. (2011). A meta-analysis of the relation of intolerance of uncertainty to symptoms of generalized anxiety disorder, major depressive disorder, and obsessive-compulsive disorder. *Clinical Psychology Review, 31*(6), 923–933.

Gruber, J., Mauss, I. B., & Tamir, M. (2011). A dark side of happiness? How, when and why happiness is not always good. *Perspectives on Psychological Science, 6*(3), 222–233.

Huta, V. (2013). Eudaimonia. In S. A. David, I. Boniwell, & A. Conley Ayers (Eds.), *The Oxford handbook of happiness* (pp. 201–214). Oxford, UK: Oxford University Press.

Huta, V., & Ryan, R. M. (2010). Pursuing pleasure or virtue: The differential and overlapping Well-being benefits of hedonic and eudaimonic motives. *Journal of Happiness Studies, 11*(6), 735–762.

James, W. (1902). *The varieties of religious experience: A study in human nature*. New York, NY: Longman, Green.
Johnson, S. L. (2005). Mania and dysregulation in goal pursuit: A review. *Clinical Psychology Review, 25*(2), 241–262.
Kashdan, T. B. (2010). Psychological flexibility as a fundamental aspect of human health. *Clinical Psychology Review, 30*(7), 865–878.
Kesebir, P., & Diener, E. (2008). In pursuit of happiness: Empirical answers to philosophical questions. *Perspectives on Psychological Science, 3*(2), 117–125.
Keyes, C. L. M., Shmotkin, D., & Ryff, C. D. (2002). Optimizing well-being: The empirical encounter of two traditions. *Journal of Personality and Social Psychology, 82*(6), 1007–1022.
King, L. A., Richards, J. H., & Stemmerich, E. (1998). Daily goals, life goals and worst fears: Means, ends, and subjective well-being. *Journal of Personality, 66*(5), 713–744.
Koerner, N., & Dugas, M. J. (2008). An investigation of appraisals in individuals vulnerable to excessive worry: The role of intolerance of uncertainty. *Cognitive Therapy and Research, 32*(5), 619–638.
Kuppens, P., Realo, A., & Diener, E. (2008). The role of positive and negative emotions in life satisfaction judgment across nations. *Journal of Personality and Social Psychology, 95*(1), 66–75.
Linley, P. A., Joseph, S., Harrington, S., & Wood, A. M. (2006). Positive psychology: Past, present, and (possible) future. *The Journal of Positive Psychology, 1*(1), 3–16.
Lyubomirsky, S. (2008). *The how of happiness: A scientific approach to getting the life you want*. New York, NY: Penguin Press.
Lyubomirsky, S., Dickerhoof, R., Boehm, J. K., & Sheldon, K. M. (2011). Becoming happier takes both a will and a proper way: An experimental longitudinal intervention to boost well-being. *Emotion, 11*(2), 391–402.
Lyubomirsky, S., Sheldon, K. M., & Schkade, D. (2005). Pursuing happiness: The architecture of sustainable change. *Review of General Psychology, 9*(2), 111–131.
MacInnes, D. (2004). The theories underpinning rational emotive behaviour therapy. *International Journal of Nursing Studies, 41*(6), 685–695.
MacInnes, D. L. (2006). Self-esteem and self-acceptance: an examination into their relationship and their effect on psychological health. *Journal of Psychiatric and Mental Health Nursing, 13*(5), 483–489.
Maddux, J. (2002). "Stopping the madness". Positive psychology and the deconstruction of the illness ideology and the DSM. In C. R. Snyder & S. J. Lopez (Eds.), *Handbook of positive psychology* (pp. 13–25). New York, NY: Oxford University Press.
Martin, R. C., & Dahlen, E. R. (2005). Cognitive emotion regulation in the prediction of depression, anxiety, stress, and anger. *Personality and Individual Differences, 39*(7), 1249–1260.
Maslow, A. H. (1950). Self-actualizing people: A study of psychological health. In W. Wolff (Ed.), *Personality symposia: symposium 1 on values* (pp. 11–34). New York: Grune & Stratton.
Maslow, A. H. (1973). Self-actualizing people: A study of psychological health. In R. J. Lowry (Ed.), *Dominance, self-esteem, self-actualization: Germinal papers of A. H. Maslow* (pp. 177–201). Monterey, CA: Brookes/Cole (Original work published in 1950).
Mauss, I. B., Savino, N. S., Anderson, C. L., Weisbuch, M., Tamir, M., & Laudenslager, M. L. (2012). The pursuit of happiness can be lonely. *Emotion, 12*(5), 908–912.
Mauss, I. B., Tamir, M., Anderson, C. L., & Savino, N. S. (2011). Can seeking happiness make people happy? Paradoxical effects of valuing happiness. *Emotion, 11*(4), 807–815.
McEvoy, P. M., & Mahoney, A. E. J. (2012). To be sure, to be sure: Intolerance of uncertainty mediates symptoms of various anxiety disorders and depression. *Behavior Therapy, 43*(3), 533–545.
Möller, A. T., & De Beer, Z. C. (1998). Irrational beliefs and marital conflict. *Psychological Reports, 82*(1), 155–160.

Möller, A. T., Rabe, H. M., & Nortje, C. (2001). Dysfunctional beliefs and marital conflict in distressed and non-distressed married individuals. *Journal of Rational-Emotive & Cognitive-Behavior Therapy, 19*(4), 259–270.

Oltean, H. R., & David, D. (2018). A meta-analysis of the relation between rational beliefs and psychological distress. *Journal of Clinical Psychology, 74*, 883–895.

Peterson, C., Park, N., & Seligman, M. P. E. (2005). Orientations to happiness and life satisfaction: The full life versus the empty life. *Journal of Happiness Studies, 6*(1), 25–41.

Peterson, C., Ruch, W., Beernann, U., Park, N., & Seligman, M. E. P. (2007). Strengths of character, orientations to happiness, and life satisfaction. *The Journal of Positive Psychology, 2*(3), 149–156.

Rogers, C. R. (1961). *On becoming a person*. London, UK: Constable.

Ryan, R. M., & Deci, E. L. (2001). On happiness and human potentials: A review of research on hedonic and eudaimonic well-being. *Annual Review of Psychology, 52*, 141–166.

Ryff, C. D., & Singer, B. H. (2006). Know thyself and become what you are: A eudaimonic approach to psychological well-being. *Journal of Happiness Studies, 9*(1), 13–39.

Schooler, J. W., Ariely, D., & Loewenstein, G. (2003). The pursuit and assessment of happiness may be self-defeating. In J. Carillo & I. Brocas (Eds.), *The psychology of economic decisions* (pp. 41–70). Oxford, UK: Oxford University Press.

Schwartz, C., Meisenhelder, J. B., Ma, Y., & Reed, G. (2003). Altruistic social interest behaviors are associated with better mental health. *Psychosomatic Medicine, 65*(5), 778–785.

Seligman, M. E. P. (2002). *Authentic happiness: Using the new positive psychology to maximize your potential for lasting fulfillment*. New York, NY: Free Press.

Seligman, M. E. P. (2011). *Flourish: A visionary new understanding of happiness and well-being*. New York, NY: Free Press.

Seligman, M. E. P., & Csikszentmihalyi, M. (2000). Positive psychology. An introduction. *American Psychologist, 55*(1), 5–14.

Shannon, H. D., & Allen, T. W. (1998). The effectiveness of a REBT training program in increasing the performance of high school students in mathematics. *Journal of Rational-Emotive and Cognitive-Behavior Therapy, 16*(3), 197–209.

Sheldon, K. M., Abad, N., Ferguson, Y., Gunz, A., Houser-Marko, L., Nichols, C. P., & Lyubomirsky, S. (2010). Persistent pursuit of need-satisfying goals leads to increased happiness: A 6-month experimental longitudinal study. *Motivation and Emotion, 34*, 39–48.

Sheldon, K. M., & Elliot, A. J. (1999). Goal striving, need satisfaction, and longitudinal well-being: The self-concordance model. *Journal of Personality and Social Psychology, 76*(3), 482–497.

Sheldon, K. M., & Houser-Marko, L. (2001). Self-concordance, goal attainment and the pursuit of happiness: Can there be an upward spiral? *Journal of Personality and Social Psychology, 80*(1), 152–165.

Sheldon, K. M., & King, L. (2001). Why positive psychology is necessary. *American Psychologist, 56*(3), 216–217.

Sheldon, K. M., Ryan, R. M., Deci, E. L., & Kasser, T. (2004). The independent effects of goal contents and motives on well-being: It's both what you pursue and why you pursue it. *Personality and Social Psychology Bulletin, 30*(4), 475–486.

Şoflău, R., & David, D. (2017). A meta-analytical approach of the relationship between the irrationality of beliefs and the functionality of automatic thoughts. *Cognitive Therapy and Research, 41*, 178–192.

Stuewig, J., Tangney, J. P., Heigel, C., Harty, L., & McCloskey, L. (2010). Shaming, blaming and maiming: Functional links among the moral emotions, externalization of blame and aggression. *Journal of Research in Personality, 44*(1), 91–102.

Szentágotai, A., & David, D. (2013). Self-acceptance and happiness. In M. Bernard (Ed.), *The strength of self-acceptance* (pp. 121–137). New York, NY: Springer.

Szentágotai, A., & Jones, J. (2010). The behavioral consequences of irrational beliefs. In D. David, S. J. Lynn, & A. Ellis (Eds.), *Rational and irrational beliefs. Research, theory and clinical practice* (pp. 75–97). New York, NY: Oxford University Press.

Szentágotai-Tătar, A., & Miu, A. C. (2016). Individual differences in emotion regulation, childhood trauma and proneness to shame and guilt in adolescence. *PLoS One, 11*(11), e0167299. https://doi.org/10.1371/journal.pone.0167299

Tracy, J. L., Cheng, J. T., Robins, R. W., & Trzesniewski, K. H. (2009). Authentic and hubristic pride: The affective core of self-esteem and narcissism. *Self and Identity, 8*, 196–213.

Tracy, J. L., & Robins, R. W. (2004). Putting the self into self-conscious emotions: A theoretical model. *Psychological Inquiry, 15*(2), 103–125.

Tracy, J. L., & Robins, R. W. (2007). The psychological structure of pride: A tale of two facets. *Journal of Personality and Social Psychology, 92*(3), 506–525.

Vella-Brodrick, D. A., Park, N., & Peterson, C. (2008). Three ways to be happy: Pleasure, engagement and meaning - Findings from Australian and US samples. *Social Indicators Research, 90*, 165–179.

Vîslă, A., Flückiger, C., grosse Holtforth, M., & David, D. (2015). Irrational beliefs and psychological distress: A meta-analysis. *Psychotherapy and Psychosomatics, 85*, 8–15.

Waterman, A. S. (1993). Two conceptions of happiness: Contrasts of personal expressiveness (eudaimonia) and hedonic enjoyment. *Journal of Personality and Social Psychology, 64*(4), 678–691.

Weinrach, S. G., DiGiuseppe, R., Wolfe, J., Ellis, A., Bernard, M. E., Dryden, W., et al. (2006). Rational emotive behavior therapy after Ellis: Predictions for the future. *Journal of Rational-Emotive & Cognitive-Behavior Therapy, 24*(4), 199–214.

Wicker, F. W., Brown, G., Hagen, A. S., Boring, W., & Wiehe, J. A. (1990). Interactions of irrational beliefs with goal pursuit. *Journal of Rational-Emotive & Cognitive-Behavior Therapy, 8*(3), 147–158.

Yook, K., Kim, K.-H., Suh, S. Y., & Lee, K. S. (2010). Intolerance of uncertainty, worry, and rumination in major depressive disorder and generalized anxiety disorder. *Journal of Anxiety Disorders, 24*(6), 623–628.

Ziegler, D. J. (2003). The concept of psychological health in rational emotive behavior therapy. *Journal of Rational-Emotive and Cognitive-Behavior Therapy, 21*(1), 21–36.

Chapter 12
REBT in Coaching

Oana David

REBT Theory, Research and Practice Relevant for Coaching

While initially used in the sports field, coaching is currently considered a domain at the intersection of various disciplines (e.g., andragogy, psychology, behavioral sciences, consulting), which is defined by different theories (e.g., adult learning theories, counseling, psychotherapeutic approaches, and positive psychology). Coaching is primarily conceptualized as an adult learning strategy, using focused conversations between a coach and coachee, where the coach acts as a catalyst for the coachee's learning process in relation to their goal/issue. Change processes are facilitated by the coach through the use of effective questioning – derived from counseling - meant to assist the coachee in order to formulate realistic goals, overcome obstacles and implement effective steps in reaching their goals.

Coaching is nowadays flourishing as one of the fastest growing industries. One of the main reasons for its rapid growth is that it addresses the personal and professional development needs of people, without the stigma associated with psychotherapeutic interventions. Most psychotherapeutic approaches have started from a deficit model, based on the pressures to find cures for psychopathology, this being one of the criticisms when their theories were transferred into the coaching field. Compared to psychotherapy, coaching has been conceptualized as being sought by people without mental health problems/psychopathology or severe distress, and with a high level of functioning; thus, the focus of coaching is on helping people attain their goals in terms of personal or professional

O. David (✉)
International Coaching Institute, Kent, WA, USA

Department of Clinical Psychology and Psychotherapy, Babes-Bolyai University, Cluj-Napoca, Romania
e-mail: oanadavid@psychology.ro

© Springer Nature Switzerland AG 2019
M. E. Bernard, W. Dryden (eds.), *Advances in REBT*,
https://doi.org/10.1007/978-3-319-93118-0_12

fulfillment. Coaching can be however conceptualized both as a specific intervention or an intervention sequence, case in which it can be part of another intervention or program, as a learning or change strategy.

Rational Emotive Behavioral Therapy (REBT) is the first cognitive-behavioral approach (Bernard & David, 2018) that is devoted to approaching life goals in a directive and active way, having at least as much a promotion orientation as curative focus. Albert Ellis demonstrated REBT during live sessions at the Albert Ellis Institute, events originally known as *"Problems of Everyday Living"* and then named *"Friday night live"*, during which he applied REBT to life problems/goals brought by the participants who were seeking help in overcoming personal obstacles but not mental health problems seeking his advice about how they could achieve their life goals in different areas. As a result of Ellis' demonstration of life coaching, REBTers interested in coaching over the past two decades have conceptualized coaching using the REBT framework, under the name of Rational Emotive Behavior Coaching (REBC) (Dryden, 2010, 2011; Neenan & Dryden, 2001).

This chapter will answer the following questions: What is REBC? What are the common grounds and distinctive features of REBT and REBC? Which REBT based programs, goals, models, processes and tools are used in REBC? What are the main applications of REBC? What is the empirical status of REBC and future directions?

What Is REBC?

REBC is a form of coaching developed (see Anderson, 2002; Kodish, 2002) based on the theory and practices of REBT (Ellis, 1962), aimed at assisting people in reaching well-being, stress management and performance-related goals. The field of RECB coaching has been comprehensively described (theory, processes/techniques, applications) in Bernard and David (2018). REBC emphasizes the role of thinking, and more specifically rational beliefs (RBs), in attaining personal growth or professional development goals and overcoming emotional/behavioral obstacles. REBC aims at raising awareness about irrational beliefs (IBs) and changing them into RBs, in order to alleviate clients' emotional barriers to goal attainment, and increasing their psychological resilience, well-being and performance.

REBC is a specific form of cognitive-behavioral coaching (CBC; like cognitive coaching or behavioral coaching), which is defined as an integrative approach to coaching, using a cognitive-behavioral framework for making sense of client's goals/problems, and addressing them by making use of various cognitive, behavioral, solution focused and problem-solving strategies (e.g., Palmer & Szymańska, 2007). REBC sits within the CBC framework with its focus on strengthening rational beliefs and removing emotional/practical barriers for goal attainment as a fundamental mechanism for well-being and productivity (see also Bernard & David, 2018).

REBC can be focused towards helping coachees to address their problems, be they practical or emotional. When focused on emotional problems, REBC identifies and modifies the irrational beliefs (Gyllensten & Palmer, 2005), challenging and replacing them with rational beliefs, in order to remove obstacles (e.g., stress, procrastination) for goals such as happy and productive living.

Types of cognitions addressed for removing or lessening emotional obstacles are: (a) Demandingness, as main rigid, absolutist, dogmatic and illogical beliefs (e.g., "I must be appreciated at work") to be replaced with Preferences as flexible, realistic and logic beliefs concerning own desires (e.g., "I prefer to be appreciated at work but this does not mean that I must be").The other three types of beliefs are considered derivatives of demandingness (Montgomery, David, DiLorenzo, & Schnur, 2007), (b) Awfulizing, when events are exaggeratedly evaluated as catastrophic (e.g., "It is awful to not be appreciated for my efforts.") to be replaced with Badness type of rational beliefs, case in which negative events are assessed realistically (e.g., "It is bad, but not awful if I am not appreciated for my efforts"), (c) Frustration intolerance, when the person considers that she/he cannot tolerate the frustration or discomfort connected with the situation faced (e.g.,"I cannot stand to not be appreciated"), to be replaced with Frustration tolerance beliefs, when the person considers the negative situation/emotions tolerable ""I do not like this situation but I can tolerate it and move forward") and (d) Depreciation or global evaluation of self/others/life, when the person uses global negative evaluations (e.g., "My manager is totally hopeless"), to be replaced with unconditional acceptance beliefs, when the person considers herself/others/life acceptable without conditions, and commits towards changing specific aspects that could make them more successful/enjoyable (e.g., "I accept my manager as fallible human being and try to check the reasons for his lack of appreciation regarding my efforts").

Ellis (1972) and colleagues (e.g., Gavita & Duta, 2013; Palmer, 2009) proposed the following key IBs that can trigger stress in employees: "I must do better", "You must treat me better", "My working conditions must be better", and "People must like me". Based on these primary beliefs, the following derivative beliefs are involved in stress: "I won't do well and that would be awful", "I can't stand my working conditions", "If people don't like me, I am worthless".

REBT and REBC: Common Grounds and Distinctive Features

here are important misunderstandings in the coaching field regarding the differences between coaching and psychotherapy, which are delineated considering as prototype psychodynamic therapies. REBC shares however the same essential characteristics with REBT, such as being active and dynamic, collaborative, psychoeducational, structured, time-limited, present focused, problem/solution oriented, motivational and change oriented, integrative, culturally informed, cognitively appropriate, supportive and empirically oriented.

REBC provides coaches with advanced accurate empathy – the ability to understand the problems of coachees, including IBs that lead to problematic Cs. REBT is hypothetic-deductive and involves practitioners testing out their hypotheses concerning IBs –using at the same time a collaborative style of guided discovery. REBC makes use of the REBT tested tools for change, such as: Socratic questioning, a time-limited and goal-directed framework, using self-awareness emotions and beliefs based on the REBC theory. REBC can be used for a variety of life or workplace issues such as procrastination, enhancing performance, problem-solving, assertiveness, dealing with criticism, stress management.

Both REBT and REBC have the common goals of equipping clients with effective psychological tools (e.g., cognitive disputation) they can use to change their life philosophies needed for living a rational life and solve not only the current problem but also problems for the rest of their lives. Other common foci are staying in the present, seeking cognitive change but also emotional and behavioral change, establishing and implementing between-session goal-oriented tasks, organizing and setting an agenda in every session, seeing the relationship as a partnership for collaborating in achieving the goal, and adopting an experimental, curious approach to change. Both REBT and REBC emphasize the important role for sustained effort and commitments in reaching the goals as opposed to quick fixes, which require implementing behavioral changes between the sessions.

There are also distinctive features between REBT and REBC, including the setting where intervention takes place, which in coaching is, oftentimes, the client's office; while in therapy the clients sets own personal goal, coaching is oftentimes contracted by the organizations and thus the goal can be pre-established.

Criddle (2007a, 2007b) and Neenan (2008) identified a few qualitative changes of REBT that are needed in order to make it more suitable for coaching. Among the most important is the fact that REBC needs to offer simple answers to the questions of people coming from business, given the short-term contracts and high time pressures of this population. Based on the same argument, the REBC process is expected to direct the clients towards finding effective solutions that will bring immediate results, based on a brief contract (i.e., between one and six sessions; Dryden, 2017). Generally, clients involved in REBC are high functioning, who, oftentimes, know what they want but are searching for ways to get there or are stuck in some point of action implementation. This population is searching for effective tools that they can access quickly when getting stuck.

When using REBC especially in the business field, there are important lexical changes necessary for the REBT terminology (Criddle, 2007a), such as:

- Replacing the homework name, due to its connections with an authoritarian relationship developed in school settings, with the action plan terminology, which is often used as development tool in organizations;
- Changing the focus from emotions to behaviors, which are more salient for the performance and target oriented field of the organizations;

- Using adjusted concepts when talking about adaptive or maladaptive behavioral, affective or cognitive reactions, like productive versus counterproductive behaviors, healthy versus unhealthy emotions, performance interfering thoughts (PITS) versus performance enhancing thoughts (PETS; Williams, Edgerton, and Palmer (2010), flexible versus rigid thinking etc.). Criddle (2007a, 2007b) suggests even replacing the irrational processes with usual terms in order to make them more familiar, like using instead of rational beliefs the term management principles that work, or mastery of the emotional muscle (Grieger, 2007; Grieger & Fralick, 2007).

Professional training of coaching practitioners in REBC and that of REBC practitioners, is currently a topic of concern due to the lack of agreed professional standards for coaches, the lack of regulations of coaching practice and, thus, the existence of a large mass of practitioners having poor training. The situation is maintained because coaching is also an activity part of the job description of professionals in various fields – like managers. There are general bodies (e.g., International Coach Federation) and specific ones (i.e., the International Association of Cognitive Behavioral Coaching; ACBC) that have made important steps of offering professional standards, training, and professional certification for the practice of coaching, respectively REBC. For example, the IACBC offers two paths for becoming certified practitioner in REBC, one for psychologists/psychotherapists (e.g., REBT) and the other for other professionals, licensed in related fields (e.g., medical doctors, social workers etc). REBT professionals need to complete additional specific training in using coaching in order to be able to practice REBC.

REBT Applications and Programs Relevant to the Coaching Field

Historically, REBT was the first CBT approach which developed a series of positive programs designed specifically for applying its principles and models in various fields for promoting individual adjustment, happiness, and performance. Two of the most prolific programs were meant to teach children life skills, respectively to enhance work effectiveness. Rational Emotive Education (Knaus, 1974) was developed for promoting mental health in schools and Rational Effectiveness Training (Ellis & DiMattia, 1991) was developed for promoting well-being and performance in organizations. Another important resource for the development of the REBC field was the self-help REBT literature for personal development.

There is a vast REBT based self-development literature. Ellis wrote many self-help books with specific applications. The books, *A Guide to Rational Living* (Ellis & Harper, 1961), A *New Guide to Rational Living* (Ellis, Powers, & Harper, 1975), *A Guide to Personal Happiness* (Ellis, Powers, & Becker, 1982), *How to Make Yourself Happy and Remarkably Less Disturbable* (Ellis, 1999) are some of the most relevant for the life coaching field, since they nicely synthetize the main philosophy of REBT, using case studies and practical examples. These books serve as guides for coaching thinking habits that can make people happier and help them change their irrational beliefs in order to deal with adversities. Another REBT based self-coaching program is *Stage climbing: the shortest path to your highest potential* developed by Broder (2012). This program combines the REBT theory with Maslow's theory of motivation and uses a seven -level category system for assessing the change stage of the person. Based on this, it offers rational thinking tools for moving to their next change level, considering main life areas in which improvements are needed.

Interest in adapting REBT theory and practice to the workplace dates back to1967, when Ellis and Blum wrote the article *Rational Training: A New Method of Facilitating Management and Labor Relations*, and continued in 1972, with Ellis's book on *Executive Leadership: A Rational Approach*. Before explicitly talking about REBC (Kodish, 2002), REBT was documented for bringing positive results as employee assistance program (Klarreich, DiGiuseppe, & DiMattia, 1987), and as RET for the workplace (Ellis & DiMattia, 1991; DiMattia & IJzermans, 1996).

RET was developed by Dominic DiMattia (1990) as a comprehensive REBT based model for workplace emotional change. The goal of RET is to create a personal development experience for emotional growth which would bring the person closer to attaining their personal and professional goals. More specifically, RET aims at identifying the causes of unproductive behaviors (e.g., emotional blocks), and modifying them in order to increase performance, teamwork, communication skills, and work satisfaction (David, 2016). RET was conceptualized both as a development focused approach, based on a series of rational principles for workplace, and a model of emotional management, using strategies and steps for overcoming psychological blocks for performance. The principles of this model will be detailed when presenting how REBC can be applied for creating a rational organizational culture.

REBC Goals, Models, Process and Tools

REBC serves two types of major goals: (1) personal/professional development and (2) Solving practical or emotional problems (Dryden, 2018a, 2018b). Thus, REBC can be development focused or problem focused, depending on its goals.

Development-Focused REBC

Development-focused REBC is employed by a coach when coaching is sought for growth and improvement purposes related to living a happier and more productive life. In this case, the coachee is having a high level of general functioning (personal or professional), and the coach can assist her/him in growing in specific areas of their lives (e.g., outstanding performance for executives or athletes). More specifically, the coach can assist the coachee in selecting achievable goals/refining their goals, developing appropriate action plans for attaining goals, and finding effective ways to implementing the changes. Strategies used in this type of REBC are directed towards building a *rational mindset for living a fulfilled life* based on the principles of rational living (Ellis & Harper, 1961; Bernard, 2011), and can be complimented with other techniques (i.e., derived from positive psychology; see Bernard, 2011, 2013).

When assisting a coachee in finding or refining their goals, it is important that the coach help the coachee explore her/his values in order to make sure that the specified development goals are aligned to them. (e.g., to accept a new job offer that involves staying extra time at work). This alignment is important in terms of coachee's commitment for attaining their goals and having the positive impact that they expect in their lives. Then, there are a series of rational principles derived from Ellis writings which can serve as powerful strategies for attaining specific growth goals. Bernard (2011) has extracted 11 rational principles for living a happy life based on Ellis work: (1) Self-interest, (2) Social Interest, (3) Self-direction, (4) Self-acceptance, (5) Tolerance of Others, (6) Short-term and Long-term Hedonism, (7) Commitment to Creative, Absorbing Activities and Pursuits, (8) Responsible Risk-taking and Experimenting, (9) High Frustration Tolerance and Willpower, (10) Problem Solving, (11) Scientific Thinking and Flexibility. When incorporated in the living mindset, these strategies are meant to build a new rational living philosophy that helps the coachee to be more happy and productive.

Thus, the development-focused REBC aims at assisting the coachee to improve its behaviors, performance, well-being, by making use of the rational living principles and change models for helping the coachee to implement changes.

The GRAPE Model of Development-Focused REBC

A model with a developmental focused approach is the **GRAPE model** developed by Bernard (2018). The model has four steps:

Step 1: **G**OALS – in which the coachee is assisted in identifying professional goals for coaching sessions;

Step 2: **R**EFLECTION – in which the coachee is assisted in reflecting on different areas of their current approach to their life areas/work;

Step 3: **A**CTION **P**LANNING – in which the coachee is assisted to develop an action plan to activate beliefs, to strengthen commitments, use behavioral strengths, and remove blockers;

Step 4. **E**VALUATION – in which the coachee is assisted to evaluate and revise the action plan.

Problem-Focused REBC

Problem-focused REBC refers to assisting coachees in solving their practical or emotional (non-clinical though) problems with which they are confronted. Clients often seek coaching when they feel stuck regarding a specific life area or work related problem, but are generally highly functional in the various domains of their lives (e.g., family, social, professional).. Strategies used in this type of REBC are directed towards developing a *problem-solving mindset in life*, using various models (e.g., the ABCDEFG model, the PRACTICE model), depending on the type of the problem, emotional or practical.

In order to determine if the coachee has an emotional problem, the coach will assess if the emotion is blocking the coachee in reaching her/his goal and if the client is not able to address it by her/himself. Then the coach needs to establish if an emotional problem solving coaching is suitable for the client (not psychotherapy), the coach can use a series of criteria (Dryden, 2018a): (1) emotional problem is recent and intermittent; (2) is limited to specific contexts/situations; (3) is associated with mild to moderate distress; (4) is recognized by the coachee; (5) the client is willing to change it.

The ABCDEFG Model for Solving Emotional Problems

The ABC(DEF) model (Ellis, 1956, 1962, 1991, 1994) is a core explanatory framework of REBT which states that our reactions (Cs – emotional, behavioral or physiological consequences) are determined in a great part not by the negative situations (As – Activating events) but by the Beliefs we hold about them (Bs). This model was further developed in order to specify change steps for the coaching field into ABCDEFG (Dryden, 2018a, 2018b), with the G step being focused towards setting a Goal for change (the new adaptive C), the D step being Disputing or restructuring coachee's irrational thinking, E referring to the effective new approach or rational beliefs, and the F standing for Functional consequences or a new philosophy of life.

There are three disputing strategies (DiGiuseppe et al., 2014) that can be used in this process:

(a) Logical disputing – by asking whether the belief held by the coachee is logical;
(b) Empirical disputing, by questioning if the belief held by the coachee has empirical evidence; and
(c) Pragmatic/functional disputing, by questioning whether the belief held by the coachee is helpful.

In the end, the coachee is expected to learn to adopt a flexible rational problem-solving mindset in order to be their own coach when facing adversities. The ABC(DEF) model can integrate problem solving models for changing the As (such as the PRACTICE model) or can be integrated in other models, depending on client goals/needs.

The PRACTICE Model of Solving Practical Life Problems

The PRACTICE model of coaching was developed by Palmer (2008, 2009; see also Neenan & Palmer, 2012) based on the problem-solving theory and is meant to address practical problems or activating events (As) based on the ABC model.

The PRACTICE model includes the following steps: **P**roblem identification, **R**ealistic, relevant goal development, **A**lternative potential solutions generated, **C**onsequences of potential solutions considered, **T**argeting most feasible potential solution, **I**mplementing the chosen solution, **C**onsolidation of the chosen solution, and **E**valuation. The first step in the process refers to identifying and putting the problem in perspective, while the second step refers to setting specific and realistic goals for solving the problem. In the next phase, a brainstorming process is supported by the coach and afterwards potential solutions are considered based on their anticipated consequences and the most adequate solution is selected. The next phase consists of developing an action plan and implementing it based on selected solution, while offering lose monitoring and assessment of the success of solving the problem in the end. The PRACTICE model is meant to make use of the ABC model at any step if an emotional problem is identified.

Tools and Techniques Used in REBC

Comprehensive Assessment The field of coaching suffers from the lack of valid instruments meant to measure its outcomes, CBC and REBC fields have been informed from their therapeutic tradition that supports the importance of using valid assessment (e.g., guided by the ABC model; see David & Breightmeyer, 2018). There are a few instruments developed in the REBC paradigm for measuring irrational/rational beliefs in various settings: Managerial Rational and Irrational Beliefs Scale (David, 2013); Employee Rational and Irrational Beliefs Scale (Gavita & Duta, 2013), Parent Rational and Irrational Beliefs Scale (Gavita et al., 2011). There are also technological developments that allow the momentary assessment of functional/dysfunctional emotions and beliefs based on the REBC theory – the MoodWheel app (David, 2013).

Structured Formulation and Process Based on Models REBC formulation and change process are making use of the ABC generic model adapted to the type of the goal/problem (see Fig. 12.1; David & Bernard, 2018).

REBT and CBT have underlined the importance of using a case formulation and of the client accepting it. Thus, REBC uses a validated model that helps to explain to client's the mechanisms that need to be changed for reaching their goals. Afterwards, as described above, the situational ABCDEFG model is used to guide the process of change.

Elegant Solution to Life Problems REBC is interested in pursuing what Ellis has called the elegant solution for helping people grow and overcome their emotional

Components/ Tools	A Activating events and context		B Beliefs-Strengths and weaknesses		C Consequences: Behaviors, emotions, physiology, cognitions	
Assessment focus and conceptualization	Opportunities, threats Environment: Context, roles, culture, changes		Strengths, weaknesses Schemas, Beliefs, Mindset, Perspectives, Values, Personality characteristics		Behaviors, Emotions, Physiology, Cognitions Meaning and motivation	
Coaching focus	Goal	Problem	Goal	Problem	Goal	Problem
G - Examples goals/problems per area	"I want more friends", "I would like to go out more often", "I want to be more engaged in pleasant activities"	"I do not have friends", "I spend too much time on FB", "I do not like what I do for living"	"I want more meaning in my life", "I want to find work-life balance", "I want to build a healthier life perspective"	"I have lost my life meaning", "My work-life areas are in conflict", "My life perspective is that is not worth the effort"	"I want to feel happier" "I want to have higher performance in my work" "I want to relate better with my team"	"I feel stressed at work" "My performance at work has declined" "I have problems relating with my team"
Main coaching strategy*	Solution focused/Development focused	Practical problem solving	Development focused	Cognitive restructuring	Development focused	Behavior change, Emotional problem-solving, Skills building
Model selection (example)	GROW/GRAPE	PRACTICE	Generic, GRAPE	ABCDEFG	Generic, GRAPE	ABCDEFG

Fig. 12.1 The ABC model use for guiding REBC assessment and conceptualization

disturbances. This refers to producing philosophical changes by building a rational mindset and restructuring core beliefs by strengthening rational beliefs. It is a unique feature, since rational beliefs are considered proximal to emotional reactions. More specifically, REBC proposes the elegant solution to the self-esteem problem, by teaching unconditional self-acceptance (USA) as an essential mechanism that eliminates any type of self-rating. The USA philosophy refers to unconditionally accepting oneself as an imperfect human, whether or not the person is doing well or poorly, and whether or not others love or hate them.

Socratic Questioning REBC makes use of Socratic questioning as a powerful method of guided discovery, known as the cornerstone of REBT. The aim of Socratic questioning (Neenan, 2008) is to cultivate awareness and reflection and improve problem-solving thinking strategies. Thus, it is a method of guided discovery where the coach uses questions in order to support clients to identify and examine their thinking objectively in terms of accuracy (logical and empirical) and usefulness. This way, the coachee is encouraged in reaching own conclusions rather than the coach telling what they should be.

Addressing Secondary Emotions REBC is addressing secondary dysfunctional emotions (e.g., anxiety about anxiety) that can create emotional problems in time or exacerbate the existing ones. It is now accepted that the beliefs that people hold about their emotional difficulties are important mechanisms for their distress and are involved in maintaining these difficulties. One distinctive strategy that REBT used from the beginning was to initially address the secondary emotional problems and only then the primary emotional problems. In other words, in emotional problem focused REBC the coach will first assess the existence of a secondary emotional problem (being upset about being upset) and address that problem first in order to build effective emotion-regulation strategies.

Collaborative Empiricism REBC is based on developing a collaborative coach-coachee relationship as basis for co-investigating, problem solving and long-lasting change. While there are many ingredients for a successful coach-coachee relationship (e.g., empathy, trust, respect), the main ingredient emphasized in REBC and supported by scientific evidences (Grant, 2014) is collaboration. This collaborative relationship refers to agreeing the goals for coaching and the tasks that need to be accomplished in order to attain them. The collaborative empiricism refers to the partnership taken by the coach and coachee in identifying and testing coachees' beliefs as a means for change.

Action Plans REBC incorporates action plans, which in REBT are called homework, for supporting the autonomy of the client in implementing the agreed changes to reach their goals. Setting development plans is an essential tool of both CBT and REBT/REBC, which was recently found (deHaan, Duckworth, Birch, & Jones, 2013) as a component of the coach-coachee relationship correlated with positive coaching outcomes.

Close Monitoring and Feedback REBC discussion cultivates self-awareness of coachee's psychological blocks to change and emphasizes the essential role that close monitoring play is for approximating the changes. Thus, the coach is taking an active stance for monitoring the agreed tasks and offering close feedback (e.g., using the ABC form when working on emotion problems) and refining the plan accordingly.

Experiential Framework REBC employs an experiential framework based on designing development tasks that can give coachee the opportunity to try new experiences, to practice courage, and in the end to adopt different perspectives and change their mindset. Based on the behavioral experiments prescribed, the coachee is then encouraged during the sessions to derive conclusions and is supported to try new experiments which can help in reaching the agreed goals.

Empirical Basis of the REBC

While the coaching field used to rely on anecdotal evidence for its support (e.g., based on success stories and testimonials), the empirical data grew in time, evolving from low quality designs (case studies and within subjects) towards stronger designs (between group and randomized clinical trials). Developmental cognitive-behavioral coaching (having a solution-focused approach) has been the most commonly employed in the research and existing studies are documenting its effectiveness both in terms of life coaching and organizational/workplace coaching (Green et al., 2006) for enhancing goal attainment, psychological resilience and workplace well-being. Also, recent quantitative meta-analyses (de Meuse, Dai, & Lee, 2009; Jones, Woods, & Guillaume, 2016; Theeboom, Beersma, & van Vianen, 2014) document the effectiveness of CBC in the workplace, with small to high effect sizes, depending on the quality of the design (low effect sizes for better controlled designs) and type of the outcome (strong effect sizes for individual level performance and medium for the others).

In terms of its evidence base, REBC has a strong advantage given by the empirical support received by REBT and its positive applications relevant to coaching, such as REE, RET and REBT for the workplace (see David & Szamoskozi, 2011). The meta-analysis of David and Szamoskozi (2011) showed that among cognitive-behavioral interventions in the workplace, REBT had the larger effect sizes. This meta-analysis revealed high effect sizes for changes in irrationality and medium changes for emotional distress, and for measures of distress consequences after participating in workplace REBT.

There are a few studies that have investigated the effectiveness of REBC, focusing mostly on the workplace related outcomes. Palmer and Gyllensten (2008) describe a case study using REBC when they used multiple techniques to raise self-awareness of emotional reactions and to tackle procrastination, which in turn had effects on preventing a client's depressed mood. In another study, Gyllensten and Palmer (2005) used a quasi-experimental design in order to investigate the effects of REBC on stress. Thirty one employees from a UK finance organization participated in this study and they were randomly assigned to a coaching or wait-list condition. Participants in the REBC reported decreased anxiety and stress compared to the control condition after the intervention. However, no significant effect was found for depression.

We investigated the effectiveness of the newly developed Rational Managerial Coaching Program (David & Matu, 2013; Ratiu, David, & Baban, 2017) and Rational Leadership Program (David, Ionicioiu, Imbarus, & Sava, 2016) and found positive results in terms of positive effects on performance, stress, rational mindset, and leadership. Moreover, preliminary analyses showed that the rational mindset and mood improvements are functioning as mechanisms of change, supporting REBT/REBC theory.

Ogbuanya et al. (2017) investigated the effect of REBC on occupational stress and work ability among electronics workshop instructors. 108 electronics workshop instructors in technical colleges were included in the study, who were randomly assigned in two groups, one group received REBC, the other instructors were assigned to a wait-list control group. Results showed that participants the REBC group reported a significant reduction in occupational stress, work-related irrational beliefs, and an increase in work ability compared to participants in the waitlist control group. Most importantly, the improvements registered in the REBC group were maintained at 3-month follow-up. Since this study was conducted in Nigeria, the studies presented above in Romania, and most of the studies on REBT effectiveness in workplace in the USA and UK, we can conclude that there is preliminary evidence for cross-cultural suitability of the REBC.

Effectiveness of the REBC models presented above (e.g., ABC, PRACTICE) when used in coaching interventions has also been investigated. The effectiveness of the generic ABC(DEF) model was investigated in the self-coaching or personal development module of students taking a REBC course (David & Cobeanu, 2015). The ABC(DEF) model was presented during the courses and students used afterwards the ABC(DEF) form for monitoring and carrying out action plans. Results have shown that after taking the course participants (N = 105) reported lower levels of depressed mood, as well as improvements in their work performance. Their improvements in emotion–regulation skills and the quality of their homework tasks was found as mechanisms of change for their outcomes.

David, Matu, Pintea, Cotet, and Nagy (2014) explored the most effective components of the ABC(DEF) model in a qualitative study. The forms of the students were collected (340 forms) and coded by external raters in accordance with the REBC theory. Results showed that students used the forms more often for managing own anxiety and anger. Demandingness, Awfulizing and Global Evaluation were most frequently reported when forms are used for anxiety, while low frustration tolerance is associated with anger. The beliefs themes most often reported when monitoring anxiety were comfort, affiliation, achievement, while fairness theme was most frequently identified when using forms for dealing with anger. Pragmatic cognitive restructuring was the most frequently used by trainees. This study offers evidence for supporting the use of the ABC(DEF) model in personal development and were in line with the theoretical predictions form the cognitive model of REBT.

In order to answer the question as to the importance of a positive approach in coaching (e.g., solution-focused), such as claimed in the coaching field, we investigated in a recent study (Comsa & David, 2018) the comparative efficacy of the GROW model – solution-focused model- versus the PRACTICE - REBT based-model in coaching. This study supported the efficacy of both models and we could not find any significant difference between them. Thus, the superiority of solution focused models is not supported by empirical data. Based on the data presented above, we can say that REBC is a form of coaching that is using evidence-based theoretical models and programs.

Applications of REBC

REBC is suitable for use in many contexts (see Bernard & David, 2018), with life coaching being the most popular for personal growth; other close fields to clinical psychology are health coaching (Palmer, 2004) or parenting and family coaching (David et al., 2017), but also in organizational field (Criddle, 2007a, 2007b), executive and managerial coaching (David et al., 2016; Grieger & Fralick, 2007; Kirby, 1993). More recently, in order to better adapt REBT to the coaching field, brief versions of REBC were proposed (1–6 sessions; Dryden, 2017) and also technology based REBC tools (PsyPills app; David, Soflau, & Matu, 2018).

Life REBC

REBC-based life coaching addresses coachees' life goals. When approaching life practical or emotional problems, the coach can use one of the models presented above (e.g., the ABCDEFG model; see Dryden, 2010, 2018a). When adopting developmental coaching, the coach needs to make use of the 11 rational principles for living a happy life described by Bernard (2011) that we mentioned above.

In developmental life coaching, the goal is to build a new rational living philosophy based on incorporating these principles in the living habits of the coachee. In order to do this, the coach works collaboratively with the coachee in a series of steps (see the GRAPE model) that allow (1) selecting a development goal based on an in depth analyze of client's personal values, then(2) Identifying the rational principles that support the growth goal, then(3) Developing an action plan for implementing specific changes in line with the identified rational principles, then (4) Identifying personal strengths, resources, and obstacles for implementing the changes, and in the end (5) Monitoring implementation and evaluating the goal attainment, using specific techniques described above and others (e.g., based on positive psychology).

REBC in Organizations

RET offers the first REBT program for applying REBT principles in the workplace, including strategies for dealing with specific issues that might be encountered, such as participant resistance (see DiMattia, 1990). Subsequently, there were other models and programs which specify the applications of REBT in the leadership development and workplace (Kirby, 1993; Grieger & Fralick, 2007).

DiMattia proposed a set of principles of rationality in organizations that would need to be internalized by the managers and employees when applying developmental REBC, such as: Self-knowledge; Flexibility; Realism and reality acceptance:; Unconditional self-acceptance and self-confidence:; Respect for self and others; Discomfort and frustration tolerance; Aiming at long term benefits; Taking calculated risks; Being balanced; Taking responsibility for own emotions and behaviors; Self-directedness and involvement.

DiMattia's (1990) REBC approach consists of four main steps, that can be used both in individual or group work: Step 1: identifying the problems faced by clients; Step 2: establishing goals for change; Step 3: addressing behavioral, emotive and cognitive obstacles that interfere with the goals; Step 4: analyzing the above mentioned three components, with the behavioral one being primarily addressed. The effectiveness of the REBT based workplace interventions, (i.e., in the form of EAPs or counseling) was documented and the results of a recent quantitative meta-analysis (David & Szamoskozi, 2011) synthesizing these studies is showing that it brings high level benefits.

Performance REBC: High Performance Mindset at Work (HPMW; Bernard, 2018)

Bernard identified a set of positive psychological capacities for high work performance based on various positive psychological theories, in the form of rational beliefs, character strengths, psychological capital, mindfulness, authenticity, self-efficacy, optimism etc. He then categorized the psychological capabilities into a *high-performance capability framework* or the *architecture of the high performance mindset* (Bernard, 2013) and organized them in a self-survey that can be used during coaching for their assessment (see chapter in this book, REBT in the Workplace). In order to describe the process of HPMW coaching Bernard uses the four-step *Grape Model* described above.

Executive REBC

Ellis (1972) proposed the *rational model of leadership,* in which he emphasized the importance of rational sensitivity, concentration, discipline, rational decisions, effective communication and unconditional acceptance in this model. Grieger and Fralick (2007) further developed these components under the name of *the tree of extraordinary leadership*, using the categories of results, means and source. In this model, results are located at the top of the tree, where fruits grow, and can consist of strengths that contribute to profit, such as teamwork, relationships with employees, employee satisfaction.

The Freeman-Gavita Prescriptive Executive Coaching model (Gavita, Freeman & Sava, 2012) is an integrative and multi-modal framework based on an initial assessment multi-source survey for executives and using the REBC principles for developing problematic areas and capitalizing on the strengths of the executives. Various REBC tools presented before can be used for teaching the executives about how their mindset and beliefs are influencing their behaviors, performance and work relationships, and how to adopt a more effective mindset based on cognitive and behavioral rehearsal.

The Rational Leadership Program is a REBC model of executive coaching that was developed based on the theories and techniques presented above by the author. The Rational Leadership Program consists of a 5 h workshop focused on managerial performance mindset, managerial coaching, leadership, and self-regulation strategies. The program was tested by David et al. (2016) in a multinational banking group. 59 executive managers participated in the program during the financial crisis and completed questionnaires regarding their emotion management, performance and irrational/rational beliefs. Results showed that the Rational Leadership Program was effective in reducing executives' depressed mood, irrational beliefs, strengthening their rational beliefs and managerial skills considered as performance indicators. Mechanisms of change analyses found that strengthening executives' rational beliefs based on their rational mindset was responsible for reducing their depressed mood. Fairness demanding beliefs were identified as mechanisms of change for improvements registered after the program in executives' managerial skills.

Managerial Coaching

Managerial coaching is considered a development tool based on effective leadership practices which is meant to facilitate the learning processes of the employees for being more effective in their roles. More and more companies are investing in teaching their managers on how they can use coaching for empowering their subordinates to gain skills that make them capable to solve problems and make decisions. This way, the manager invests more time and energy in the short run but gains more in the long run in terms of both performance and time to solve complex problems.

The Rational Managerial Coaching Program (**rMCP**; David & Matu, 2013; Ratiu et al., 2017) is a program using REBT models and rational leadership theory for developing leaders in their managerial coaching roles. The program consists of three main modules: (1) a group workshop session of 4 h, where the basics of managerial coaching are discussed, (2) an individual coaching session with each manager, (3) a shadowing individual coaching session, (4) a group coaching and observational assessment of managerial behaviors/skills during a managerial coaching simulated session. The workshop is focused on (a) using a model for managerial coaching (the PRACTICE/GRAPE/GROW model), (b) efficient communication and feedback skills, (c) motivating and empowering employees, and (d) self-coaching for building emotional muscle. The workshop makes use of experiential learning strategies of the managerial coaching behaviors/skills and managerial soft-skills (e.g., role-plays); each manager is asked to develop their own action plan to be followed during the individual coaching sessions. The rMCP proved to be effective in improving managerial coaching skills based both on self-report but also on observation, improving performance and satisfaction with the team and building their rational beliefs, reducing manager's distress and irrational beliefs (David & Matu, 2013). Moderation analyses showed that managers showing a higher level of optimism reported higher emotional improvements following the program, even when faced with a major life event, like being fired.

Future Directions in the REBC Field

Although coaching is nowadays considered a suitable intervention for achieving personal or work-related goals, there are important questions that need to be answered in coaching in general and also in REBC, with the most important one being concerned with growing its evidence-based status level based on sound research methodologies. Most of the studies conducted to date for testing the effectiveness of REBC have used within-subject designs and, thus, we cannot draw definite conclusions based on them. Future studies need to use controlled designs and adequate measures in order to be able to provide strong support for its effects – both efficacy and effectiveness. However, we need to note that due to the characteristics of both coaching and its clients (high costs, status, organizational contracts) there are difficulties in conducting well powered and designed studies and this makes the progress of the scientific knowledge in the field slower. However, it was suggested (Stober & Grant, 2006) that the methods specific to the clinical field might not be the most adequate for the coaching field and thus specific methods need to be used and developed, such as social network analysis etc.

Another important future direction of the REBC and coaching field in general is related to investigating its mechanisms of change and responding to the question how does coaching work. Only preliminary studies have been conducted in this direction, analyzing mainly moderators or using weaker designs. Our studies (David & Matu, 2013; David & Cobeanu, 2015; David et al., 2016) have confirmed the role of reducing irrational beliefs and strengthening rational thinking in building psychological resilience, reducing stress, and enhancing performance. Future studies will need to use stronger methodologies and also investigate general factors as mechanisms of change (e.g., collaborative relationship, motivation etc.).

An important question that needs to be answered is concerned with the role of the model used. REBC has used the ABC(DEFG) model and this is a generalized model of change which received adequate support for personal improvement goals and workplace related goals (David & Matu, 2013; David & Cobeanu, 2015; David et al., 2016). There is a debate however in the coaching field regarding the solutions focus that this field needs to have based on its positive approach. REBC has We have investigated the comparative efficacy of the PRACTICE and GROW model and we did not find any differences between them. Future studies will need to extend this research and establish the most effective models, approaches (DF vs PF) and techniques for specific goals that clients bring in REBC.

REBC is especially suited for being delivered based on technology developments, which have the potential to best serve coaching clients which are frequent users of technology. Palmer (2004) describes a case study in which he successfully used blended REBC, with face to face, telephone and online coaching. Incorporating technology in REBC carries the potential of improving its efficacy. A few examples in this direction express differently are the PsyPills app, the REThink serious online game, the online Rational Positive Parenting Program. Also, assessment, monitoring and feedback during action plan can benefit from being mediated by mobile phones, using experience sampling methods. The PsyPills app is a mobile (IOS based) lifestyle application that give rational thinking prescriptions to users in the form of psychological pills and can be also used for assessment and monitoring (with the free MoodWheel version only for assessment). The app was tested preliminary and results support its effectiveness (David & David, in preparation). Future studies need to test the efficacy and cost-effectiveness of technology mediated coaching together with client satisfaction.

An important line of REBC study is concerned with tracking brain changes following participation in coaching, using neuroimaging methods. While neuroscience folk language is often used by practitioners of pseudoscientific forms of coaching in order to suggest a scientific approach to the naïve client, the field of neuroscience has expanded dramatically during the last decades and so did the research concerning neural changes following CBT/REBT which can be used as source of information in REBC research. There are studies (e.g., Toepper et al., 2010) exploring the key brain areas mediating learning which are of key importance for the coaching field. Data can be used as informant for the neural changes that are correlated with subjective, behavioral and cognitive changes brought by REBC. Dias et al. (2015) discusses the benefits of such research, including using brain imaging as a tool to predict coaching effectiveness or as a means to detect its effectiveness. There are also challenges of conducting such studies though given the time pressures and performance demands of the population that requests coaching.

References

Anderson, J. P. (2002). Executive coaching and REBT: Some comments from the field. *Journal of Rational-Emotive & Cognitive-Behavior Therapy, 20*, 223–233.

Bernard, M. E. (2011). *Rationality and the pursuit of happiness: The legacy of Albert Ellis*. London: John Wiley & Sons.

Bernard, M. E. (2013). *The high-performance mindset at work* (2nd ed., p. 140). Southbank, Australia: The Bernard Group.

Bernard, M. E. (2018). Coaching high workplace performance. In M. E. Bernard & O. A. David (Eds.), *Coaching for rational living. Theory, techniques and applications*. New York, NY: Springer Press.

Bernard, M. E., & David, O. A. (2018). *Coaching for rational living. Theory, techniques and applications*. New York, NY: Springer Press.

Broder, M. S. (2012). *Stage climbing: The shortest path to your highest potential*. Philadelphia, PA: Media Psychology Associates.

Comsa, L., & David, O. A. (2018). GROW or PRACTICE in coaching? That is the question. Manuscript under review.

Criddle, W. D. (2007a). Adapting REBT to the world of business. *Journal of Rational-Emotive & Cognitive-Behaviour Therapy, 25*, 87–105.

Criddle, W. D. (2007b). The transition from therapist to executive coach. *Journal of Rational-Emotive & Cognitive-Behaviour Therapy, 25*, 121–141.

David, A. R., & Szamoskozi, S. (2011). A meta-analytical study on the effects of cognitive behavioral techniques for reducing distress in organizations. *Journal of Cognitive and Behavioral Psychotherapies, 11*(2), 221–236.

David, O. A. (2013). Prescriptive index: Development and validation of the mood wheel and manager-rational and irrational beliefs scale. *Romanian Journal of Applied Psychology, 15*(2), 41–50.

David, O. A. (2016). The foundations and evolution of cognitive behavioral coaching in organizations: An interview with Dominic DiMattia. *Journal of Rational-Emotive and Cognitive-Behavioral Therapy, 34*, 282–288.

David, O. A., & Bernard, M. E. (2018). Coaching for rational living: Rational-emotive, cognitive-behavioral perspectives. In M. E. Bernard & O. A. David (Eds.), *Coaching for rational living. Theory, techniques and applications*. New York, NY: Springer Press.

David, O. A., & Breightmeyer, A. (2018). Assessment, case formulation and intervention models. In M. E. Bernard & O. A. David (Eds.), *Coaching for rational living. Theory, techniques and applications*. New York, NY: Springer Press
David, O. A., Capris, D., & Jarda, A. (2017). Online coaching of emotion-regulation strategies for parents: Efficacy of the online rational positive parenting program and attention bias modification procedures. *Frontiers in Psychology, Special Issue Emotion Science, 8*. https://doi.org/10.3389/fpsyg.2017.00500
David, O. A., & Cobeanu, O. (2015). Evidence-based training in cognitive-behavioural coaching: Can personal development bring less distress and better performance? *British Journal of Guidance & Counselling, 44*, 12–25.
David, O. A., Ionicioiu, I., Imbarus, C. A., & Sava, F. A. (2016). Coaching banking managers through the financial crisis: Effects on stress, resilience, and performance. *Journal of Rational-Emotive and Cognitive-Behavioral Therapy, 34*(4), 267–281.
David, O. A., Matu, A., Pintea, S., Cotet, C., & Nagy, D. (2014). Cognitive-behavioral processes based on using the ABC analysis by trainees' for their personal development. *Journal of Rational-Emotive and Cognitive-Behavioral Therapy, 32*(3), 198–215.
David, O. A., & Matu, S. A. (2013). How to tell if managers are good coaches and how to help them improve during adversity? The managerial coaching assessment system and the rational managerial coaching program. *Journal of Cognitive and Behavioral Psychotherapies, 13*, 259–274.
David, O. A., Soflau, R., & Matu, S. (2018). Technology and coaching. In M. E. Bernard & O. A. David (Eds.), *Coaching for rational living. Theory, techniques and applications*. New York, NY: Springer Press.
De Meuse, K. P., Dai, G., & Lee, R. J. (2009). Evaluating the effectiveness of executive coaching: Beyond ROI? *Coaching: An International Journal of Theory, Research and Practice, 2*(2), 117–134.
deHaan, E., Duckworth, A., Birch, D., & Jones, C. (2013). Executive coaching outcome research: The contribution of common factors such as relationship, personality match, and self-efficacy. *Consulting Psychology Journal: Practice and Research, 65*, 40–57.
DiMattia, D. (1990). *Rational effectiveness training: Increasing productivity at work*. New York, NY: Institute for Rational Emotive Therapy.
DiMattia, D., & IJzermans, T. (1996). *Reaching their minds: A trainer's manual for rational effectiveness training*. New York, NY: Institute for Rational – Emotive Therapy.
Dryden, W. (2010). Dealing with Clients' Emotional Problems in Life Coaching: A Rational-Emotive and Cognitive Behaviour Therapy (RECBT) Approach. London, UK: Routledge.
Dryden, W. (2011). *First steps in using REBT in life coaching*. New York, NY: Albert Ellis Institute.
Dryden, W. (2017). *Very brief, cognitive behavioural coaching*. Hove, UK: Routledge.
Dryden, W. (2018a). Life coaching. In M. E. Bernard & O. A. David (Eds.), *Coaching for rational living. Theory, techniques and applications*. New York, NY: Springer Press.
Dryden, W. (2018b). *Rational emotive behavioural coaching: Distinctive features*. New York, NY: Routledge.
Dias, G.P., Palmer, S., O'Riordan, S., de Freitas, S.B., Habib, L.R., do Nascimento Bevilaqua, M.C., & Nardi, A.E. (2015). Perspectives and challenges for the study of brain responses to coaching: Enhancing the dialogue between the fields of neuroscience and coaching psychology. *The Coaching Psychologist 11*(1), 21–29.
Digiuseppe, R. A., Doyle, C. A., Dryden, W., and Backx, W. (2014). A Practitioner's Guide to Rational Emotive Behavior Therapy, 3rd Ed. New York, NY: Oxford University Press.
Ellis, A. (1956). The ABC model of rational emotive therapy. Paper presented at the *American Psychological Association (APA) Convention*, Chicago, IL.
Ellis, A. (1962, 1994). *Reason and emotion in psychotherapy* (re. ed.). Secaucus, NJ: Birch Lane.
Ellis, A. (1972). *Executive leadership: A rational approach*. New York, NY: Institute for Rational Living.
Ellis, A. (1991). The revised ABC's of rational-emotive therapy (RET). *Journal of Rational-Emotive & Cognitive-Behavior Therapy, 9*(3), 139–172.

Ellis, A. (1999). *How to make yourself happy and remarkably less disturbable*. Atascadero, CA: Impact Publishers.

Ellis, A., & Harper, R. A. (1961). *A guide to rational living*. Englewood Cliffs, NJ: Prentice-Hall.

Ellis, A., & DiMattia, D. (1991). Rational effectiveness training: A new method for facilitating management and labor relationships. New York, NY: Institute for rational emotive therapy.

Ellis, A., Powers, & Harper, R. A. (1975). *A new guide to rational living*. Englewood Cliffs, NY: Prentice-Hall.

Ellis, A., Powers, M., & Becker, I. (1982). *A guide to personal happiness*. Hollywood, CA: Wilshire Book Company.

Gavita, O. A., DiGiuseppe, R., David, D. & DelVecchio, T. (2011). The development and validation of the Parent Rational and Irrational Beliefs Scale. Procedia of Social and Behavioral Sciences, 30, 2305 – 2311.

Gaviţa, O. A., & Duţă, T. (2013). The employee rational and irrational beliefs scale: Preliminary validation. *Transylvanian Journal of Psychology, 14*(1), 19–39.

Gavita, O. A., Freeman, A., & Sava, A. F. (2012). The development and validation of the Freeman-Gavita Prescriptive Executive Coaching (PEC) Multi-Rater Assessment. *Journal of Cognitive and Behavioral Psychotherapies, 12*(2), 159–174.

Grant, A. M. (2014). Autonomy support, relationship satisfaction and goal focus in the coach –coachee relationship: Which best predicts coaching success? *Coaching: An International Journal of Theory, Research and Practice, 7*(1), 18–38.

Green, L. S., Oades, L. G., & Grant, A. M. (2006). Cognitive-behavioural, solution-focused life coaching: Enhancing goal striving, well-being and hope. *Journal of Positive Psychology, 1*, 142–149.

Grieger, R. (2007). One REBTers model for business consulting. *Journal of Rational-Emotive & Cognitive-Behavior Therapy, 25*, 107–120.

Grieger, R., & Fralick, F. (2007). The use of REBT principles and practices in leadership training and development. *Journal of Rational-Emotive and Cognitive-Behavior Therapy, 25*, 143–154.

Gyllensten, K., & Palmer, S. (2005). Can coaching reduce workplace estress: A quasi-experimental study. *International Journal of Evidence Based Coaching and Mentoring, 3*, 75–85.

Jones, R. J., Woods, S. A., & Guillaume, Y. R. (2016). The effectiveness of workplace coaching: A meta-analysis of learning and performance outcomes from coaching. *Journal of Occupational and Organizational Psychology, 89*, 249–277.

Kirby, P. (1993). RET counseling: Application in management and executive development. *Journal of Rational-Emotive & Cognitive Behavior Therapy, 11*, 7–18.

Klarreich, S. H., DiGiuseppe, R., & DiMattia, D. J. (1987). Cost effectiveness of an employee assistance program with rational-emotive therapy. *Professional Psychology: Research and Practice, 18*(2), 140–144.

Knaus, W. J. (1974). *Rational-emotive education: A manual for elementary school teachers*. New York, NY: Institute for Rational Living.

Kodish, S. P. (2002). Rational emotive behavior coaching. *Journal of Rational-Emotive & Cognitive Behavior Therapy, 20*, 235–246.

Montgomery, G. H., David, D., DiLorenzo, T. A., & Schnur, J. B. (2007). Response expectancies and irrational beliefs predict exam-related distress. *Journal of Rational-Emotive and Cognitive-Behavior Therapy, 25*(1), 17–34.

Neenan, M. (2008). From cognitive behaviour therapy (CBT) to cognitive behaviour coaching (CBC). *Journal of Rational-Emotive & Cognitive-Behavior Therapy, 26*, 3–15.

Neenan, M., & Dryden, W. (2001). *Life coaching: A cognitive-behavioural approach* (p. 2014). Hove, UK: Routledge.

Neenan, M., & Palmer, S. (Eds.). (2012). *Cognitive behavioural coaching in practice: An evidence-based approach*. Hove, UK: Routledge.

Ogbuanya, T. C., Eseadi, C., Orji, C. T., Ohanu, I. B., Bakare, J., & Ede, M. O. (2017). Effects of rational emotive behavior coaching on occupational stress and work ability among electronics workshop instructors in Nigeria. *Medicine, 96*(19), e6891.

Palmer, S. (2004). Health coaching: A developing field within health education. *Health Education Journal, 63*(2), 189–191.
Palmer, S. (2008). The PRACTICE model of coaching: Towards a solution-focused approach. *Coaching Psychology International, 1*(1), 4–8.
Palmer, S. (2009). Rational coaching: A cognitive behavioural approach. *The Coaching Psychologist, 5*, 12–19.
Palmer, S., & Gyllensten, K. (2008). How cognitive behavioural, rational emotive behavioural or multimodal coaching could prevent mental health problems, enhance performance and reduce work related stress. *Journal of Rational-Emotive & Cognitive-Behavior Therapy, 26*, 38–52.
Palmer, S., & Szymańska, K. (2007). Cognitive behavioural coaching. An integrative approach. In S. InPalmer & A. Whybrow (Eds.), *Handbook of coaching psychology. A guide for practitioners* (pp. 86–117). London, UK: Routledge.
Ratiu, L., David, O., & Baban, A. (2017). Developing managerial skills through coaching: Efficacy of a cognitive-behavioral coaching program. *Journal of Rational-Emotive Cognitive-Behavior Therapy, 35*, 88–110. https://doi.org/10.1007/s10942-015-0225-8
Stober, D. R., & Grant, A. M. (Eds.). (2006). *Evidence based coaching handbook: Putting best practices to work for your clients*. Hoboken, NJ: John Wiley & Sons Inc.
Theeboom, T., Beersma, B., & van Vianen, A. E. (2014). Does coaching work? A meta-analysis on the effects of coaching on individual level outcomes in an organizational context. *Journal of Positive Psychology, 9*(1), 1–18.
Toepper, M., Gebhardt, H., Beblo, T., Thomas, C., Driessen, M., Bischoff, M., … Sammer, G. (2010). Functional correlates of distractor suppression during spatial working memory encoding. *Neuroscience, 165*(4), 1244–1253.
Williams, H., Edgerton, N., & Palmer, S. (2010). Cognitive behavioural coaching. In E. Cox, T. Bachkirova, & D. Clutterbuck (Eds.), *The complete handbook of coaching*. London, UK: Sage.

Chapter 13
Rational Emotive Behavior Education in Schools

Ann Vernon and Michael E. Bernard

Albert Ellis pioneered the application of rational-emotive behavior therapy (REBT) to the treatment of children and adolescents in the mid 1950s, and it has a long-standing history of application in schools. As Ellis stated, "I have always believed in the potential of REBT to be used in schools as a form of mental health promotion and with young people experiencing developmental problems" (Ellis & Bernard, 2006, p. ix). Many years ago Ellis stressed the importance of a prevention curriculum designed to help young people "help themselves" by learning positive mental health concepts that will benefit them in the present as well as in the future (Ellis, 1972).

The educational derivative of REBT, rational-emotive behavior education (REBE) can be applied with children and adolescents individually, in classrooms and small groups, and in consultation with parents, teachers, and other school personnel (Vernon, 2007, 2009). There are now a number of "best practice" school-based programs that address social-emotional development based on REBT, including *rational emotive education* (Knaus, 1974), the *Thinking, Feeling, Behaving* curricula (Vernon, 2006a, 2006b), and *You Can Do It! Education* (Bernard, 2006a, 2006b, 2007, 2018a, 2018b). These programs all support Bernard's contention (Ellis & Bernard, 2006) that teaching children social and emotional competence is essential not only for their social and emotional well-being, but also for their academic achievement, success in life, self-management, and sense of social responsibility.

REBE's distinctiveness as a prevention, promotion and intervention approach is focused on emotional and behavioral self-awareness, self-management and

A. Vernon (✉)
University of Northern Iowa, Cedar Falls, IA, USA

M. E. Bernard
Melbourne Graduate School of Education, University of Melbourne, Parkville, VIC, Australia

California State University, Long Beach, Long Beach, CA, USA

© Springer Nature Switzerland AG 2019
M. E. Bernard, W. Dryden (eds.), *Advances in REBT*,
https://doi.org/10.1007/978-3-319-93118-0_13

change. It teaches children and adolescents rational thinking including the strengthening of rational beliefs (e.g., self-acceptance, high frustration tolerance, other-acceptance, non-approval seeking, responsible risk taking), how to challenge and re-structure irrational beliefs employing a variety of cognitive, emotional and behavioral change methods. REBT and REBE has for many years been used with parents (e.g., Çekiç, Akbas, Turan, & Hamamcı, 2016; Joyce, 1995) and teachers in a consultative role (e.g., Forman & Forman, 1980), where the emphasis is on helping them deal with their own irrational beliefs and unhealthy negative emotions that negatively impact their ability to interact appropriately with children and prevent them from being effective role models. The premise is that by helping adults deal with their own problems they in turn will be more effective parents and teachers as well as model and teach rationality to their children.

In this chapter, a brief rationale for social-emotional education programs is addressed, with specific emphasis on REBT principles that enhance development. Examples of core concepts and implementation guidelines will be described, along with a specific lesson to illustrate the process. In addition, the *You Can Do It! Education* program will be reviewed, with supporting research, theory, and practice. Finally, we'll briefly review the use of REBT and REBT as a form of stress management that is employed by school counselors and psychologists.

The Rationale for Social-Emotional Education Programs

We live in a complex, rapidly-changing world that poses multiple challenges for children and adolescents as they are faced with circumstances and decisions that are often beyond their developmental capacity to deal with. Years ago psychologist David Elkind (1988) contended that youth are growing up too fast, too soon, which is much more of a reality in this contemporary society where the Internet and the media, as well as day-to-day experiences, expose youth to adult issues that they may not be far beyond their capacity to fully comprehend. A compounding factor is that children and many adolescents have not achieved formal operational thinking, which has significant ramifications for how they perceive events and predisposes them to irrational thinking in the form of overgeneralizations, frustration intolerance, demanding, and self/other downing (Vernon, 2007, 2009).

For increasing numbers of young people, dealing with typical developmental issues is overshadowed by the more serious situational problems they face, such as being victims of bullying or cyber bullying, living with increasing anxiety due to the high prevalence of violence throughout the world, or dealing with varying forms of family dysfunction including abuse and neglect, separation and divorce, substance abuse, and various types of loss. Depression, anxiety, suicide or suicide ideation, eating disorders, and substance abuse result when young people are not unsuccessful in dealing with their problems (Henderson & Thompson, 2011; Vernon, 2009).

Unfortunately, many youth will not receive mental health services, which further exacerbates the problems. Even if there is treatment, it may be costly or ineffective. For these reasons, a proactive, preventive approach is imperative. If implemented systematically in schools, all children can learn in an environment that promotes social and emotional growth, giving them "tools" that equip them to better handle life's challenges. These types of programs help children "grow up before they give up."

The important role and effcts of social and emotional learning skills (SELs) in student learning and well-being has been well documented (Durlak, Weissberg, Dymnicki, Taylor, & Schellinger, 2011). The Collaborative for Academic, Social, and Emotional Learning (CASEL), a leading international organization promoting theory, research, intervention, and policy-advocacy related to SEL, identifies SEL as encompassing the following five sets of competencies ("SEL Competencies," n.d.).

- Self-awareness: The ability to accurately recognize one's emotions and thoughts and their influence on behavior. This includes accurately assessing one's strengths and limitations and possessing a well-grounded sense of confidence and optimism.
- Self-management: The ability to regulate one's emotions, thoughts, and behaviors effectively in different situations. This includes managing stress, controlling impulses, motivating oneself, and setting and working toward achieving personal and academic goals.
- Social awareness: The ability to take the perspective of and empathize with others from diverse backgrounds and cultures, to understand social and ethical norms for behavior, and to recognize family, school, and community resources and supports.
- Relationship skills: The ability to establish and maintain healthy and rewarding relationships with diverse individuals and groups. This includes communicating clearly, listening actively, cooperating, resisting inappropriate social pressure, negotiating conflict constructively, and seeking and offering help when needed.
- Responsible decision making: The ability to make constructive and respectful choices about personal behavior and social interactions based on consideration of ethical standards, safety concerns, social norms, the realistic evaluation of consequences of various actions, and the well-being of self and others.

CASEL further defines SEL as encompassing a set of interventions at all levels of a school, designed to promote the development of those skills in continuous and coordinated ways (Collaborative for Academic, Social, and Emotional Learning, 2013).

Today, throughout many states in the United States and in many countries (e.g., Singapore, Scotland, Australia), school-based programs that teach all students that learning and acting with SEL is the norm rather than the exception ("State Standards," n.d.; http://enseceurope.org/).

REBE is one of the oldest social and emotional learning programs (e.g., Knaus, 1974) with extensive research attesting to its effectiveness and qualifying it as a best, evidence-based practice (e.g., Bernard, 2006a; Gonzalez et al., 2004; Hajzler

& Bernard, 1991). Overall findings of this research were summarized by Trip, Vernon, and McMahon (2007) as follows:

> REE has a powerful effect on lessening irrational beliefs and dysfunctional behaviors, plus a moderate effect concerning positive inference making and decreasing negative emotions. The efficiency of REE appeared to not be affected by the length of applied REE. Rather, the REE effect was strong when participants were concerned with their problems. Types of psychometric measure used for irrational beliefs evaluation affected the results. Effect sizes increased from medium to large when the subjects were children and adolescents compared to young adults.

More recent research supports the positive impact of REE on a variety of negative emotions, behaviors and irrational beliefs (e.g., Caruso et al., 2018; Lupu & Iftene, 2009; Mahfar, Aslan, Noah, Ahmad, & Jaafar, 2014).

Rational-Emotive Behavioral Education (REBE)

The basic premise of REBE is that a systematic, structured curriculum based on REBT principles can empower young people to take charge of their lives to the degree that this is possible, learning how to think, feel, and behave in self-enhancing rather than in self-defeating ways. REBT is uniquely suited for a prevention program because the principles can be easily transferred into specific developmentally-appropriate lessons, the concepts can be adapted to various age groups, ethnicities, and intelligence levels, and there are numerous cognitive-behavioral techniques that can employed in creative ways, making it much easier for them to comprehend what it being presented. This skills-oriented approach helps children deal more effectively with the problems of daily life in the present as well as in the future, and these "life lessons" better equip them to apply cognitive, emotive, and behavioral strategies to lessen the severity and intensity of problems that can impede their development and their success in life.

In addition, REBT reinforces goals compatible with educational goals: critical thinking skills, problem-solving and decision-making skills, practice and persistence, self-reliance and self-responsibility, and goal setting, all, which promote achievement. As will be discussed later in this chapter, achievement is what schools are all about. Implementing REBE in schools promotes achievement by reducing emotional upset which can interfere with learning, and by teaching children and adolescents specific skills such as persistence/frustration tolerance, goal setting, rational thinking, and self-acceptance which impact their achievement.

Core REBE Concepts

The basis on an REBE program emanates from REBT principles; namely, the interrelatedness of thoughts, feelings, and behaviors. Teaching young people that they can control their emotions and behaviors by changing the way they think is a powerful first step in helping them learn how to reduce emotional disturbance. As they learn that it is not the event itself that "makes" them feel or behave in unproductive ways, they also need to be taught how to change their thoughts by differentiating between facts and assumptions, identifying distorted cognitions and irrational beliefs, and learning how to dispute these faulty thinking patterns. The goal is to help them think more rationally, replace unhealthy negative emotions with healthy negative emotions, and reduce or eliminate self-defeating behaviors.

The following basic concepts can be developed into specific grade-level lessons as reflected in the *Thinking, Feeling, Behaving* curriculums (Vernon, 2006a, 2006b):

Self Acceptance In REBE, we distinguish between self-esteem and self-acceptance. Self-esteem implies putting a value on oneself as a good or bad person, for example. In contract, self-acceptance implies accepting oneself as a worthwhile human being who has strengths as well as weaknesses. Clearly this idea should be promoted in schools, helping students understand that as they learn new things, they will make mistakes. This doesn't mean that they are stupid; they can learn from their mistakes and set goals for self-improvement, but they should never equate their self-worth with their performance (Vernon, 2009)

Emotional and Behavioral Consequences As mentioned, a fundamental aspect of REBT is the emotions and behaviors result not from the event itself, but from the way one thinks about the event. It is important, therefore, that children and adolescents learn to identify how they feel and how they behave in relation to the feeling, always reinforcing the notion that they can change the way they feel and behave by changing their thoughts. Young people will need specific help in developing a feeling vocabulary, but feelings can also be inferred by helping them identify how they behaved in relation to a specific situation (Vernon, 2009).

Beliefs Children and adolescents need to learn how to differentiate between rational and irrational beliefs. Rational beliefs are consistent with reality and are flexible and self-enhancing. They help people achieve their goals and typically result in constructive behaviors and healthy negative emotions. Irrational beliefs are illogical, rigid, and result in unhealthy negative emotions and self-defeating behaviors. Irrational beliefs manifest themselves in the forms of demands (the absolute expectation that events or people must be the way an individual wants them to be), awfulizing (exaggerating the negative consequences of a situation), frustration intolerance (things should be easy, life should be comfortable), and global evaluation of human worth (individuals can be rated and some people are worthless) (DiGiuseppe, Doyle, Dryden, & Backx, 2014). Conveying these concepts to young people can be rather difficult, so it is essential to be creative and introduce these concepts in developmentally-appropriate ways as reflected in the *Thinking, Feeling, Behaving* curriculums (Vernon, 2006a, 2006b) and other social-emotional education programs.

Disputing Beliefs Disputing is the cornerstone of REBT, where irrational beliefs are replaced with rational beliefs. There are many different kinds of disputes that can be employed with children and adolescents. In addition to functional, logical, and empirical disputes, practitioners are strongly encouraged to incorporate disputational techniques into different types of developmentally-appropriate methods and reinforcing the new rational beliefs in numerous ways. For example, suppose that in a previous lesson third graders learned that everyone has strengths as well as weaknesses and that it is important not to rate themselves as an "all good or all bad." In a follow-up lesson on disputing, the facilitator might engage them in a puppet play, where one puppet is really down on himself because he missed two spelling words on his test. The other puppet will say things like: "just because you missed two doesn't mean you are stupid. Maybe you just didn't study enough, or maybe you do better in other subjects." After modeling this type of dialogue, the facilitator can ask for volunteers who will role play a different problem and "dispute" the irrational beliefs. When done in a developmentally-appropriate way, even younger children can grasp the essence of the concept, which will then be reinforced throughout the curriculum.

Implementation Guidelines

REBE can be implemented in several ways within the school setting: through social-structured emotional education lessons, integration into the curriculum, the teachable moment, and integration into the total school environment. While each has its merits, the structured emotional education lesson sequence is the "gold standard" – the preferred method – because REBE concepts are specifically taught so that children learn the theory and how to put it into practice. The other three methods are excellent ways of reinforcing these principles. In order to deliver a comprehensive program of this nature, it is imperative that teachers and other school personnel clearly understand the REBE philosophy, so teacher in-service is essential.

Structured REBE Lessons These lessons can be presented in classrooms or in small-group psycho-education counseling sessions. The lessons should be presented in a sequential manner so that the core concepts are introduced in grade 1 and then re-introduced and reinforced throughout elementary, middle school and high school, with the lessons reflecting developmentally-appropriate ways of presenting the ideas. These lessons should be engaging, creative, and experiential, with a great deal of student involvement and group interaction. This increases the likelihood that children will develop a good understanding of the concepts because they are presented and reinforced in various ways to appeal to auditory, visual, and kinesthetic learners.

Having a well-developed lesson is essential, and I (AV) recommend the following:

(a) Develop 2–3 specific objectives, which are grade-level appropriate for each lesson.

(b) Present a short stimulus activity to introduce the content and engage learners in the lesson. Examples of stimulus activities include games, art and music activities, writing and worksheets activities, drama, experiments, bibliotherapy, or role playing. The stimulus activity presents the content of the lesson that corresponds to the objectives identified for the lesson.

(c) Process the stimulus activity by engaging students in a discussion based on two types of questions: content questions and personalization questions. Content questions refer to the concepts that were presented in the stimulus activity. For example, if the facilitator had read a book to elementary-age children about anxiety, What If It Never Stops Raining? (Carlson, 1992), the questions would reflect the content of the book: "What did the boy in the story worry about? Did all of things he worried about actually occur? And if they did, was it as bad as he thought it would be? What did the boy in the story learn about worrying so much?" Personalization questions help them apply the concepts to their own lives. For example, "Do you ever worry a lot like the character in this story? Do the things you worry about usually come true? If they come true, are they as bad as you thought they would be? What are some of the things you do or could do to help you deal with your worries?" The emphasis in on practical application of the concepts, so it is important to allow adequate time for discussion.

An example of a lesson for middle school students is described below to give readers a better idea of an emotional education lesson on the topic of irrational beliefs, entitled *Rose Colored Glasses* (adapted from Vernon, 2006a, pp. 241–244).

Objective: To identify the effects of rational versus irrational thinking.
Materials needed: Two pair of glasses, one with the lenses covered in black construction paper and the other pair in pink paper.
Procedure/Stimulus Activity:

1. Review the concept of rational versus irrational thinking and explain that when we think irrationally, we often fail to differentiate facts from assumptions and we overgeneralize and awfulize, making things seem worse than they actually are. It is like "doom and gloom" thinking, where everything seems bad. Then contrast that with rational thinking characterized by looking at the facts and thinking logically and realistically, which can result in a positive as opposed to a negative perspective.
2. Divide the students into two groups and give one group the rose colored glasses (and have a volunteer put them on) and do the same for the group with the dark glasses. Inform them that you will be describe an event and in their groups, they are to generate responses about how they might think, feel, and behave relative to that event, based on the glasses they are wearing.
3. Read examples such as the following, but before moving to the next example, have each group share and compare their responses with regard to thoughts, feelings, and behaviors. Examples include: your best friend doesn't sit by you at lunch; your parents won't let you invite a particular friend over to spend the

night; you don't get a good grade on an assignment; your sister refuses to do her share of chores and you get blamed for it.

4. Discuss the content questions:

   - Do you see a difference between the way you think, feel and act when you have the dark glasses on as opposed to the rose-colored ones? What were some of the differences?
   - Which kind of thinking is more helpful? Why?

   Discuss the personalization questions:

   - Which kind of thinking do you typically practice?
   - What have been your experiences with the effects of irrational thinking?
   - If you wanted to change the way you think, how would you go about doing it? What do you think would be the results? What did you learn from this activity?

Integration into Subject Matter This is another viable way to reinforce principles learned from the structured lessons. With this approach, teachers integrate rational concepts into subject matter curriculum. For example, topics for writing assignments could include what it is like to make a mistake, what they consider to be personal strengths and weaknesses, or an example of a time when they thought through consequences of their behavior versus a time they did not. Vocabulary and spelling lessons could include feeling-word vocabularies and definitions. Social studies lessons could focus on facts versus assumptions as they relate to political campaigns or to the concept of fairness as it relates to oppressed groups throughout history. Frustration tolerance can be addressed by reading about how soldiers struggled during wars or by discussing examples from current events. As noted, although this is a less direct approach, the integration of these concepts into the regular curriculum has numerous benefits.

The Teachable Moment The assumption here is that teachers (and hopefully parents) will take advantage of teachable moments to introduce or reinforce rational concepts. This can be done with individuals, a small group, and an entire classroom. For example, when my son was playing his first football game in middle school, the team anticipated winning, but they lost. When I picked him up after the game he said that everyone felt terrible and that some boys were even crying because they thought it was their fault that the team lost. I asked what the coach did or said on the bus on the way back to the school, and he said that he didn't say a word. This would have been an ideal teachable moment, asking the boys how they felt, helping them understand that this was a team effort and not the fault of one or two individuals, that it was their first game and so it was likely that they would make some mistakes but could learn from them, and that one loss didn't mean that they were a horrible team. This might have taken all but 5 minutes but could have had a major impact on how they responded to the next loss!

The "teachable moment" approach can be used in many different ways. Suppose you are a teacher and you are giving your class a test. Just before the students put away their books and get ready to take the exam you ask for a show of hands as to how many are nervous about taking this test and then how many aren't that anxious. Contrast the two positions by asking what the students who are anxious are thinking versus those who are not as anxious. Briefly explore these thoughts and help them see that if they don't think catastrophically (I won't pass, it will be terrible) or put themselves down if they do poorly (if I don't pass it proves that I'm an idiot) they will be less anxious and can do a better job concentrating on the exam. Although this is a short intervention, it is very helpful. Or, suppose you are walking down the hall and you see two students arguing in the hallway. As you approach them you hear one student berate the other, calling her a loser and a liar. Suddenly this girl hauls off and hits the name caller, and she in turn starts hitting back, spewing out more unsavory names. You pull them aside and ask the girl who was called "loser and liar" how she felt about being called names. She said she was angry and that the other girl shouldn't have called her a name. You agree with her, noting that it is a school rule, but asking her if people sometimes break rules? And even if she didn't like being called names, is she really a loser and a liar? After processing this for awhile and diffusing the fight, you can also help the "victim" see that she even though she didn't like being called names, she had a choice about how to think about it, helping her see how her thinking impacted her feelings and her behavior. You also work with the bully to help her examine her behavior – would she like it if others called her names? And what did she gain from doing it since she had to serve detention for breaking a rule? Short intervention such as these introduce and/or reinforce rational principles.

To use this approach, teachers have to have a good understanding of REBT concepts and rather lecture students, they engage them in a discussion which helps students learn to think more rationally, which in turn impacts their feelings and their behaviors and promotes more effective problem-solving.

Total School Environment It is important that the key concepts previously described are reflected in the total school environment so that there is congruence between what is being presented in the social-emotional education curriculum and what is reinforced through school practices and procedures. For example, many schools give awards for best performance, but to be consistent with REBT, it is important to have a variety of awards, not only for good performance, but also for persistence and practice, most improved performance, and so forth. Another example would be to de-emphasize competition and the "winner/loser" notion in games, focusing instead on things each team did well and what they could do to improve, which reinforces the notion that everyone has strengths as well as weaknesses. An additional way to reinforce these concepts would be for teachers in each classroom to nominate a "student of the week," someone who demonstrated good behavior management, anger management, or problem-solving skills. The nominated students could be acknowledged at a school-wide assembly each month and the 4 students per class could make rational posters and banners to present at the assembly with words or phrases describing what they did to deserve the nomination and what rational thoughts helped them demonstrate good behavior management and problem-solving skills.

REBT has always championed an educative, preventative focus, which is particularly relevant for use in schools. The importance of a social-emotional education curriculum cannot be stressed enough, and the research clearly connects healthy development to school achievement.

You Can Do It! Education

You Can Do It! Education is one of a number of social-emotional learning programs that derive in part from the theory and practice of rational emotive education. As can be see in Fig. 13.1, Bernard (e.g., 2013), the theory of You Can Do It! Education identifies 12 irrational beliefs referred to as Negative Habits of the Mind (Attitudes) that give rise to five social-emotional blockers (feeling very angry/misbehaving, not paying attention/disturbing others, procrastination, feeling very worried, feeling very down) and 12 rational beliefs called Positive Habits of the Mind (Attitudes)

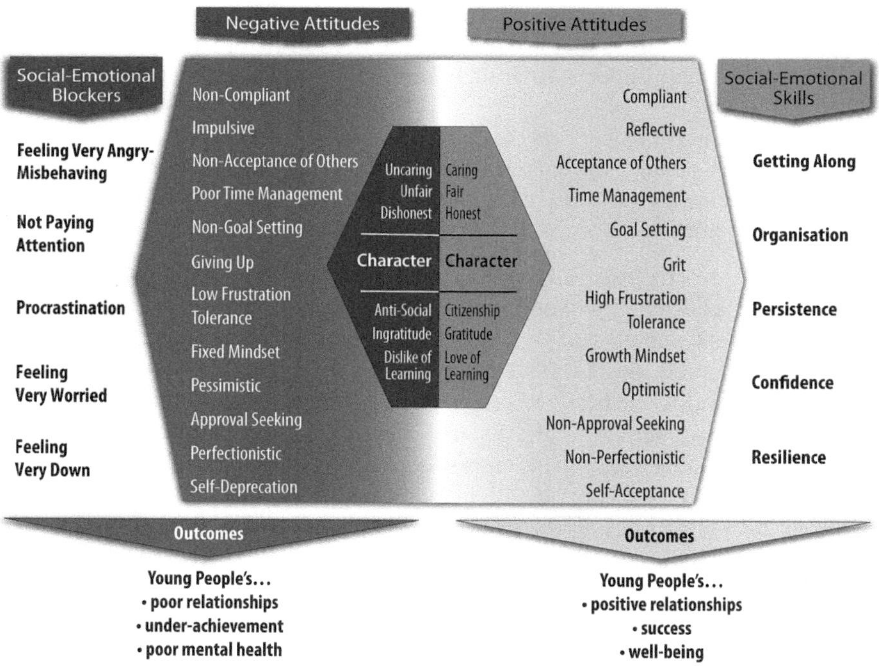

Fig. 13.1 You Can Do It! Education's social and emotional learning framework (Bernard, 2007)

that are associated with five social-emotional skills (confidence, persistence, organization, getting along, resilience).

There are a number of different ways that the 5 Social-Emotional Skills and the 12 Attitudes are taught in YCDI including: YCDI curricula programs, YCDI classroom and school-wide practices, and YCDI parent education. Of particular interest are the YCDI curriculum programs for students in pre-school and grades 1–12 that teach students depending on their developmental level the ABCs of REBT, how to distinguish, challenge and change irrational beliefs to rational beliefs as well as additional emotional and problem solving skills

YCDI Curricula Programs

There are four YCDI! Education social-emotional curricula that are used extensively in schools.

1. The *You Can Do It! Education Early Childhood Program* (ages 4–7) (Bernard, 2018a) that is used in over 2500 kindergarten and year 1 classrooms.
2. *Program Achieve* (ages 6–18) (Bernard, 2018b) is a curriculum series used in over 4000 primary and secondary schools.
3. *Bullying: The Power to Cope* (ages 9–16) (Bernard, 2016b) is A four-part program designed to be taught by teachers and mental health practitioners to classroom groups of students between grades 4–9.
4. *The You Can Do It! Education Mentoring Program* (Bernard, 2014) consists of activities that are designed to be presented to a student by a coach, mentor or teacher. The activities are designed to strengthen the student's core social-emotional skills (confidence, persistence, organization, getting along and resilience).

YCDI Classroom- and School-Wide Practices

In addition to teachers presenting lessons and activities from YCDI's curricula programs, over the years a number of different teaching practices have been identified that help develop students' knowledge and use of the 5 Foundations and the 12 Habits of the Mind (see Bernard, 2006b). Some of these practices include:

Practice 1. Have Discussions with Students About Each of the 5 Foundations

It is important for teachers to have conversations about each of the 5 Foundations and how important each is to everyone's success and well-being. Teachers should engage students in a discussion of the Foundations asking them for their views/definitions and making sure that at the end of the discussion, a definition is provided.

Practice 2. Describe to Students Examples of Behaviours to Be Practised that Reflect Each Foundation

After discussion, teachers should display on a poster a list of examples of behaviours of each of the 5 Foundations that students will need to practise in order to develop the Foundations (e.g. practicing times tables, spending time doing research in the library, practicing spelling, spending time reading). Teachers encourage students to practise these behaviours.

Practice 3a. Teach Students about the Important Role of Thinking/Self-Talk to Their Feelings and Behaviour

One of the important ideas to impart to students is that it is not what happens to

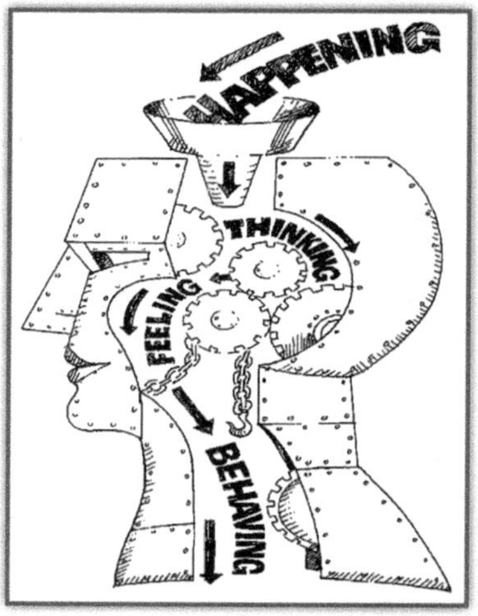

Metal man illustration--"Thinking Makes It So"

them that determines how successful and happy they are. This idea has been around for some time. Epictetus, a Stoic-Roman philosopher, wrote in the second century A.D. that 'People are not affected by events, but by their view of events.' Shakespeare wrote that 'Things are neither good nor bad, but thinking makes them so.'

Practice 3b. Discuss with Students the Positive Habits of the Mind that Support Each of the 5 Foundations

Teachers will want to provide students with opportunities to learn the meaning of 12 positive Habits of the Mind and how they support the 5 Foundations. Teachers will want to illustrate through discussion and role-play how a positive Habit of the Mind can help someone to practise positive behaviour.

Practice 4. Provide Students with Behaviour-Specific Feedback When They Display Examples of the Behaviours that Reflect the 5 Foundations

When teachers catch a student practicing a behaviour that reflects the Foundation they are teaching, teachers should acknowledge the student verbally, non-verbally, or in a written comment (e.g. 'You were confident.' 'You tried hard and did not give up. That's persistence.' 'Doesn't it feel good to be organised?' 'You are getting along very well when working together.' 'You stayed calm in a difficult situation. That's resilience.').

Practice 5. Teach Students Not to Blow Things out of Proportion

This is a very popular teaching practice that helps develop students' resilience. Teachers discuss with students how there are different degrees of 'badness'. Some things are 'a bit bad', some things are 'bad', some things are 'very bad', and some things are 'awful and terrible'. Teachers explain to students that when 'bad' things happen to them, they should use their thinking to mentally place the negative events in the correct category of 'badness' and not to blow the badness of the event out of proportion.

Practice 6. Integrate YCDI in the Academic Curriculum

The more teachers can incorporate the Foundations and the Habits of the Mind in other activities of their class or in one-to-one mentoring discussions, the more rapidly students will internalise them. A popular activity in Language Arts is for students to identify a character from a book they are reading or a movie they have seen and conduct a character analysis using key YCDI concepts.

Practice 7. Integrate YCDI in Art, Music and Drama

YCDI should be expressed in the artwork and music that is found in school. Art classes can design murals and posters that illustrate the 5 Foundations and which can then decorate the school. Students create their own songs and plays to bring the YCDI themes to life. There are a range of YCDI songs created by Kevin Hunt and myself that communicate different social-emotional skills and rational attitudes taught in YCDI ('I'm feeling confident today'; 'I'll be persistent') for elementary-age students and a series for young children (e.g. 'I'm Connie Confidence').

Here is a list of recommended actions that experience has shown will build the critical mass needed for YCDI to become an intrinsic part of school culture so that all students are influenced.

1. Awards. Existing awards for student behaviour (classroom, school-wide) can be modified so that students are 'caught' and acknowledged by their teachers for displaying confidence, persistence, organisation, getting along and resilience.

2. Assemblies. Assembly time can be used to invite speakers to talk to students about the importance of the 5 Foundations and 12 Habits of the Mind in their lives.
3. Excursions. Adults who take students on excursions can prepare students for successful outings by reviewing in advance with students how the different YCDI Foundations can make their excursion a success.
4. Celebration of Student 'Success' Stories. These stories should be shared on a regular basis at staff meetings.
5. School/Classroom Signage. The five YCDI Foundations can be displayed in the library, reception area, corridors, and inside/outside walls and in select spots around the school grounds. These can be creative contributions made by school parents or teachers.
6. Assessment. For students and staff to take YCDI seriously, it is good practice for students to be formally assessed by their teachers on the school's report card in terms of their display of their social and emotional learning skills.

Summary of Research on You Can Do It! Education

Over two decades of published research studies show that You Can Do It! Education is a proven, "best-practice" set of programs for enhancing the achievement and well-being of young people.

- When You Can Do It! Education was implemented throughout seven primary schools where positive attitudes and social-emotional skills were taught using a variety of classroom and whole-school practices including the *Program Achieve* social-emotional learning curriculum, the social-emotional well-being of students improved in comparison with students enrolled in similar schools where You Can Do It! Education was not implemented (Bernard & Walton, 2011).
- Four evaluation studies (3 in primary schools; 1 in high school) that examined the effects of You Can Do It Education in a whole school, multiple classrooms, in tutorial groups and in an after-school coaching showed positive effects on the grades, effort and quality of homework and school attendance (Bernard, Ellis, & Terjesen, 2006).
- When the *You Can Do It! Education Early Childhood Program* was taught to grade 1 students with a focus on strengthening confidence, persistence, organization, getting along and resilience, a positive impact was found on students' well-being, social skills and reading comprehension (students in lower 50% of class) in comparison with students who were not taught the program (Ashdown & Bernard, 2012).
- When You Can Do It! Education's program, *Bullying: The Power to Cope* designed to teach positive attitudes and coping skills was taught to students in primary schools, the impact of bullying (cyber-, verbal, physical, isolation) on their emotions and thinking (cognitive) was much less severe in comparison with students who are not taught the program (Markopolous & Bernard, 2015).

- When You Can Do It! Education's curriculum, *Program Achieve*, was taught to students with achievement, behavioral, social and/or emotional challenges, these 'at risk' students show strengthened resilience in comparison to a group of 'at risk' who did not participate (Bernard, 2008).
- When the You Can Do It! Education program, *Attitudes and Behaviours for Learning* (AB4L), was taught by teachers to students who are in the lower 50% of their class in reading, their reading achievement improved in comparison with the reading level of students not taught the program (Bernard, 2017b).

REBT and Teacher Stress

Since the 1980s (e.g., Bernard, Joyce, & Rosewarne, 1983), 1990s (Forman, 1994) and continuing to the present day (e.g., Bernard, 2017a; Warren & Hale, 2016). REBT has been deployed in professional development for teachers, in individual coaching programs and in pre-service teacher education programs (e.g., Nucci, 2002; Steins, Haep, & Wittrock, 2015) to help manage stress.

Bernard devised The Teacher Irrational Belief Scale (TIBS) (see Bora, Bernard, & Decsei-Radu, 2009) that revealed strong associations between irrationality and high amounts of teacher stress (Bernard, 2016a). Employing a sample of 850 primary and secondary teachers in Australia, Bernard, 2016a conducted an exploratory factor analysis of the TIBS that resulted in four distinct factors: Self-Downing, Authoritarianism, Demands for Justice, and Low Frustration Tolerance. In a second study, 140 teachers and 26 teachers retired from teaching because of stress completed the TIBS and a measure of teacher stress. Teachers retired from teaching due to stress scored higher on sub-scales of Self-Downing and Low Frustration Tolerance than teachers still teaching.

Professional development stress management programs that incorporate REBT teach the basic ABC including how to recognize, challenge and change irrational beliefs. What follows is an example of such a program offered by consultants (school psychologists, counselors) (from Warren & Hale, 2016):

Session 1 Topic: Introduction to Rational Emotive Behavior Therapy

Objectives: To gain an understanding of the history of REBT; to become aware of the efficacy of REBT; to build an awareness of the value of utilizing counseling theory in classroom; to learn principle basic principles of REBT and how they apply to classroom situations

Session 2 Topic: Rational-Emotive Philosophy and Theory

Objectives: To gain awareness of knowing verses thinking; to understand the values and goals of REBT; to learn and apply the concepts presented related to rational and irrational beliefs

Session 3 Topic: Rational-Emotive Behavior Therapy

Objectives: To become aware of the three major "musts" and their derivatives; to explore the belief-consequence connection; to learn the ABC Model of Emotional Disturbance; to apply the ABC Model to personal and professional situations

Session 4 Topic: The ABC Model Expanded

Objective: To learn the expanded version of the ABC Model; to learn the value of disputing irrational beliefs; to acquire cognitive techniques and strategies for challenging irrational beliefs; to implement and practice the strategies provided

Session 5 Topic: Disputing Irrational Beliefs

Objectives: To learn additional cognitive challenges for irrational beliefs; to learn emotional and behavioral disputes; to apply strategies and techniques for challenging irrational beliefs

Session 6 Topic: Classroom Applications of REBT

Objectives: To further learn how to apply REBT to classroom situations; to learn cognitive-behavioral strategies and techniques specific to classroom scenarios.

Conclusion

The theory and practice of rational emotive behavior therapy and its application in the form of rational emotive behavior education and consultation for stress management continues to benefit student and teacher outcomes. It can be seen from this chapter that rationality is a precious human commodity that when under-developed is associated with a myriad of social and emotional difficulties of students as well as stress in teachers. We hope that the evident benefits of strengthening rationality a well as the relatively straightforward methods for doing so will encourage educators and mental health practitioners who teach and consult in schools to promote *rationality for all.*

References

Ashdown, D. M., & Bernard, M. E. (2012). Can explicit instruction in social and emotional learning skills benefit the social-emotional development, well-being, and academic achievement of young children? *Early Childhood Education Journal, 39*, 397–405.

Bernard, M. E. (2006a). *Providing all children with the foundations for achievement, well-being and positive relationship* (3rd ed., p. 286). Oakleigh, VIC, Australia: Australian Scholarships Group; Priorslee, Telford (ENG): Time Marque.

Bernard, M. E. (2006b). It's time we teach social-emotional competence as well as we teach academic competence. *Reading and Writing Quarterly, 22*, 103–119. https://doi.org/10.1080/10573560500242184

Bernard, M. E. (2007). *Program achieve. A social and emotional learning curriculum* (3rd ed.). (Primary Set, six vols.: Ready Set, You Can Do It!, Confidence, Persistence, Organisation, Getting Along, Resilience). Oakleigh, VIC, Australia: Australian Scholarships Group; Priorslee, Telford (ENG): Time Marque, pp. 1200.

Bernard, M. E. (2008). The effect of You Can Do It! Education on the emotional resilience of primary school students with social, emotional, behavioral and achievement challenges. *Proceedings of the Australian Psychological Society Annual Conference, 43*, 36–40.

Bernard, M. E. (2013). You Can Do It! Education: A social-emotional learning program for increasing the achievement and well-being of children and adolescents. In K. Yamasaki (Ed.),

School-based prevention education for health and adjustment problems in the world. Tokyo, Japan: Kaneko Shobo.
Bernard, M. E. (2014). *The You Can Do It! Education mentoring program* (p. 180). Oakleigh, VIC, Australia: Australian Scholarships Group; Priorslee, Telford (ENG): Time Marque.
Bernard, M. E. (2016a). Beliefs and teacher stress. *Journal of Rational-Emotive & Cognitive-Behavior Therapy, 34*, 209–224. https://doi.org/10.1007/s10942-016-0238-y
Bernard, M. E. (2016b). *Bullying: The power to cope*. Oakleigh, VIC, Australia: Australian Scholarships Group.
Bernard, M. E. (2017a). *Stress management for teachers and school principals*. Oakleigh, VIC, Australia: Australian Scholarships Group.
Bernard, M. E. (2017b). Impact of teaching attitudes and behaviors for learning on the reading achievement of students falling behind. *International Journal of Learning, Teaching and Educational Research, 16*, 51–64.
Bernard, M. E. (2018a). *Program achieve. A social emotional learning curriculum for young children*. Melbourne, VIC, Australia: The Bernard Group.
Bernard, M. E. (2018b). *The NEW program achieve. Attitudes and social-emotional skills for student achievement, behaviour and wellbeing*. Melbourne, VIC, Australia: The Bernard Group.
Bernard, M. E., Ellis, A., & Terjesen, M. (2006). Rational-emotive behavioral approaches to childhood disorders: History, theory, practice, and research. In A. Ellis & M. E. Bernard (Eds.), *Rational emotive behavioral approaches to childhood disorders: Theory, practice and research* (pp. 3–84). New York, NY: Springer.
Bernard, M. E., Joyce, M. R., & Rosewarne, P. (1983). Helping teachers cope with stress. In A. Ellis & M. E. Bernard (Eds.), *Rational-emotive approaches to the problems of childhood* (pp. 415–466). New York, NY: Plenum Press.
Bernard, M. E., & Walton, K. E. (2011). The effect of You Can Do It! Education in six schools on student perceptions of wellbeing, teaching-learning and relationships. *Journal of Student Well-being, 5*, 22–37.
Bora, C., Bernard, M. E., & Decsei-Radu, A. (2009). Teacher irrational belief scale – Preliminary norms for Romanian population. *Journal of Cognitive and Behavioral Psychotherapies, 9*, 211–220.
Carlson, N. (1992). *What if it never stops raining?* New York, NY: Penguin Books.
Caruso, C., Angelone, L., Abbata, E., Ionni, V., Biondi, C., Agostino, C. D., … Mezzaluna, C. (2018). Effects of a REBT based training on children and teachers in primary school. *Journal of Rational-Emotive & Cognitive-Behavior Therapy, 36*, 1–14.
Çekiç, A., Akbas, T., Turan, A., & Hamamcı, Z. (2016). The effect of rational emotive parent education program on parents' irrational beliefs and parenting stress. *Journal of Human Sciences, 13*, 1. https://doi.org/10.14687/ijhs.v13i1.3729
Collaborative for Academic, Social, and Emotional Learning. (2013). *2013 CASEL guide: Effective social and emotional learning programs: Preschool and elementary school edition*. Chicago, IL: Collaborative for Academic, Social, and Emotional Learning.
DiGiuseppe, R., Doyle, K. A., Dryden, W., & Backx, W. (2014). *A practitioner's guide to rational emotive behavior therapy* (3rd ed.). New York, NY: Oxford University Press.
Durlak, J., Weissberg, R., Dymnicki, A., Taylor, R., & Schellinger, K. (2011). The impact of enhancing students' social and emotional learning: A meta- analysis of school- based universal interventions. *Child Development, 82*, 474–501. https://doi.org/10.1111/j.1467-8624.2010.01564.x
Elkind, D. (1988). *The hurried child: Growing up too fast too soon*. Reading, MA: Addison-Wesley.
Ellis, A. E. (1972). Emotional education in the classroom: The living school. *Journal of Child Psychology, 1*, 19–22.
Ellis, A. E., & Bernard, M. E. (2006). *Rational emotive approaches to the problems of childhood* (2nd ed.). New York, NY: Springer.
Forman, S. (1994). Teacher stress management: A rational-emotive therapy approach. In M. E. Bernard & R. D. DiGiuseppe (Eds.), *Rational-emotive consultation in applied settings*. Hillsdale, NJ: Lawrence Erlbaum.

Forman, S. G., & Forman, B. D. (1980). Rational-emotive staff development. *Psychology in the Schools, 17*, 90–95.
Gonzalez, J. E., Nelson, J. R., Gutkin, T. B., Saunders, A., Galloway, A., & Shwery, C. S. (2004). Rational emotive therapy with children and adolescents: A meta-analysis. *Journal of Emotional and Behavioral Disorders, 12*, 222–235.
Hajzler, J. D., & Bernard, E. M. (1991). A review of rational-emotive education outcome studies. *School Psychology Quarterly, 6*, 27–49.
Henderson, D. A., & Thompson, C. L. (2011). *Counseling children*. Belmont, CA: Brooks/Cole.
Joyce, M. R. (1995). Emotional relief for parents: Is rational-emotive parent education effective? *Journal of Rational-Emotive and Cognitive-Behavior Therapy, 13*, 55–75.
Knaus, W. J. (1974). *Rational emotive education: A manual for elementary school teachers*. New York, NY: Institute for Rational Living.
Lupu, V., & Iftene, F. (2009). The impact of rational emotive behaviour education on anxiety in teenagers. *Journal of Cognitive and Behavioral Psychotherapies, 9*, 95–105.
Mahfar, M., Aslan, A. S., Noah, S. M., Ahmad, J., & Jaafar, W. M. W. (2014). Effects of rational emotive education module on irrational beliefs and stress among fully residential school students in Malaysia. *Procedia-Social and Behavioral Sciences, 114*, 239–243.
Markopolous, Z., & Bernard, M. E. (2015). Effect of the bullying: The power to cope program on children's response to bullying. *Journal of Relationships Research, 6*, 1–11.
Nucci, C. (2002). The rational teacher: Rational-emotive behavior therapy in teacher education. *Journal of Rational-Emotive & Cognitive-Behavioral Therapy, 20*, 15–32.
Steins, G., Haep, A., & Wittrock, K. (2015). Technology of the self and classroom management – A systematic approach for teacher students. *Creative Education, 6*, 2090–2104. https://doi.org/10.4236/ce.2015.619213
Trip, S., Vernon, A., & McMahon, J. (2007). Effectiveness of rational-emotive education: A quantitative meta-analytical study. *Journal of Cognitive & Behavioral Psychotherapies, 7*(1), 81–93.
Vernon, A. (2006a). *Thinking, feeling, behaving: An emotional education curriculum for children* (2nd ed.). Champaign, IL: Research Press.
Vernon, A. (2006b). *Thinking, feeling, behaving: An emotional education curriculum for adolescents* (2nd ed.). Champaign, IL: Research Press.
Vernon, A. (2007). Application of rational emotive behavior therapy to groups within classrooms and educational settings. In R. W. Christner, J. L. Steward, & A. Freeman (Eds.), *Handbook of cognitive-behavior group therapy with children and adolescents: Specific settings and presenting problems* (pp. 107–127). New York, NY: Routledge.
Vernon, A. (2009). *More what works when with children and adolescents: A handbook of individual counseling techniques*. Champaign, IL: Research Press.
Warren, R., & Hale, R. W. (2016). The influence of efficacy beliefs on teacher performance and student success: Implications for student support services. *Journal of Rational-Emotive and Cognitive-Behavior Therapy, 34*, 187–208.

Chapter 14
REBT in Sport

Martin J. Turner

Advances in REBT Theory, Research and Practice

Sport is tough. Amidst the highly demanding environment of competitive sport (Reardon & Factor, 2010), and the growing concern for the psychological wellbeing of athletes (MacIntyre et al., 2016), effective interventions for promoting mental health in athletes is a major concern in applied research literature. Sport psychology involves the application of psychological theory and methods to the understanding and enhancement of athletic performance and athlete wellbeing. The practice of sport psychology historically draws mostly from cognitive-behavioural approaches to psychotherapy. Known as "the canon", the most prevalently reported techniques used in sport psychology are imagery, relaxation, goal setting, and self-talk. All four have obvious cognitive-behavioural routes, but rarely are the origins of these techniques recognized and referenced in sport psychology literature. Also, these techniques are often used as isolated "mental skills" in the absence of full CBT procedures. Therefore, whilst CBT *should* occupy a prominent place in the investigation and application of sport and exercise psychology, there is actually a dearth in literature reporting the effects of CBT with athletes.

Recent developments in sport psychology research indicate that CBT, and specifically REBT, may be an effective framework for promoting mental health and wellbeing in athletes. Indeed, there is a growing corpus of research (see Turner, 2016a, for a review) reporting the effects of REBT with athletes, which although still sparse, represents a significant advance in the application of REBT. This chapter discusses the advances being made in the field of REBT as applied to sport, commenting on how the theory, research, and practice, of REBT are interpreted, and in some cases adapted, in order to help athletes to maximize short- and long-term

M. J. Turner (✉)
School of Life Sciences and Education, Staffordshire University, Stoke-on-Trent, UK
e-mail: m.turner@staffs.ac.uk

© Springer Nature Switzerland AG 2019

M. E. Bernard, W. Dryden (eds.), *Advances in REBT*,
https://doi.org/10.1007/978-3-319-93118-0_14

athletic potential. It is important to state, prior to continuing this chapter, that REBT as applied to sport could really be considered as Rational Emotive Behavioural Coaching (REBC; e.g., Kodish, 2002), since *therapy* does not necessarily take place. However, given the literature-base referring to REBT in sport, I will remain consistent and refer to REBT rather than REBC throughout.

Research in Sport

To understand the recent developments in the investigation of REBT in sport, it is first appropriate to provide a brief outline of the work published to date. At the time of writing, there have been approximately fifteen articles (including peers reviewed papers and book chapters) that report the use of REBT with athletes. The participating athletes in these studies represent female and male youth and adult athletes, across a range of sports and competitive levels. Most articles are case-study reflections and single-case designs.

One case-study article demonstrates the effective use of REBT with Australian Rules Football players (Bernard, 1985), where athletes were better able to control their thoughts to directly influence performance as a result of REBT education, concentration training and goal setting. Marlow (2009) took a similar approach with a youth ten-pin bowler, reporting enhanced performance and adaptive behavioural changes as a result of a psychological skills programme that included REBT. Another study focused on helping an Olympic table tennis athlete to reduce his LFT beliefs (Si & Lee, 2008) using REBT and mental skills training, finding that the athlete was more able to control frustration, was less perfectionistic, and experienced performance improvements. More recently, a detailed case-study reporting the use of a seven-session REBT intervention with a county-level archer led to increases in self-efficacy, perceived control, and objective competitive performance scores (Wood, Barker, & Turner, 2016). Wood and colleagues also report a case study with a 42-year-old Paralympic athlete (Wood, Turner, & Barker, 2018) where a five-session REBT intervention was met with short-term and maintained reductions in irrational beliefs, enhanced competition concentration and less distraction, and greater emotional control. Furthermore, another case-study with a 15-year old cricketer (batsman) using six REBT sessions helped the athlete to develop greater ability to control emotions during challenging moments, an improvement validated by the athlete's father (Wood, Barker, & Turner, 2017).

Single-case designs have been employed frequently in the investigation of REBT with athletes. Compared to case-studies, single-case designs offer specific procedures with which to determine intervention effectiveness and efficacy (Barker, Mellalieu, McCarthy, Jones, & Moran, 2013). Elko and Ostrow (1991) applied a single-case design to examine the use of REBT with six gymnasts, with results showing reductions in anxiety in five and improved performance in three of the participants. More recently, Turner and Barker (2013) applied a three-session REBT intervention with four elite youth cricketers, helping the athletes reduce their cognitive performance anxiety. However, no performance markers were obtained. In a rare investigation into the psychological approach of Mixed Martial Arts (MMA) athletes, Cunningham and Turner (2016) found that a three-session REBT intervention reduced self-depreciation beliefs and increased unconditional self-acceptance (USA) beliefs in two of the three semi-professional MMA athletes. One of the athletes was resistant to changing his irrational beliefs, which is certainly a valuable potential future research focus.

New research has applied a five-session REBT intervention with eight elite Paralympic athletes (Wood, Barker, Turner, & Sheffield, 2017). At post-REBT, five of the eight athletes showed reductions in irrational beliefs, matched by enhanced athletic performance, and reductions in resting Systolic Blood Pressure. The athletes also reported adopting functional self-talk, reductions in negative cognitions, and improved concentration during competitions, which may explain the positive performance effects. In addition, one study explored the use of REBT in five elite Malaysian squash athletes using five REBT sessions (Deen, Turner, & Wong, 2017). The REBT intervention also included the application of the Athlete Rational Resilience Credo (ARRC; Turner, 2016b) for the first time in research, adapted from Dryden's original Rational Resilience Credo (Dryden, 2007). Using complex visual analysis, results revealed that all athletes reported a substantial reduction in irrational beliefs, and an increase in self-reported resilience (three of whom demonstrated substantial increases).

Some research studies have applied what is best described as rational emotive education (REE; Knaus, 2006), where REBT is delivered educationally to a group of athletes. Two studies (Turner, Slater, & Barker, 2014, 2015) showed that interactive REBT education sessions led to significant reductions in irrational beliefs in elite youth soccer athletes. However, REE applied using a single session yielded short-term reductions in irrational beliefs (Turner et al., 2014), whilst three sessions of REE led to longer-term reductions in irrational beliefs (Turner et al., 2015), which suggests REE is not a quick fix and dose effects may be important to consider. In both studies, athletes felt that REE helped them to improve their emotional control and performances, but no objective markers of performance were sought by the authors. Finally, Vertopolous and Turner (2017) employed REE (four sessions) with 20 Greek athletes, ten of whom also received Rational Emotive Personal Disclosure Mutual Sharing (REPDMS) after REE. This study, which is the first to explore the effects of REPDMS, revealed that REE led to reductions in irrational beliefs and increases in rational beliefs in all athletes, but those who received REPDMS after the REE demonstrated further reductions in irrational beliefs and a maintained elevation in rational beliefs. Athletes who received REE only showed an increase in irrational beliefs and a decrease in rational beliefs in a follow-up phase.

The application of REBT in sport with athletes offers advancements in the breadth of contexts in which REBT can be successfully used. Indeed, REBT has been examined across clinical and nonclinical populations, in youths and adults, across education, military, and business contexts; sport reflects a relatively new and exciting avenue for future REBT research and development. But apart from simply a novel understanding of REBT in a new context, the growth of research and applied reflections detailing the use of REBT in sport has begun to offer advancements in how REBT is investigated, 'packaged', and delivered in sport settings. The use of REBT within sport is growing, and with this comes some realization about how REBT can best be implemented in what is a constantly changing and unpredictable environment.

Adapting REBT for Sport

Perhaps many sport psychology practitioners use REBT within their practice, but do not report their work empirically. Recently, the first volume of REBT-practitioner case stuides with athletes has been published (Turner & Bennett, 2018), and what is clear from the chapters therein, and the work being published reporting the application of REBT in sport, is that REBT can be delivered within the often time-constrained (typically using five sessions of around 45-min duration) and ever-changing context of sport. This is important because practitioners working in sport will sometimes get minimal time with athletes, and will be required to adapt their preferred ways of working to suit the culture of the sport within which they are working. The application of REBT in such time-restricted circumstances creates the potential need for brief, sometimes single-session, REBT interventions that have been operationally described and defined by Dryden (2016) as single-session integrated cognitive behavior therapy, or if the work is more focused on helping the client to get more out of themselves (i.e., personal development), very brief cognitive-behavioral coaching (VBCBC; Dryden, 2016). In particular, VBCBC fits well within the environments that sport psychology practitioners may find themselves working in, where performance and personal growth towards goal attainment is usually salient. In reality, the idea of 10 weeks of consecutive one-to-one 60-min counseling sessions is not feasible for many practitioners working in sport, and as such, an approach such as REBT that can be delivered briefly (as VBCBC for example), flexibly, and cost-effectively, is appealing. The choice to apply REBT briefly and flexibly must obviously be considered alongside the individual athlete's presenting issues, as a more long-term approach may be required depending on the case.

In addition, many of the studies applying REBT within sport adopt a group psycho-educational mode of delivery (e.g., Turner et al., 2015), akin to REE (Knaus, 2006). REE in sport boasts time and cost efficiency for sporting organizations and athletes, because more than one athlete can receive REE at any one time. But caution should be exercised because research suggests that positive effects experienced by athletes participating in REE can be short-lived (Turner et al., 2014). Limitations notwithstanding, by engaging sports teams in group-level REBT (REE) it is possible to create a shared understanding of REBT principles that live and grow within the team. By adapting REBT to be delivered practically within sport environments practitioners are able to integrate REBT principles into training. For example, to facilitate the interactive and ongoing disputation of awfulizing beliefs, a technique sport psychology practitioners will often use is hanging a badness or 'catastrophe' scale (Ellis, Gordon, Neenan, & Palmer, 1997) poster on the wall of the changing room. Athletes, and coaches, can write down 'bad' events on post-it notes and add them to the badness scale between 0% (*not at all bad*) and 100% (*worst thing possible*), encouraging debate about how bad the event really is. In sport, it is important to take therapeutic principles out of the consulting room or classroom, and into the performance environment, for maximal transferability to performance.

As well as testing, and reflecting upon, the traditional modes of REBT delivery where the focus is predominantly on ABCDE framework, research has also begun to offer novel advancements in how REBT can be operationalized in a sport context. The ARRC (Turner, 2016b) adopted in Deen et al. (2017) is an example of how a technique conceived outside of sport (Dryden, 2007) has been developed for use within sport, and offers the first empirical examination of such a technique. In addition, the REPDMS technique utilized by Vertopolous and Turner (2017) offers a merger of REBT and PDMS to create a new group-based activity to enhance the effects of REBT. Thus, by adapting current REBT practices and by creatively engineering new techniques, sport is offering potential new ways in apply REBT that fit the contextual needs of the athletic environment. This adaptation could be broadened too, with REBT techniques such as rational emotive imagery (Maultsby, 1971) sharing similarities with certain types of imagery advocated for use with athletes (e.g., motivational-general mastery; Martin, Moritz, & Hall, 1999), where the adverse event is the chief subject of the imagery conducted.

Assessment of Irrational Beliefs

Amidst the growth of research investigating REBT in sport, authors have identified the need for a psychometric that measures performance-specific irrational beliefs. Indeed, situational perception is important for psychometrics (Ziegler & Horstmann, 2015), so that a more accurate understanding of the specific conditions or subpopulation with which a tool works best in can be gained. To this end, the irrational Performance Beliefs Inventory (iPBI; Turner et al., 2018a; Turner & Allen, 2018) was developed as a brief (28-item) psychometric for use in performance settings such as sport, academia, business, and the military, and reflects current manifestations of REBT theory and measures only beliefs, not emotional and or behavioural outcomes (Terjesen, Salhany, & Sciutto, 2009). The iPBI has subsequently been used in published research in sport (Deen et al., 2017), but further research is needed to fully validate the measure across various samples and across time. Also, psychometrics are not panaceas for the assessment of irrational beliefs, as many people are not sufficiently aware of their irrational beliefs without experiencing their activating event in the real (Churchman, 2018), and self-report measures should be supplemented with a full ABC assessment and observation of the athlete if possible. However, the development of the iPBI represents a sport (or more accurately 'performance') specific tool that can advance the research and application of REBT in sport.

More broadly, the assessment of athlete issues often takes place very briefly, and because of the nature of sport, can be very focussed. That is, athletes often seek the advice of sport psychologists due to a specific performance-limiting issue(s) that with further exploration may turn out to be a more complex psychological issue. By the same token, the presenting issue may not be very complex and initial assessments of client As, Bs, and Cs may not reveal irrational beliefs, and therefore the practitioner can help the athlete to solve whatever seems to be effecting their performance quite directly. For example, an athlete may present with some concern (healthy C) about meeting the requirements for a new fitness test (A). On assessment, the athlete may reveal rational beliefs regarding the fitness test (B), and as such, may have a healthy approach to the test, but all the same, they are unsure about their ability to perform well. The practitioner can then help the athlete to plan for the testing and draw upon current strengths pertaining to fitness. However, the athlete may present with anxiety (unhealthy C) concerning the fitness test (A), evident through a desire to self-handicap and purposely underprepare for the test. On assessment, the athlete may hold irrational beliefs (B) regarding the test (or perhaps about the introduction of a new test) that is leading to the self-limiting intention to self-handicap. With specific issues, it is possible to conduct a meaningful, but brief, ABC assessment because little time is lost figuring out why the athlete is sat before you. This occurrence also places great importance on the accuracy of assessment, and if deeper issues are identified, follow-up work should take place.

One of the challenges of applying REBT with athletes is that the notion of between-session homework is not always met with enthusiasm. This is perhaps because of educational or academic connotations, which suggest a distinction between training and REBT homework. This poses a problem because adherence to homework assignments is a vital part of REBT (Ellis & Dryden, 1997). One can of course call 'homework assignments' whatever one wishes to call them, be it 'between-session tasks', 'mental training', or 'self-help' to assuage academic connotations. Another way to enhance the appeal of homework assignments with athletes is to use modern technology to engage the athletes on familiar terms. For example, the use of Smartphone Apps for psychotherapeutic gains is receiving growing attention, and recently an App has been developed that helps clients to more deeply understand the ABCDE framework (Turner & Wood, 2016). The digitisation of the ABCDE framework helps to educate the client in the early stages of REBT, and also allows for remote long-term monitoring of As, Bs, and Cs experienced by clients. Ultimately, by more accurately assessing athlete adversities, beliefs, and consequences, a practitioner can better tailor REBT to the athlete's needs.

'Smarter Thinking' and Rational Emotive Behavioural Coaching (REBC)

The aforementioned potentially negative connotations attached to 'homework' in sport settings can be overcome quite simply. But within sport, there are also negative connotations attached to REBT (and CBT in general) due to the word 'therapy'. Indeed, recent reports indicate that athletes may be discouraged from seeking mental health support due to the potential stigma attached to mental illness and treatment, and this stigma can extend to mental skills training in the absence of mental illness (Gulliver, Griffiths, & Christensen, 2012; Thompson & Sherman, 2007). Further, some sport psychologists may be deterred by REBT's clinical connotations (Marlow, 2009), and negative perceptions from some cognitive-behavioral therapists (e.g., Trower & Jones, 2001). Therefore, psychologists working in sport have adopted the term 'Smarter Thinking' (Turner, 2014) instead of 'REBT'. Of course, the principles and techniques of REBT are retained in Smarter Thinking, but are more accepted as part of athlete mental skills training rather than being seen as therapy.

Sporting organisations will often want to know what they are getting for their investment (of time, energy, and money), and how the work will be structured. As such, Smarter Thinking also offers a clear cyclical process (see Fig. 14.1) born from REBT, but packaged to appeal to sporting organisations, coaches, and athletes. As can be seen in Fig. 14.1, the first stage ('recognise') involves a full assessment of the athlete's ABCs and a significant amount of education and discussion concerning the ABC elements of REBT. The next three steps ('evidence, logic, pragmatics') are encapsulated by the disputing (D) stage of REBT. Steps five and six are encapsulated by the effective rational beliefs (E) stage of the REBT process, and involve encouraging the individual to adopt and commit to rational beliefs.

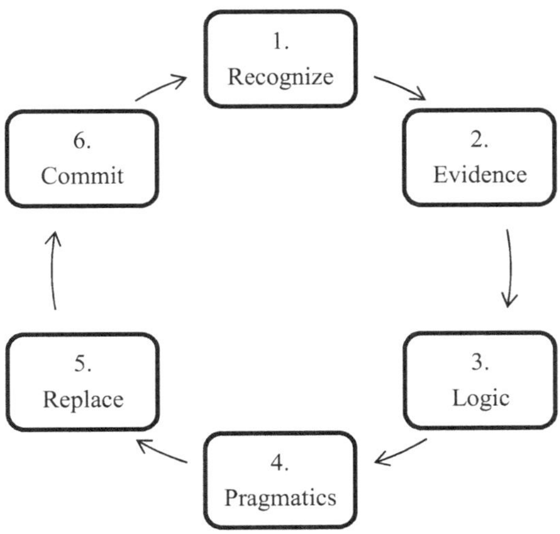

Fig. 14.1 A six-step REBT process (Smarter Thinking; Turner, 2014)

Importantly, the Smarter Thinking framework can be applied at an individual, and group level, can be delivered didactically, interactively, or loosely, as an underpinning framework for conversations about how beliefs can influence emotions, behaviours, and sports performance. If delivered at a team level, as part of step 6 'commit' the practitioner would ideally work with the coach and support staff (e.g., physiotherapist, strength and conditioning coach, sport scientist) to help encourage the athletes to refine and strengthen their newly developed rational philosophies. I will make specific comments later in the chapter on the importance of coaches and the social support of athletes in the effectiveness of REBT.

REBT as applied to sport, by sport psychologists, is usually not 'therapy' and, therefore the goals of REBT with athletes are more closely aligned to the goals of rational emotive behavioural coaching (REBC) coined by Kodish (2002) and Neenan and Dryden (2002). REBC's focus on coaching, as opposed to therapy, reflects the development of strengths within athletes, rather than remedially dealing with problems and issues (as may be perceived by some about 'therapy'). Sporting organisations and coaches may be more open to 'coaching' compared to 'therapy', and in any case, REBC is more closely aligned with the professional boundaries of many sport psychologists who are not qualified to provide therapy for mental illness. REBC can be considered a direct and pragmatic coaching approach for enhancing human functioning and improving behavioral health (Ogbuanya et al., 2017); a purpose that fits with the role of sport psychologists working with athletes. Further, a critical appraisal of the REBT in sport research to date (see Turner, 2016a) reveals that 'therapy' has not taken place. Researchers have ensured high REBT standards and rigorous adherence to REBT practices, but have actually conducted REBC, because the goals of the intervention have been to augment sporting performance (e.g., Wood et al., 2016). REBC needs to be further examined in sport, as it offers a promising approach to promoting and applying REBT within performance settings.

The Education of Sport Coaches in REBT

Coaches are fundamental to the generation and the fostering of rational and irrational beliefs in athletes. Coaches are a vital source of information for athletes to model themselves on, and in times of stress, are important sources of social support (Lu et al., 2016), which is an important coping strategy for the pressure of competitive sport (Reeves, Nicholls, & McKenna, 2009; Skinner & Zimmer-Gembeck, 2007). Coaches can influence the coping of athletes via informational support (e.g., House, 1981) for example, which can contribute to enhanced coping by encouraging more functional cognitive appraisals of stressors (e.g., Aspinwall & Taylor, 1997; Festinger, 1954). As such, athletes looking to coaches for information on how to react to adversity require a role model who can react well to adversity. In sum, coaches have an important influence on the emotional well-being of their athletes

(Reinboth, Duda, & Ntoumanis, 2004), and can offer a vital source of social support for athletes facing adversity.

It is because of the coach's influence on the psychology of their athletes that practitioners should include coaches in their sport psychology provision where possible. This includes getting 'buy-in' from the coach for the nature and the focus of the work done with athletes. Not only can coaches reinforce what the athletes have learned with regard to sport psychology, coaches can also develop their own psychosocial skills with a view to providing more effective coaching to their athletes. For example, research shows that coaches who struggle to cope with stress, are more likely to adopt controlling behaviours and are less able to attune to their athletes' thoughts and feelings, which can damage the coach-athlete relationship and negatively impact athlete motivation (Mageau & Vallerand, 2003). Coaching is a stressful activity (e.g., Gould, Greenleaf, Guinan, & Chung, 2002) and highly stressed coaches are more likely to experience burnout (specifically emotional exhaustion) and a need to distance themselves from others (Frey, 2007; Kelley, Eklund, & Ritter-Taylor, 1999) and withdraw social support (Dixon, Turner, & Gillman, 2017). Therefore, a coach's ability to regulate their own emotions can influence theirs and their athletes' experience of competitive sport.

Thusly, one potentially important advancement in the provision of REBT with athletes is the effective engagement of coaches in the imbedding of REBT principles into the athletic environment. Due to the often time-restricted circumstances within which sport psychologists work with athletes, educating and working with coaches on REBT principles and how to pass these principles onto athletes, can be a very effective way of exposing athletes to REBT. As sport psychologists we do not have as much contact with athletes as the coach does, and therefore the education of coaches in REBT principles can enable them to reinforce REBT work completed with athletes, and also help them to use REBT techniques in their coaching.

A Case Example In my work, I undertake coach education frequently, and sometimes never meet the athletes who will (hopefully) benefit from my work with coaches. To best illustrate how I typically approach this work, it is perhaps most useful to provide a brief case-illustration for a coach education workshop delivered to a group of Olympic coaches (I have withheld the sport in which the coaches work to preserve their anonymity) over a single 4-h period. As the reader will notice, the following is a brief account of how coaches ($n > 60$) within a REBT educational workshop can be introduced to fundamental REBT concepts such as the ABC framework (specifically the B-C connection), the notion of healthy and unhealthy negative emotions, and disputation of irrational beliefs (Ellis & Dryden, 1997; Turner & Barker, 2014). To be clear, the aim was not to fully and comprehensively train the coaches in REBT; this would be impossible in a single workshop, and I am not qualified as an REBT trainer. Instead, the objective was to help the coaches to understand the mechanics behind how healthy and unhealthy negative emotions and behaviours arise, and how their coaching language can be more aligned with rational beliefs to encourage more adaptive emotional and behavioural responding in athletes. It was also hoped that by raising the coaches' awareness of fundamental REBT concepts (such as the ABC framework), that the coaches could better control their own emotions in adverse situations, as well as helping their athletes.

Discovering the Adversity (A) With the coaches, before I introduced any REBT concepts explicitly, the first thing I asked them to do was to answer a simple question: What is adversity for you and your athletes? I organised the larger group into smaller units, and asked each unit to arrive at a one-sentence definition of adversity. After this, I then asked the coaches to list the adversities that they and their athletes might experience in the short and long-term. Here I was looking for the coaches to explore A and to recognise the vast number and variety of adversities salient within the competitive environment. These As included performance-related events such injury, failure, deselection, poor treatment, and poor officiating decisions, and non-performance-related events such as family issues, illness, friendship sacrifices, relationship break-ups, and financial constraints. It was important here for the coaches to recognise that for athletes, the coach can also be a source of various As. For example, when I run similar activities with athletes, deselection is usually mentioned, which is (usually) ultimately a coaching decision and is typically communicated by the coach to the athlete. It was also important that the coaches recognised their own As, and in particular, how similar their As were to their athletes (e.g., failure is as salient for a coach as it is for an athlete). At the end of this activity, coaches had a good idea of important As for themselves and their athletes.

Discovering the Emotional and Behavioural Consequences (C) The initial recognition of As was important because it helped orient the coaches towards situations in which they should be aware of theirs and their athletes' emotions and behaviours. To explore C, I used two main activities. In the first task, I asked the coaches to write down on separate post-it notes five emotions that may arise from an A (they could choose an A previously discussed). Coaches completed this task alone, and were encouraged to think about feelings and emotions, not thoughts and behaviours. Coaches were then invited to the front of the room to place their post-it notes on a white board. The white board had a line down the centre, and to the right of the line I asked coaches to place emotions that they thought were helpful for performance, and to the left, emotions that were unhelpful for performance. Some emotions such as anxiety and anger were placed in both columns. That is, some coaches felt that anxiety and anger could be helpful, while others felt that anxiety and anger could be unhelpful. This opened up a discussion around the functionality of emotions. I challenged the group to decide when emotions were helpful and when they were not, and what was the major factor determining when an emotion is helpful vs. not helpful. The group decided it is the behaviour associated with the emotion that is crucial. I used the example of performing under pressure to further illustrate this point. Here I contrasted an athlete who is anxious and wanting to avoid challenges with an athlete who was concerned and spends extra time preparing for the competition, tying this notion into the concepts of healthy vs. unhealthy negative emotions, stressing the point that negative emotions are not necessarily detrimental to performance, it depends on the associated behaviours. The coaches then went back to their adversity notes and aligned each adversity to a functional emotional response, and a dysfunctional emotional response. This helped to contextualise the emotions within the performance context.

Introducing the Beliefs-Consequences (B-C) Connection At this point, the coaches had discussed A and C, and the connection between A and C was very apparent. Pursuing the REBT tradition, the B-C connection was introduced, and the A-C connection dissuaded. At the start of this process, coaches were given two narratives that portrayed an athlete who had underperformed under pressure. The narratives were identical, apart from the self-talk the athlete used. In narrative 1 the athlete used irrational self-talk ("I must not underperform, it is terrible to let people down, I can't stand failing, this failure makes me a complete failure") and in narrative 2 the athlete used rational self-talk ("I would like not to underperform, it is bad but not terrible to let people down, I can stand failing and it is worth it to do so, this failure does not make me a complete failure"). In response to these narratives, coaches were asked to discuss the differences between the two, and to predict what emotions and behaviours may arise in each. Coaches reflected that compared to narrative 2 (rational) the athlete in narrative 1 (irrational) was very negative and self-defeating, and that they would most likely experience UNEs, suffer limited motivation, and would be less likely to bounce back from the underperformance. I made the point that the only difference between the two narratives was the self-talk used by the athlete, which led onto some discussion around how B rather than A is the major determinant of C. This then progressed nicely onto the next section, which provided some detail around B.

Discovering the Beliefs (B) This was the most didactic element of the workshop, because I wanted to be very clear with the coaches as to the nature of irrational and rational beliefs. With the coaches it was important that I detail the core irrational and rational beliefs in enough detail that they could recognise them in themselves, and also in others if verbalised by athletes around them. The coaches were educated in the differences between irrational and rational beliefs including the primary and secondary beliefs, and asked to reflect on when they have noticed and used these beliefs in the past. To introduce some interaction into this section, coaches completed a sorting task where they were provided with 10 beliefs (5 irrational and 5 rational) scrambled with no order. In pairs they were asked to group the irrational beliefs together, and then the rational beliefs together. They also had to provide justifications for why each belief was either irrational or rational. This led to conversations around logic and evidence, which I encouraged. This activity can be used prior to B education to see if the coaches intuitively know which are rational or irrational, but here I wanted to use it as a formative assessment of their understanding of the key differences. Once I was happy that all the coaches realized the differences, I moved on to some low-level disputation advice.

Low-Level Disputation While the recognition and understanding of the ABC framework can be an effective intervention in itself, I wanted to leave the coaches with some ideas of how they could challenge and dispute irrational beliefs. Therefore the workshop finished with me detailing some "quick wins" that the coaches could implement, born from REBT philosophy, that may help encourage RBs in their athletes. I call this "low-level" because I am not rigorously teaching the coaches the full evidence, logic, and pragmatic arguments. This included three pieces of advice.

1. *Ask yourself and your athletes: "What are you saying to yourself about the situation, that is leading to your emotions?"* This reinforces the B-C connection over the erroneous A-C connection (Dryden, 2009).
2. *Challenge irrational language when you hear it from others, or when you hear it inside your own mind. Its ok to encourage athletes to realise that failure isn't fatal!* This is instilling some assertiveness in the coaches to start to change the performance lexicon around the athletes.
3. *Provide opportunities for athletes to create their own evidence that they can tolerate discomfort and adversity*. This is really a behavioural activity (Ellis & Dryden, 1997) as I am challenging the coaches to set up real situations in which athletes experience discomfort in a safe supportive environment, so that athletes realise that they can actually tolerate such circumstances.

The purpose of the workshop was to develop the coach's understanding and practical knowledge of REBT so that they can implement some REBT principles with their athletes. Conducting a workshop in this way relies on strict aims and objectives and the recognition that there is only so much you can do in a single 4-h session. By keeping my aims modest, I was able to cover some in-depth information and lead some useful discussion around core themes. In addition, coaches left with enough information to make some small changes that may make a difference to their athletes.

It is important to more formally (in research) to explore ways in which REBT can be taught to coaches, and how they can translate what they have learned to the athletes they coach. There is huge untapped potential to influence a great many young athletes via coaches, because they spend a significant amount of time with their athletes, and the coach-athlete relationship is so important for athlete development (Jowett & Cockerill, 2003).

Why Is the Interest in Using REBT in Sport Growing?

Thus far in the chapter, I have discussed the research work that has been published applying REBT, in its various forms, in sport. I have also detailed how REBT has been adapted and packaged for delivery with athletes and coaches. The need to think about how REBT can be best delivered in sport has arrived due to increasing interest in how REBT applies to sport. My first reflections on the use of REBT in sport (Turner & Barker, 2014) were triggered by observations that irrational beliefs were prevalent in the athletes I worked with, and that the sporting environment seemed especially promoting of irrational beliefs. As I have continued to use REBT in my work with athletes and coaches, I have since realized that there are various reasons why REBT is particularly applicable within sport. I believe that the spike in interest in REBT as applied within sport can be attributed to at least two main reasons. Both of these reasons will be expanded upon henceforth.

Sport May Promote and Propagate Irrational Beliefs There is a realization amongst some practitioners that sport may promote and propagate irrational beliefs, and does very little to dissuade A-C thinking. Therefore, sport and exercise psychologists have begun to explore REBT as a solution to irrational beliefs and A-C thinking. We often forget that the idea of ABC is very powerful, as it can foster autonomy over how people emote and behave in the face of adversity. Simply helping an athlete to realize that by controlling their beliefs they can control their emotions can empower the athlete to take responsibility for their emotional wellbeing. In essence, helping athletes to take charge of their thoughts requires the athlete developing and refining meta-cognitive skills, particularly 'thinking about thinking'. Ellis (2003) once said "Humans, unlike just about all the other animals on earth, create fairly sophisticated languages which not only enable them to think about their feeling, their actions, and the results they get from doing and not doing certain things, but they also are able to think about their thinking and even think about thinking about their thinking" (p. 220). It is impossible to conceive of an effective REBT intervention with an athlete without the athlete being able to think about thoughts, not least because the disputation process involves critical thinking about irrational and rational beliefs. However, key stakeholders of athlete wellbeing and performance working in sport will inadvertently promote A-C thinking by suggesting that pressure competition "makes" you anxious, or that poor officiating decisions "makes" me angry.

Aside from A-C thinking, sport may actually promote irrational beliefs (Turner, 2016a). For example, irrational beliefs appear in how the media report on sport, to the extent that the media would have us believe that success is a must and failure is fatal. For example, Louis van Gaal (Manchester United Football Club manger) described a Boxing Day match against Stoke City Football Club "must-win" stating that "When you have lost three times in a row to you need to win." He remarked "We have to focus on that match and we have to win that match." Manchester United lost 2–0, which apparently was a "must-win" (Sheen, 2015). More recently Antonio Conte (2017; Chelsea Football Club manager) gave his views on how the severity of failure in the English Football Premier League is dependent on the status and goals of the team. He said:

> If [Spurs] don't win the title, it's not a tragedy…if they don't arrive in the Champions League, it's not a tragedy. If they go out in the first round of the Champions League, it's not a tragedy. If they go out after the first game that they play in the Europa League, it's not a

> tragedy. Maybe for Chelsea, Arsenal, Manchester City, Manchester United and – I don't know – Liverpool, it is a tragedy. You must understand the status of the team. Every team has to understand what their ambitions are. If their ambitions are to fight for the title or win the Champions League.

Conte is suggesting here that whether failure is awful or not is dependent on one's ambition, simultaneously taking a swipe at Spurs by suggesting that they should perhaps lower their expectations. The use of language in sport media is very powerful, and managers often wage war using words, to try to gain a psychological victory of the opponent before a ball has been kicked, and can inflate the importance of success and severity of failure very easily. In contrast, Claudio Ranieri on his way to winning the English Football Premier League with Leicester City Football Club, stated that "We play without pressure because we don't have to win the league". Further, Jurgen Klopp after failing to win in his first three matches in charge of Liverpool Football Club in 2015 said:

> This is not the end of the world…We conceded a goal near the end, and it felt like the end of the world, but it is not the end of the world…I hope I'm not the only person in the stadium who thought: 'This is not the end of the world.' We can work on this…Of course, it is not the best moment for us, because we wasted a lot of energy. Southampton haven't lost away from home, so we had to work hard…You score the goal and you want to win, but it didn't happen for us today. Football is not a fairytale. Sometimes we can write stories like this but it doesn't always happen. (Agence France-Presse, 2015)

The issue here is not what coaches believe per se, and it should be considered that what coaches utter in the media might not reflect their actual core beliefs. But a more important point is that common cultural stereotypes in our language play a part in developing rational and irrational beliefs (Digiuseppe, Doyle, Dryden, & Backx, 2014). In other words, the language used in sport media may or may not reflect irrational beliefs, but a greater concern is the role sport media may play in the development of irrational beliefs in consumers of sport media. Youth athletes, for example, navigate a complex social world of coaches, teammates, support staff, opponents, supporters (and non-supporters), the media, and of course friends and family. From these sources, athletes gather information about how to develop an athletic career through formal and informal communication and interaction, and since people are influenced by language used in communication with others and oneself, when imprecise language is used (such as the verbal expression of rigid, extreme, and illogical beliefs) this can augment imprecise thinking (Dryden, 2015).

Ellis (1987) recognized that societal and cultural irrationalities are driven by the teachings of significant others, and that we internalize and perpetuate these irrationalities. Irrational beliefs are exacerbated by those around us whom we look to for guidance on how to live our lives (Sharf, 1996). Ultimately, society drives irrationality, and we as humans develop irrational beliefs as a function of our biological tendency to do so. Even if we take the stance that media representations of sports personalities do not accurately reflect core beliefs, the communication of irrational beliefs attributed to these personalities may contribute to the beliefs of young athletes. Indeed, it is often evident that sporting clubs organizations communicate in absolutes. For example, recently Pep Guardiola (Manager of Manchester City

Football Club) commented on the congested fixture schedule stating that "we are going to kill them" (PA Sports, 2018). Communicating in this way could be done so to make an impact, on The Football Association in this case, sometimes with tongue in cheek. However, decontextualized and taken as a sound bite, a tactic often employed by the media, the utterances of high-profile leaders in sport echo rigid, extreme, and frankly unsubstantiated, attitudes.

Therefore, practitioners working within sport are advised to as often as possible look beyond the beliefs of individual athletes within the sporting organization, and examine the language and cultural norms of the organization itself. In my experience, an athlete's development of irrational beliefs often stems from a top-down organizational structure where mantras and values are irrational or imprecise at inception. Indeed in a recent study (Evans, Turner, Pickerin, & Powditch, 2018) at the half-time period in a soccer match, the two competing teams were given either a "rational team talk" or an "irrational team talk". Data showed that athletes who received the "irrational" team talk reported greater avoidance goals and threat appraisal concerning the second half of the match. Examining irrational beliefs in the symbolic form of language offers an achievable examination of irrational beliefs and also allows for overt and direct manipulation (Dryden, 2015) compared to deeper level beliefs (e.g., schemas; David, Schnur, & Belloiu, 2002). In other words, if irrational beliefs and A-C thinking are challenged at a cultural and organizational level within the sport, then the propagation of irrational beliefs in young athletes can be moderated. Cultural changes within organizations have the potential to have long-lasting and broader effects (KatzenbachI, Steffen, & Kronley, 2012) on a large number of athletes.

The Importance of Athlete Mental Health The mental health and wellbeing of athletes is thankfully garnering growing interest and attention. A recent Frontiers in Psychology special issue (MacIntyre et al., 2016) progressed the scientific understanding of athlete mental health by bringing the current understanding of athlete mental health into focus. This interest in athlete mental health is perhaps unsurprising given that some (Hughes & Leavey, 2012) consider athletes to be at greater risk of mental illness due to the contextual demands of sport (e.g., requirement for high effort, great investment of time, and high exertion of energy; Cresswell & Eklund, 2007). Recent research indicates that athletes may be vulnerable to depressive symptoms (dysphoria), due to the stressful nature of being an athlete (Frank, Nixdorf, & Beckmann, 2015). Current thinking intimates that contextual factors can increase the risk of depression, such as injuries, overtraining, excessive stress, competitive failure, and ageing (e.g., Nixdorf, Frank, & Beckmann, 2016; Reardon & Factor, 2010), tournament frequency, important tournaments, and chronic stress (Nixdorf, Frank, & Beckmann, 2015). Therefore, psychotherapeutic methods that fit within the difficult context of sport, that can promote and maintain athlete mental health and psychological wellbeing, are valuable. REBT with its vast evidence-base represents a potentially important strategy for athlete welfare.

Only two published research studies have shown that irrational beliefs are associated with poorer wellbeing in athletes (Turner, Carrington, & Miller, 2018; Turner

& Moore, 2016). Turner and Moore had Elite Gaelic footballers ($N = 46$) complete a measure of burnout at six timepoints across 8 weeks of a competitive season, and an irrational beliefs questionnaire at the beginning and end of the 8 weeks. Irrational beliefs significantly predicted increased emotional and physical exhaustion, a dimension of burnout, across the season. Turner et al. (2018) found that greater irrational beliefs in a wide sample of athletes was related to greater anxiety, depression, and anger. They also found that secondary irrational beliefs were more proximal to anxiety, depression, and anger than primary irrational beliefs, supporting the REBT-Model I hypothesis (DiLorenzo, David, & Montgomery, 2007) in athletes. But despite the dearth of research in sport, much research outside of sport has demonstrated that irrational beliefs are associated with dysfunctional emotions and behaviours (Browne, Dowd, & Freeman, 2010), including a recent meta-analysis (Visla, Fluckiger, Grosse Holtforth, & David, 2015). In addition, the extant literature shows that REBT is effective in reducing emotional dysfunction, including three meta-analyses (Engels, Garnefski, & Diekstra, 1993; Gonzalez et al., 2004; Lyons & Woods, 1991). Therefore, the importance of REBT theory and practice in the understanding and promotion of athlete mental health is clear. However, literature lacks studies examining whether and what extent irrational beliefs are a risk factor for mental illness in athletes, and there is a dearth in research demonstrating mental health and wellbeing outcomes of REBT use in sport.

One construct that is growing in popularity in the sport literature, but has been recognized for a while in clinical literature (e.g., Davydov, Stewart, Ritchie, & Chaudieu, 2010), is resilience. The American Psychological Association (APA) considers resilience to be a process of adapting well in the face of adversity, trauma, tragedy, threats or significant sources of stress. In addition, sport specific conceptualizations of resilience recognize that emotional distress is very much a part of becoming resilient (see Sarkar, Fletcher, & Brown, 2015). It is also important to recognize that coming back from adversity is not necessarily an immediate occurrence (Dryden, 2007), in contrast to some notions that resilience is akin to “bouncing back” (Neenan, 2009).

According to Dryden (2007) and Neenan (2009) some symmetry exists between REBT and resilience whereby those who are able to react to adversity with rational beliefs are more likely to evidence resilience. In fact, in theory REBT offers a potentially very effective method for promoting resilience. Fletcher and Sarkar (2012) assert, “educational programs in challenge appraisal and meta-reflective strategies, such as evaluating personal assumptions, minimizing catastrophic thinking, challenging counterproductive beliefs, and cognitive restructuring, should form a central part of resilience training” (p. 676). REBT achieves all of these assertions because it endorses meta-cognition, aims to minimize catastrophic thinking, challenges counterproductive beliefs, and teaches cognitive-restructuring. In addition, irrational beliefs are related to threat cognitive appraisals (Dixon et al., 2017), which are counter to challenge cognitive appraisals (Jones, Meijen, McCarthy, & Sheffield, 2009). One study in sport has shown that REBT can increase resilient qualities in athletes, whilst also reducing irrational beliefs (Deen et al., 2017), and some consider rational beliefs to be “protective factors” (David, Freeman, & DiGiuseppe,

2010, p. 197). However, the role of irrational and rational beliefs, and the application of REBT, in the resilience of athletes are yet to be fully understood.

Lessons from the Experience of REBT Scholars and Practitioners

So far in the chapter, I have introduced the work being done applying and investigating REBT in sport, and have discussed the notable advancements being made in this fledgling area of sport and exercise psychology. The remainder of the chapter covers what I have learned from my experiences using REBT with athletes. I try to maintain the academic philosophy I have applied to the previous content, although much of what comes is based on my observations in practice.

What I Have Learned About the Benefits of REBT

From the content of the chapter up until now, clearly there are many benefits of using REBT theory and practice in sport (e.g., greater psychological health and wellbeing, greater resilience). However, here I want to highlight three specific benefits that I have noticed in my applied work with athletes at elite and sub-elite levels.

Greater Self-Determined Motivation

One of the challenges of using REBT in sport is that there are misconceptions about the motivational significance of rational and irrational beliefs. Indeed, some feel that REBT may reduce athlete motivation to succeed (Atkinson, 2014); but this is based on a one-dimensional conception of motivation from low to high motivation, and is a misunderstanding of REBT. In my experience, I do not see athletes who have received REBT experiencing deficits in the *quantity* of motivation, but I do see the *quality* of motivation shift. Specifically, I see athletes' motivation becoming more self-determined, where the drive to succeed moves from being underpinned by self-pressure and guilt, to being underpinned by enjoyment and the satisfaction of testing themselves on the field of play. As such, I have started to understand the motivational influence of REBT from a self-determination theory (SDT; Deci & Ryan, 2000) perspective, which offers a well-grounded multidimensional and sophisticated theory of motivation.

Deci and Ryan (1985) posited three types of motivation that capture the different reasons for individual engagement in achievement situations; intrinsic motivation (autonomous), extrinsic motivation (controlling), and amotivation. Intrinsic motivation refers to engaging in behaviours because they are personally rewarding.

Extrinsic motivation lies at the other, more controlling end of the self-determination continuum and refers to behaviours prompted by external sources, such as rewards or constraints imposed by the self and others. Amotivation is when individuals experience feelings of incompetence or lack of control and they possess neither intrinsic motivation nor extrinsic motivation. Importantly for REBT, extrinsic motivation comprises four regulation sub types; external, introjected, identified, and integrated (Deci & Ryan, 2000), and it is with introjected regulation that REBT might share some theoretical similarities.

Introjected regulation reflects moderately low self-regulation, where action is controlled by self-imposed sanctions and represents contingent self-esteem (Deci & Ryan, 2000). That is, an individual engages in a particular activity not because they want to, but because they 'should' (Standage, Duda, & Ntoumanis, 2001). This is of particular interest due to its potential relationship with irrational beliefs (Turner, 2016a) and can be further characterized by an individual internalizing external regulations and having a perception that 'I should' or 'I have to' engage in an activity, echoing primary irrational beliefs. Therefore, REBT may shift an athlete's introjected regulation towards greater intrinsic motivation, which is important because more self-determined types of motivation have been related to superior performance (Gillet, Berjot, & Gobance, 2009), persistence (Sarrazin, Vallerand, Guillet, Pelletier, & Curry, 2002), and wellbeing (Gagné, Ryan, & Bargmann, 2003). In a recent research paper (Turner & Davis, 2018) triathletes who underwent REBT education reported increases in self-determined motivation, alongside reductions in irrational beliefs, as one would expect. Since less self-determined motivation reflects a sense of pressure and perceived obligation to engage in an activity (controlled motivation; Reeve, 2012), it makes sense that as irrational beliefs reduce there might be a consequent reduction in controlled motivation, captured in Turner and Davis' (2018) study by increased in self-determined motivation.

In sum, although research needs to be done to understand how REBT influences self-determined motivation, from REBT theory and my observations as a practitioner, athletes do not become less motivated by being more rational, but motivation may shift from controlling types of motivation regulation (introjected regulation) towards more autonomous types of motivation regulation (intrinsic motivation).

Greater Self-Acceptance

Competitive sport at any level is dangerous for esteem, because evaluation threat is very salient. At the elite level of sport, athletes with favorable views about themselves are called into question by others (Jordet, 2009). This 'ego threat' is likely to result in emotional distress (Baumeister, 1997). An athlete with inflated self-esteem being evaluated on something in which they consider themselves to be 'elite', in addition to performing in front of spectators with (often) unrealistically high expectations of success, is likely to be destructive for performance (Baumeister, 1997). Indeed, Jordet (2009) found that publicly esteemed soccer players performed worse in major soccer penalty shootouts than other players, suggesting that egotistical illusions render the idea of failure particularly threatening, causing self-regulatory breakdowns and choking.

One of the distinctive features of REBT is that self-esteem is not a panacea for psychological health and wellbeing, and in fact, Ellis (2005) felt that conditional self-esteem is paradoxically deleterious to psychological health and wellbeing. Self-esteem, with its focus on the rating of self-worth, causes problems because whilst it is nice to believe that when I succeed I am consequently "a success", the opposite also has to be true, that when I fail I am consequently "a failure". Since failure in sport is unavoidable (because athletes are fallible human beings, just like the rest of us), the notion of self-esteem is problematic and renders athletes vulnerable to emotional distress. If worth is dependent on performance, the athlete becomes a victim of success and failure with regards to psychological health and wellbeing. Therefore, in REBT the concept of unconditional self-acceptance (USA; Ellis, 1977) is promoted, endorsing unconditional regard for oneself despite undesirable behaviors and adverse events (Hill, Hall, Appleton, & Kozub, 2008). In addition, USA reflects the tendency to rate one's behavior and not the self as a whole (e.g., "My performance was poor in this competition" rather than "I am a failure").

With the athletes I have worked with, the promotion of USA has led to a more functional approach to pressure situations, and a more adaptive response to failure. Interestingly, Jordet (2011) suggests that to reduce choking in sport performance, practitioners should help athletes to reduce ego-threat, normalise emotional distress, and optimise self-regulation. REBT with its promotion of USA can help reduce ego-threat. REBT can help athletes to normalise emotional distress by promoting acceptance, addressing meta-emotional issues, and by using flooding to desensitise athletes to pressure. REBT can also enhance self-regulation by helping athletes to develop meta-cognitive skills in order to regulation their emotions.

Greater Meta-cognitive Skills

During the process of REBT, the athlete is encouraged to introspect on thoughts and beliefs in order to as accurately as possible assess the functionality and utility of cognitions for performance. The quality, accuracy, and efficiency, of this introspection are determined largely by the meta-cognitive skills of the athlete (Metcalfe & Shimamura, 1994). As the work progresses, and the athlete is guided by the practitioner and completes necessary homework assignments, meta-cognitive skills develop and improve. A key development is the enhancement of the athletes metacognitive knowledge, which reflects beliefs and theories about ones own thinking (Wells, 2009). The professional relationship between athlete and practitioner allows for the athlete to be led in the assessment and disputation of beliefs at first, and then as work progresses the athlete takes more responsibility for the REBT process demonstrating greater access to beliefs and greater analytical skills regarding their own beliefs. It should be recognized that for many young athletes, the idea of thinking about thinking might be alien. But this skill can be developed, and is fundamental to the application of REBT during sport psychology consultation, and even more important following the work, where the athlete must apply REBT in the real world independently.

One thing I have noticed working with athletes, is that as a consequence of enhanced meta-cognition skills, some athletes are able to engage in cognitive dissonance concerning irrational beliefs. This cognitive dissonance (Festinger, 1957) allows athletes to hold and endorse contradictory beliefs, such as irrational and rational beliefs. That is, some athletes I have worked with are capable of adopting irrational thoughts for momentary performance situations, whilst simultaneously holding rational beliefs as part of their philosophy of life. I present this as "double-think" (Turner, 2016a), the Orwellian notion of "holding two contradictory beliefs in one's mind simultaneously, and accepting both of them." (Orwell, 1949, p. 32).

For example, a triathlete in the final kilometre of the 10 km run may think "I want to get my personal best and therefore I must, and I couldn't stand it if I did not" which may inspire a final burst of enthusiasm towards the home straight. As discussed previously, irrational beliefs may be associated with extrinsic types of motivation, which may inspire effort, but are also likely to lead to greater anxiety (Ryan & Connell, 1989). Therefore, the triathlete may also harbour the core belief that "I want to get my personal best, but that does not mean I have to, and it would be tough but I could tolerate not doing so" in contrast to irrational thoughts used in the moment. When there is dissonance such as the above example the athlete can momentarily ignore the contradiction because the irrational belief is producing the desired outcome of acutely enhanced performance. The skill here is for the athlete to choose when to use irrational beliefs for the purposes of performance. This choice relies on the meta-cognitive ability to recognize the thought, decide whether the though is helpful in the moment, whilst also knowing that the thought is irrational. However, athletes who are unable to relinquish their irrational thoughts when they depart from the field of play may find it difficult to endorse rational beliefs, and therefore may at risk from the many mental health outcomes highlighted in this chapter and elsewhere (Turner, 2016a).

Performance: A Surprising Omission?

The reader might notice that "greater athletic success" does not feature in my three main benefits. This is for two chief reasons. First, success in sport is a very complex phenomenon indeed, and whist the occurrence of the three benefits I have discussed should of course influence outcomes positively, it would be imprecise to suggest that sporting success can increase following REBT. Research is currently debating this issue (e.g., Turner, Kirkham, & Wood, 2018b; Wood, Turner, Barker, & Higgins, 2017), and until more data is available, practitioners should be tentative in their assertions that REBT can improve performance outcomes. Second, my personal philosophy of practice is 'human first, performer second' (or human>performer for short) and as such, my focus with athletes is on the enhancement of the processes that contribute to performance success (e.g., their emotional control and wellbeing), rather than focusing on success itself. This fits with the REBT tradition on emotional wellbeing, and is a more long-term focused strategy for promoting career wellbeing, not just better performance tomorrow.

What I Have Learned About What Does Not *Work All That Well in Sport*

One of the main issues I have faced applying REBT within sport is the social desirability of irrational beliefs. Perhaps because of the culture of sport, where irrational language is inherent and propagated (as discussed previously in this chapter), some athletes believe that to have irrational beliefs about performance is a good thing. Athletes may feel that adopting "its bad to fail, but not the end of the world" is nonchalant and are therefore unlikely to report or openly admit to having this belief. But whatever the reason for this social desirability, it permeates the early stages of REBT when assessing the athlete's ABCs. An athlete might initially and purposely over inflate there irrational beliefs saying that "yes I absolutely have to succeed, I'd be a loser if I didn't" as a way to communicate that they care so deeply about their craft that failure is unacceptable. But in my experience, once you have an initial conversation with the athlete, these irrational beliefs fall away and you realize that they are not beliefs at all, but self-talk used to acquiesce those around them. Some coaches I have worked with would not like it if their athletes went into a performance with an "I would really like to win, but I don't have to" belief, even though this rational belief can be very strong and can reflect adaptive types of motivation.

The overall point here is that one of the things I have found not to work that well is the initial assessment of athletes irrational beliefs, because it is riddled with bias and social conformity in sport. But, this can obviously be overcome by carefully investigating if the presenting "I must" is a core belief, or just a socially desirable self-talk. This takes patience but is important because not all utterances are deeply held beliefs (Bunker, Williams, & Zinsser, 1993). Therefore, the potential for bias to affect the work a practitioner does with an athlete is really in the hands of the practitioner, to carefully assess the athlete's beliefs and take time to understand the language used by the athlete and the social influences on that language.

Bias can also permeate the disputation phase of REBT. It is challenging with some athletes to suggest that they "do not HAVE to succeed" because sport is so results driven. Many athletes have held irrational beliefs about competing in sport for many years, particular elite athletes who have often been competing since early childhood (depending on the sport). Therefore, the idea that demandingness (primary irrational beliefs) is irrational is not an easy pill to swallow for many athletes, even when this belief is hindering their wellbeing and performance. Don't get me wrong, in sport we are not on a crusade to destroy all "I must succeed" beliefs, but even when an athlete is clearly in distress because of this belief, they still hold onto demandingness very tightly. So disputing demandingness with athletes is better achieved carefully, tactfully, but at the same time, resoundingly. You can leave no doubt in the athletes mind as to why demandingness is problematic, and therefore the use of empirical, logical, and pragmatic arguments should be done collaboratively, like a joint investigation into the validity of their beliefs. If you threaten the athlete by too quickly and flippantly rejecting demandingness, the athlete may nod and agree that the belief is irrational, but will not gain much intellectual insight, never mind emotional insight.

Adjoined to the above point about disputing demandingness is the importance of recognizing conditional musts. I have in the past mistakenly pursued the disputation of a demand because I didn't fully assess the belief, and missed the fact that the must was being applied conditionally. As Dryden (2009) remarks, the unconditional vs. conditional must is a source of confusion when first using REBT, and remains a constant splinter in my mind when working in sport. For example, a soccer athlete or coach who remarks "we must win this game to get the three points" should not be challenged on the illogicality of his or her utterance. Or when an athlete says "I have to get fitter over the summer break so I can hit the ground running in pre-season", the demand should be carefully considered. We don't know whether the must is accurate or not. It might be the case that to have a good start to the next season the athlete must get fitter, as this might be a necessary for his selection and performance in pre-season. If the athlete is exhibiting UNEs about getting fitter, then it is worth exploring whether there is an unconditional must behind this conditional must. It is worth 'going down the rabbit hole' and investigating whether the athlete feels they must hit the ground running next season, which of course may open up further conditional musts, or might reveal an unconditional must that can be disputed. The point is, musts, especially in sport, can be complicated by multiple conditions that make complete sense and should not disputed if one is applying REBT. This is really important because by, for example, erroneously disputing "I have to get fitter over the summer break" you may actually harm the athlete's chances of performing well in the pre-season.

Directions for the Future of REBT

Questions Still to Be Answered in REBT The application of REBT in sport is fledgling, and therefore much research is still to be done. As a broad point, it could be argued that much of the research done outside of sport should be replicated in sport to understand the transferability of findings across contexts. Perhaps some non-sport findings hold true in sport, while other findings do not. This research should be done cross-sectionally to examine the implications of irrational beliefs on wellbeing, mental health, and performance issues. Research applying REBT across the broad spectrum of sporting populations should also be completed, so that the effectiveness of REBT across ages, sports, levels, and ability, can be determined. As such, here I echo the key questions posed in Turner (2016a, 2016b):

1. *Do irrational beliefs and rational beliefs influence the mental health of athletes?*

For me, this is the chief research question that researchers should be tackling, especially in light of growing concern for the mental health of athletes. Researchers should examine whether the four core irrational beliefs separately predict psychological ill-being so that a more precise understanding of how irrational beliefs interrelate to cause psychological distress can be achieved. Aligned to this cross-sectional approach, longitudinal research is required to assess how irrational beliefs may predict changes in psychological health over time. This may include cohort studies that are followed up over a period of years. Researchers should also engage with psychophysiological markers of psychological health to understand more objectively the impact of irrational beliefs on the biopsychosocial athlete.

2. *Do irrational beliefs and rational beliefs influence the athletic performance of athletes?*

Currently, we do not know whether and to what extend rational and irrational beliefs influence athletic performance, or whether REBT can help to enhance performance. The motivational properties of irrational and rational beliefs for sport performance need to be better understood so that we can understand how REBT may influence short vs. long-term goal attainment. Also, performance is a complex phenomenon, especially in sports where objective performance for individual athletes can be difficult to ascertain (e.g., soccer). The notion of resilience should be investigated through a REBT-lens to examine how this may affect performance across an athletic career. Further, large-scale studies are needed that represent the broad athlete population so that we can understand the prevalence of irrational beliefs, and whether higher level athletes endorse more, or less, or equal, irrational beliefs compared to lower level athletes.

3. *How are irrational beliefs developed in athletes?*

Irrational beliefs in athletes are probably a result of the biological tendency to adopt irrational beliefs, alongside the socialization of athletes into the world of sport, where imprecise language is an occupational hazard. In fact, it is argued in this chapter that sport may (sometime inadvertently) promote of irrational beliefs. But, the extant research does not indicate how athletes develop irrational beliefs, and very little research exists on this issue outside of sport. Research should first examine the nature of irrational beliefs (are they schemas?), and then investigate how irrational beliefs are developed and maintained. Understanding how irrational beliefs are developed in athletes can then guide the psychosocial development of athletes, as it may then be possible to educate and liaise with key stakeholders of athlete wellbeing to apply policy that protects against the propagation of irrational beliefs.

Conclusion

This chapter has taken a critical approach to discussing the advances of REBT in sport. Although the reported use of REBT in sport is sparse, it is growing quickly, and we are starting to understand the sport-specific considerations important for the effective use of REBT with athletes. However, this chapter, and the research it draws upon, is focused largely on the reduction of irrational beliefs as part of the ABCDE framework. But REBT has dual goals (Bernard, Froh, DiGiuseppe, Joyce, & Dryden, 2010) of helping people overcome their emotional disturbances and to help people grow and self-actualizing according to their own goals. As such, in sport REBT can support self-actualization, flourishing, and resilience (Neenan, 2009). This chapter charts an exciting time for REBT as applied to sport. Never before has REBT garnered so much research interest in sport, and as REBT becomes a more widely recognized approach to sport and exercise psychology, and graduates learn about the use of REBT on sport and exercise courses, we will see further developments and advancements in the area.

References

Agence France-Presse. (2015, October 26). It is not the end of the world: Jurgen Klopp after Liverpool's draw. *NDTV Sports*. Retrieved from http://sports.ndtv.com/english-premier-league/news/250752-it-is-not-the-end-of-the-world-jurgen-klopp-after-liverpool-s-draw

Antonio Conte: Chelsea boss questions Tottenham's ambitions. (2017, July 27). *BBC*. Retrieved from http://www.bbc.co.uk/sport/football/40736388

Aspinwall, L. G., & Taylor, S. E. (1997). A stitch in time: Self-regulation and proactive coping. *Psychological Bulletin, 121*, 417–436.

Atkinson, M. (2014, September). *The Psychologist, 27*.

Barker, J. B., Mellalieu, S. D., McCarthy, P. J., Jones, M. V., & Moran, A. (2013). Special issue on single-case research in sport psychology. *Journal of Applied Sport Psychology, 25*(1), 1–3. https://doi.org/10.1080/10413200.2012.729378

Baumeister, R. F. (1997). Esteem threat, self-regulatory breakdown, and emotional distress as factors in self-defeating behavior. *Review of General Psychology, 1*, 145–174.

Bernard, M. E. (1985). A rational-emotive mental training program for professional athletes. In A. Ellis & M. E. Bernard (Eds.), *Clinical applications of rational-emotive therapy* (pp. 227–309). New York, NY: Plenum.

Bernard, M. E., Froh, J. J., DiGiuseppe, R., Joyce, M. R., & Dryden, W. (2010). Albert Ellis: Unsung hero of positive psychology. *Journal of Positive Psychology, 5*(4), 302–310. https://doi.org/10.1080/17439760.2010.498622

Browne, C. M., Dowd, E. T., & Freeman, A. (2010). Rational and irrational beliefs and psychopathology. In D. David, S. J. Lynn, & A. Ellis (Eds.), *Rational and irrational beliefs in human functioning and disturbances: Implications for research, theory, and practice*. New York, NY: Oxford University Press.

Bunker, L., Williams, J. M., & Zinsser, N. (1993). Cognitive techniques for improving performance and building confidence. In J. M. Williams (Ed.), *Applied sport psychology* (2nd ed., pp. 225–242). Palo Alto, CA: Mayfield.

Churchman, C. (2018). Using rational emotive behavior therapy (REBT) to combat performance debilitating unhealthy anxiety in an international level karateka. In M. Turner, & R. Bennett (Eds.). *The use of rational emotive behavior theraoy in sport and exercise*. London, UK: Routledge.

Cresswell, S. L., & Eklund, R. C. (2007). Athlete burnout: A longitudinal qualitative investigation. *The Sport Psychologist, 21*, 1–20.

Cunningham, R., & Turner, M. J. (2016). Using Rational Emotive Behavior Therapy (REBT) with Mixed Martial Arts (MMA) athletes to reduce irrational beliefs and increase unconditional self-acceptance. *Journal of Rational-Emotive & Cognitive-Behavior Therapy, 34*(4), 289–309.

David, D., Freeman, A., & DiGiuseppe, R. (2010). Rational and irrational beliefs: Implications for mechanisms of change and practice in psychotherapy. In D. David, S. J. Lynn, & A. Ellis (Eds.), *Rational and irrational beliefs: Research, theory and clinical practice* (pp. 195–217). New York, NY: Oxford University Press.

David, D., Schnur, J., & Belloiu, A. (2002). Another search for the "hot" cognitions: Appraisal, irrational beliefs, attributions, and their relation to emotion. *Journal of Rational-Emotive & Cognitive-Behavior Therapy, 20*(2), 93–131.

Davydov, D., Stewart, R., Ritchie, K., & Chaudieu, I. (2010). Resilience and mental health. *Clinical Psychology Review, 30*(5), 479–495.

Deci, E. L., & Ryan, R. M. (1985). *Intrinsic motivation and self-determination in human behaviour*. New York, NY: Plenum Publishing Corporation.

Deci, E. L., & Ryan, R. M. (2000). The "what" and "why" of goal pursuits: Human needs and the self-determination of behavior. *Psychological Enquiry, 11*(4), 227–268.

Deen, S., Turner, M. J., & Wong, R. (2017). The effects of REBT and credos on irrational beliefs and resilient qualities in athletes. *The Sport Psychologist, 31*, 249–263.

Digiuseppe, R. A., Doyle, C. A., Dryden, W., & Backx, W. (2014). *A practitioner's guide to rational emotive behavior therapy* (3rd ed.). New York, NY: Oxford University Press.

DiLorenzo, T. A., David, D., & Montgomery, G. H. (2007). The interrelations between irrational cognitive processes and distress in stressful academic settings. *Personality and Individual Differences, 42*, 765–777.

Dixon, M., Turner, M. J., & Gillman, J. (2017). Examining the relationships between challenge and threat cognitive appraisals and coaching behaviours in football coaches. *Journal of Sports Sciences, 35*(24), 2446–2452.

Dryden, W. (2007). Resilience and rationality. *Journal of Rational-Emotive & Cognitive-Behavior Therapy, 25*(3), 213–226.

Dryden, W. (2009). *How to think and intervene like an REBT therapist*. London, UK: Routledge.

Dryden, W. (2015). *Rational emotive behaviour therapy: Distinctive features*. New York, NY: Routledge.

Dryden, W. (2016). *When time is at a premium: Cognitive-behavioural approaches to singel-session therapy and very breif coaching*. London, UK: Rationality Publications.

Elko, K. P., & Ostrow, A. C. (1991). Effects of a rational-emotive education program on heightened anxiety levels of female collegiate gymnasts. *The Sport Psychologist, 5*, 235–255.

Ellis, A. (1977). Psychotherapy and the value of a human being. In A. Ellis & R. Greiger (Eds.), *Handbook of rational emotive therapy*. New York, NY: Springer.

Ellis, A. (1987). On the origin and development of rational-emotive theory. In W. Dryden (Ed.), *Key cases in psychotherapy* (pp. 148–175). New York, NY: New York University Press.

Ellis, A. (2003). Early theories and practices of rational emotive behavior theory and how they have been augmented and revised during the last three decades. *Journal of Rational-Emotive & Cognitive-Behavior Therapy, 21*(3/4), 219–243.

Ellis, A. (2005). *The myth of self-esteem*. New York, NY: Prometheus books.
Ellis, A., & Dryden, W. (1997). *The practice of rational-emotive behavior therapy*. New York, NY: Springer Publishing Company.
Ellis, A., Gordon, J., Neenan, M., & Palmer, S. (1997). *Stress counselling: A rational emotive behavior approach*. London, UK: Cassell.
Engels, G. I., Garnefski, N., & Diekstra, R. F. (1993). Efficacy of rational-emotive therapy: A quantitative analysis. *Journal of Consulting and Clinical Psychology, 61*(6), 1083–1090.
Evans, A. L., Turner, M. J., Pickerin, R., & Powditch, R. (2018). The effects of rational and irrational coach team talks on the cognitive appraisal and achievement goal orientation of varsity football athletes. *International Journal of Sports Science & Coaching, 13*(3), 431–438. https://doi.org/10.1177/1747954118771183
Festinger, L. (1954). *A theory of social comparison processes*. Retrieved from hum.sagepub.com database
Festinger, L. (1957). *A theory of cognitive dissonance*. Stanford, CA: Stanford University Press.
Fletcher, D., & Sarkar, M. (2012). A grounded theory of psychological resilience in Olympic champions. *Psychology of Sport and Exercise, 13*, 669–678.
Frank, R., Nixdorf, I., & Beckmann, J. (2015). Depression among elite athletes: Prevalence and psychological factors. *Deutsche Zeitschrift Für Sportmedizin*. Retrieved from http://www.zeitschrift-sportmedizin.de/fileadmin/content/Englische_Artikel/Originalia_Frank_englisch.pdf
Frey, M. (2007). College coaches' experiences with stress—"Problem solvers" have problems too. *The Sport Psychologist, 21*, 38–57.
Gagné, M., Ryan, R. M., & Bargmann, K. (2003). Autonomy support and need satisfaction in the motivation and well-being of gymnasts. *Journal of Applied Social Psychology, 30*, 1843–1852.
Gillet, N., Berjot, S., & Gobance, L. (2009). A motivational model of performance in the sport domain. *European Journal of Sport Science, 9*(3), 151–158.
Gonzalez, J., Nelson, J., Gutkin, T., Saunders, A., Galloway, A., & Shwery, C. (2004). Rational emotive therapy with children and adolescents: A meta-analysis. *Journal of Emotional and Behavioral Disorders, 12*(4), 222–235.
Gould, D., Greenleaf, C., Guinan, D., & Chung, Y. (2002). A survey of U.S. Olympic coaches: Variables perceived to have influenced athlete performances and coach effectiveness. *The Sport Psychologist, 16*, 229–250.
Gulliver, A., Griffiths, K. M., & Christensen, H. (2012). Barriers and facilitators to mental health help-seeking for young elite athletes: A qualitative study. *Psychiatry, 12*, 157.
Hill, A. P., Hall, H. K., Appleton, P. R., & Kozub, S. A. (2008). Perfectionism and burnout in junior elite soccer players: The mediating influence of unconditional self-acceptance. *Psychology of Sport and Exercise, 9*(5), 630–644. https://doi.org/10.1016/j.psychsport.2007.09.004
House, J. S. (1981). *Work stress and social support*. Reading, MA: Addison-Wesley.
Hughes, L., & Leavey, G. (2012). Setting the bar: Athletes and vulnerability to mental illness. *The British Journal of Psychiatry, 200*(2), 95–96.
Jones, M. V., Meijen, C., McCarthy, P. J., & Sheffield, D. (2009). A theory of challenge and threat states in athletes. *International Review of Sport and Exercise Psychology, 2*, 161–180.
Jordet, G. (2009). When superstars flop: Public status and choking under pressure in international soccer penalty shootouts. *Journal of Applied Sport Psychology, 21*(2), 125–130. https://doi.org/10.1080/10413200902777263
Jordet, G. (2011). Performing under pressure: What can we learn from soccer penalty shoot outs? *Sport and Exercise Psychology Review, 7*, 11–13.
Jowett, S., & Cockerill, I. M. (2003). Olympic medallists' perspective of the athlete–coach relationship. *Psychology of Sport and Exercise, 4*, 313–331.
KatzenbachI, J. R., Steffen, I., & Kronley, C. (2012). Cultural change that sticks. *Harvard Business Review*. Retrieved from https://hbr.org/2012/07/cultural-change-that-sticks
Kelley, B. C., Eklund, R. C., & Ritter-Taylor, M. (1999). Stress burnout among collegiate tennis coaches. *Journal of Sport and Exercise Psychology, 21*, 113–130.

Knaus, W. (2006). *Rational emotive education. Theory into Practice*. New York, NY: REBT Network. Retrieved on 20th May, 2016 from https://doi.org/10.1080/00405847709542709
Kodish, S. P. (2002). Rational emotive behavior coaching. *Journal of Rational-Emotive Cognitive-Behavioural Therapy, 20*, 235–246.
Lu, J. J. H., et al. (2016). Interaction of athletes' resilience and coaches' social support on the stress-burnout relationship: A conjunctive moderation perspective. *Psychology of Sport and Exercise, 22*, 202–209.
Lyons, L. C., & Woods, P. J. (1991). The efficacy of rational-emotive therapy: A quantitative review of the outcome research. *Clinical Psychology Review, 2*, 357–369.
MacIntyre, T. E., Van Raalte, J., Brewer, B. W., Jones, M., O'Shea, D., & McCarthy, P. J. (2016). Mental health challenges in elite sport: balancing risk with reward. *Frontiers in Psychology, 8*, 1892. https://doi.org/10.3389/fpsyg.2017.01892
Mageau, G. A., & Vallerand, R. J. (2003). The coach-athlete relationship: A motivational model. *Journal of Sports Science, 21*, 883–904.
Marlow, C. (2009). Creating positive performance beliefs: The case of a tenpin bowler. In B. Hemmings & T. Holder (Eds.), *Applied sport psychology: A case based approach* (pp. 65–87). London, UK: Wiley.
Martin, K. A., Moritz, S. E., & Hall, C. R. (1999). Imagery use in sport: A literature review and applied model. *The Sport Psychologist, 13*, 245–268.
Maultsby, M. (1971). Rational emotive imagery. *Rational Living, 6*(1), 24–27.
Metcalfe, J., & Shimamura, A. P. (1994). *Metacognition: Knowing about knowing*. Cambridge, MA: MIT Press.
Neenan, M. (2009). *Developing resilience: A cognitive-behavioural approach*. East Essex, UK: Routledge.
Neenan, M., & Dryden, W. (2002). *Life coaching: A cognitive-behavioral approach*. New York, NY: Routledge.
Nixdorf, I., Frank, R., & Beckmann, J. (2015). An explorative study on major stressors and its connection to depression and chronic stress among German elite athletes. *Advances in Physical Education, 5*, 255–262. https://doi.org/10.4236/ape.2015.54030
Nixdorf, I., Frank, R., & Beckmann, J. (2016). Comparison of athletes' proneness to depressive symptoms in individual and team sports: Research on psychological mediators in junior elite athletes. *Frontiers in Psychology, 17*(7), 893.
Ogbuanya, T. C., Eseadi, C., Orji, C. T., Ohanu, I. B., Bakare, J., & Ede, M. O. (2017). Effects of rational emotive behavior coaching on occupational stress and work ability among electronics workshop instructors in Nigeria. *Medicine, 96*(19), e6891. https://doi.org/10.1097/MD.0000000000006891
Orwell, G. (1949). *Nineteen eighty-four*. London, UK: Martin Secker & Warburg Ltd.
PA Sports. (2018, 3rd January). Playing every two days is killing us and FA must act, says Guardiola. TransferMarket.com. https://www.transfermarkt.co.uk/playing-every-two-days-is-killing-us-and-fa-must-act-says-guardiola/view/news/296642. Accessed 23 March 2018.
Reardon, C. L., & Factor, R. M. (2010). Sport psychiatry: A systematic review of diagnosis and medical treatment of mental illness in athletes. *Sports Medicine, 40*, 961–980.
Reeves, C. W., Nicholls, A. R., & McKenna, J. (2009). Stressors and coping strategies among early and middle adolescent premier league academy soccer players: Differences according to age. *Journal of Applied Sport Psychology, 21*, 31–48. https://doi.org/10.1080/10413200802443768
Reeve, J. (2012). A self-determination theory perspective on student engagement. In S. L. Christenson, A. Reschly, & C. Wylie (Eds.), *Handbook of research on student engagement* (pp. 149–172). New York: Springer.
Reinboth, M., Duda, J. L., & Ntoumanis, N. (2004). Dimensions of coaching behavior, need satisfaction, and the psychological and physical welfare of young athletes. *Motivation and Emotion, 28*, 297–313. https://doi.org/10.1023/B:MOEM.0000040156.81924.b8
Ryan, R. M., & Connell, J. P. (1989). Perceived locus of causality and internalization: Examining reasons for acting in two domains. *Journal of Personality and Social Psychology, 57*, 746–761.

Sarkar, M., Fletcher, D., & Brown, D. J. (2015). What doesn't kill me . . . Adversity-related experiences are vital in the development of superior Olympic performance. *Journal of Science and Medicine in Sport, 18*, 475–479.

Sarrazin, P., Vallerand, R. J., Guillet, E., Pelletier, L. G., & Curry, F. (2002). Motivation and dropout in female handball players: A 21-month prospective study. *Journal of Social Psychology, 32*, 395–418.

Sharf, R. S. (1996). *Theories of psychotherapy and counseling: Concepts and cases*. Pacific Grove, CA: Brooks/Cole Publishing Company.

Sheen, T. (2015, December 24). Manchester United 'must win' against Stoke on Boxing Day, says under-pressure Louis van Gaal. *The Independent*, Retrieved from http://www.independent.co.uk/sport/football/premier-league/louis-van-gaal-manchester-united-must-win-against-stoke-says-under-pressure-manager-a6785446.html

Si, G., & Lee, H. (2008). Is it so hard to change? The case of a Hong Kong Olympic silver medallist. *International Journal of Sport and Exercise Psychology, 6*, 319–330.

Skinner, E. A., & Zimmer-Gembeck, M. J. (2007). The development of coping. *Annual Review of Psychology, 58*, 119–144. PubMed. https://doi.org/10.1146/annurev.psych.58.110405.085705

Standage, M., Duda, J. L., & Ntoumanis, N. (2001). A test of self-determination theory in school physical education. *British Journal of Educational Psychology, 75*, 411–433.

Terjesen, M. D., Salhany, J., & Sciutto, M. J. (2009). A psychometric review of measures of irrational beliefs: Implications for psychotherapy. *Journal of Rational-Emotive and Cognitive-Behavior Therapy, 27*, 83–96.

Thompson, R. A., & Sherman, R. T. (2007). *Managing student-athletes' mental health issues*. NCAA. Retrieved from https://www.ncaa.org/sites/default/files/2007_managing_mental_health_0.pdf

Trower, P., & Jones, J. (2001). How REBT can be less disturbing and remarkably more influential in Britain: A review of the views of practitioners and researchers. *Journal of Rational-Emotive & Cognitive-Behavior Therapy, 19*, 21–30. https://doi.org/10.1023/A:1007891115800

Turner, M., Carrington, S., & Miller, A. (2018). Psychological distress across sport participation groups: The mediating effects of secondary irrational beliefs on the relationship between primary irrational beliefs and symptoms of anxiety, anger, and depression. *Journal of Clinical Sport Psychology, 12*, 1–38.

Turner, M. J. (2014). Smarter thinking in sport. *The Psychologist, 27*(8), 596–599.

Turner, M. J. (2016a). Rational Emotive Behavior Therapy (REBT), irrational and rational beliefs, and the mental health of athletes. *Frontiers: Movement Science and Sport Psychology*. https://doi.org/10.3389/fpsyg.2016.01423

Turner, M. J. (2016b). Proposing a rational resilience credo for athletes. *Journal of Sport Psychology in Action, 7*(3), 170–181. https://doi.org/10.1080/21520704.2016.1236051

Turner, M. J., & Barker, J. B. (2013). Examining the efficacy of Rational-Emotive Behavior Therapy (REBT) on irrational beliefs and anxiety in elite youth cricketers. *Journal of Applied Sport Psychology, 25*(1), 131–147.

Turner, M. J., & Barker, J. B. (2014). Using rational emotive behavior therapy with athletes. *The Sport Psychologist, 28*(1), 75–90.

Turner, M. J., & Davis, H. (2018). Exploring the effects of Rational Emotive Behaviour Therapy (REBT) on the irrational beliefs and self-determined motivation of triathletes. *Journal of Applied Sport Psychology*. https://doi.org/10.1080/10413200.2018.1446472

Turner, M. J., & Moore, M. (2016). Irrational beliefs predict increased emotional and physical exhaustion in Gaelic football athletes. *International Journal of Sport Psychology, 47*(2), 187–201.

Turner, M. J., Slater, M. J., & Barker, J. B. (2014). Not the end of the world: The effects of rational emotive behavior therapy on the irrational beliefs of elite academy athletes. *Journal of Applied Sport Psychology, 26*(2), 144–156.

Turner, M. J., Slater, M. J., & Barker, J. B. (2015). The season-long effects of rational emotive behavior therapy on the irrational beliefs of professional academy soccer athletes. *International Journal of Sport Psychology, 5*, 429–451.

Turner, M. J., & Wood, A. (2016). *Smarter thinking app* (version 1.1) [Mobile application software]. Retrieved from https://play.google.com/store/apps/details?id=com.DKCS.SmarterThinking&hl=en

Turner, M. J., & Allen, M. (2018). Confirmatory factor analysis of the irrational performance beliefs inventory (iPBI) in a sample of amateur and semi-professional athletes. *Psychology of Sport and Exercise, 35*, 126–130. https://doi.org/10.1016/j.psychsport.2017.11.017

Turner, M. J., & Bennett, R. (2018). *Rational emotive behaviour therapy in sport and exercise*. London, UK: Routledge.

Turner, M. J., Allen, M., Slater, M. J., Barker, J. B., Woodcock, C., Harwood, C. G., & McFadyen, K. (2018a). The development and initial validation of the irrational performance beliefs inventory (iPBI). *European Journal of Psychological Assessment, 34*, 174–180.

Turner, M. J., Kirkham, L., & Wood, A. G. (2018b). Teeing up for success: The effects of rational and irrational self-talk on the putting performance of amateur golfers. *Journal of Psychology of Sport & Exercise, 38*, 148–153. https://doi.org/10.1016/j.psychsport.2018.06.012

Vertopolous, V., & Turner, M. J. (2017). Examining the effectiveness of a Rational Emotive Personal-Disclosure Mutual-Sharing (REPDMS) intervention on the irrational beliefs, rational beliefs, and emotions of Greek adolescent athletes. *The Sport Psychologist*. Accepted 24 January 2017.

Visla, A., Fluckiger, C., Grosse Holtforth, M., & David, D. (2015). Irrational beliefs and psychological distress: A meta-analysis. *Psychotherapy and Psychosomatics, 85*, 8–15.

Wells, A. (2009). *Meta-cognitive therapy for anxiety and depression*. New York, NY: The Guilford Press.

Wood, A., Barker, J. B., & Turner, M. J. (2016). Developing performance using Rational Emotive Behavior Therapy (REBT): A case study with an elite archer. *The Sport Psychologist, 31*(1), 78–87.

Wood, A., Barker, J. B., & Turner, M. J. (2017). Rational emotive behaviour therapy to help young athletes build resilience and deal with adversity. In C. J. Knight, C. G. Harwood, & D. Gould (Eds.), *Sport psychology for young athletes*. London, UK: Routledge.

Wood, A. G., Barker, J. B., Turner, M., & Sheffield, D. (2017). Examining the effects of Rational Emotive Behavior Therapy (REBT) on Performance Outcomes in Elite Paralympic Athletes. *Scandinavian Journal of Medicine & Science in Sports*. https://doi.org/10.1111/sms.12926. Accepted 5 June 2017.

Wood, A. G., Turner, M. J., & Barker, J. B. (2018). Using rational emotive behaviour therapy to promote psychological wellbeing with a paralympic athlete. In G. Breslin, & H. Leavey (Eds.). *Mental health and well-being interventions in sport: A case study analysis*.

Wood, A. G., Turner, M. J., Barker, J. B., & Higgins, S. J. (2017). Investigating the effects of irrational and rational self-statements on motor-skill and Hazard perception performance. *Sport, Exercise, and Performance Psychology*. Accepted 31 March 2017.

Ziegler, M., & Horstmann, K. (2015). Discovering the second side of the coin integrating situational perception into psychological assessment. *European Journal of Psychological Assessment, 31*, 69–74.

Chapter 15
REBT and Parenting Interventions

Oana Alexandra David, Horea-Radu Oltean, and Roxana Andreea-Ioana Cardoş

Albert Ellis pioneered the application of cognitive methods in parent education programs in the mid-1950s. Albert Ellis was interested in applying Rational-Emotive Behavior Therapy (REBT) with children, by working directly with children, or indirectly, by working with parents (Bernard, Ellis, & Terjesen, 2006). From the early 1960s with the publication of the book *'How to Raise an Emotionally Healthy, Happy Child'* (Ellis, Wolfe, & Moseley, 1966), REBT has become an important paradigm in parenting interventions, proposing that:

> *The worst care parents can provide their children is that of blaming them for their mistake making and wrongdoing. Parents or other early teachers usually help a child plummet down the toboggan slide towards disturbed feelings and behaviors by doing two things when he (child) does something that displeases them: (a) they tell him that he is wrong for acting in this displeasing manner, and (b) they strongly indicate to him that he is a worthless individual for being wrong, and that he therefore deserves to be damned and severely punished for his wrongdoing.* (Ellis et al., 1966)

The aim of this chapter is to describe the advances in the application of REBT to parenting and to illustrate some of the key ingredients of the REBT approach to parent education. First, we make a general presentation of the REBT based parent education theory, after which we describe different REBT parenting programs, history, therapeutic tools and the evidence-based status of the field. In the last part of

O. A. David (✉) · R.A.-I. Cardoş
Department of Clinical Psychology and Psychotherapy, Babeş-Bolyai University, Cluj-Napoca, Romania
e-mail: oanadavid@psychology.ro; roxana.cardos@ubbcluj.ro

H.-R. Oltean
The International Institute for the Advanced Studies of Psychotherapy and Applied Mental Health, Babeş-Bolyai University, Cluj-Napoca, Romania
e-mail: horea.oltean@ubbonline.ubbcluj.ro

© Springer Nature Switzerland AG 2019

M. E. Bernard, W. Dryden (eds.), *Advances in REBT*,
https://doi.org/10.1007/978-3-319-93118-0_15

the chapter, we discuss new directions in REBT based parent education field, focusing on developing access, efficacy and effectiveness to these programs. The chapter will thus answer the following questions:

1. What are the aspects of REBT theory that apply to parenting?
2. Types of REBT parenting interventions
3. REBT parenting interventions for parents of children with special problems
4. New directions in REBT based parent education

Application of REBT Theory to Parenting

As we mentioned above, in its earliest days, REBT was applied to the field of parent education. The pioneer work in the field was the book "*How to Raise an Emotionally Healthy, Happy Child*" (Ellis et al., 1966), which describes some of the most common child misbehaviors, points out possible causes (both genetic and environmental factors) of these problems based on the research at that time, and also recommends solutions, using both cognitive and behavioral techniques. Ellis asserted that the propensity for parents to engage in irrational thinking is 80% biological and 20% environmental.

Another early REBT application to parent education is Paul Hauck's irrational parenting styles classification (Hauck, 1967) who defined four main parenting styles based on different patterns of rational and irrational beliefs of the parents.

The irrational parenting style, *unkind and firm* implies high levels of demandingness beliefs, low frustration tolerance (e.g., "Children must always disobey to my rules"). This style has parents setting rigid rules and being excessively strict, focusing on the wrongdoing of their child and offering little praise, attacking the personality of their child. As a consequence, children will have the tendency to see themselves as worthless, experience anxiety, guilt and display avoidant or submissive behavior.

The irrational parenting styles, *kind and not firm* style, has parents who avoid frustrating their children who set very lax limits or they do not set them at all, but who are at the same time warm with children. This style is based on parent's irrational beliefs concerning their child's inability to tolerate frustration such as "My child should not be frustrated" or global self-rating ("I am a bad parent"). Children living with parents using this style may become dependent, with low frustration tolerance and low responsibility.

The irrational parenting style is the *unkind and not firm* characterized by inconsistent child rearing practices applied for misbehavior and the lack of affectionate behavior or praise for good behavior. Children experiencing this parenting style can become chronic rule breakers and display defiant behavior.

Hauck called the rational parenting style, *kind and firm*, referring to parents who show warmth based on unconditional child acceptance and who also setting firm rules for the behavior of their children. Thus, the most effective parenting style and the one promoted in REBT parent education is the *kind and firm* style, which can lead to more functional emotions and adaptive behaviors in both parents and their children.

In the following decades, REBT has been used by many parent educators (counselors, psychologists) with parents having children identified with various problems or for prevention purposes. REBT parent interventions or education can be used in two ways; namely as an indirect service to parents to assist in their management of a child with problems of adjustment including emotional difficulties or as parent mental health consultation to help parents cope with the stresses of parenting. In the first case, the child is the client and the main beneficiary of the service, with REBT parent intervention having the goals of teaching parents self-control abilities as well as to teach them how to help children deal with adversity and resultant emotional problems. In the second case, the parent and his/her problems represent the main focus of the consultation, with the aim of improving parenting skills and decrease parent stress level.

REBT parent interventions target two major categories of parents' problems: emotional and practical problems (Joyce, 1994, 2006). The main theoretical assumption of REBT parent interventions is that parents' emotional problems (i.e., anger, anxiety, guilt) are largely determined by irrational/ dysfunctional beliefs (see Fig. 15.1). Practical problems are reflected in parents not knowing how to manage their child's behavior or solve developmental issues. Practical problems are tackled by teaching parents positive parenting skills, like positive discipline, communication, while for emotional problems, techniques are aimed at changing parents' beliefs about children behavior or their role.

REBT-based parenting intervention with individual parents often involve an assessment phase (Bernard, 2004) for determining: (a) child development and functioning; (b) how supportive the parent-child relationship is; (c) which style of parenting is used and if the parent use effective child behavior management strategies; and (d) are parent's emotional problems interfering with using effective parenting strategies. Thus, assessment conducted with the parent is focused both on identifying the problems for determining the services required (education, consultation, therapy), and evaluating and analyzing the problems based on the ABC model, parenting styles and practices for determining the mechanisms and main focus of the intervention. Thus, a beginning point for work with parents is to help them realize that their emotional and behavioral reactions may be contributing to their child's issues and is key factors for getting their child to change.

Parent Irrational and Rational Beliefs

According to REBT, parent's irrational beliefs are categorized in four main categories: (1) demandingness (e.g., "My child must be compliant all the time"); (2) awfulizing/catastrophizing (e.g., "It will be awful if my child does not obey to me"); (3) low frustration tolerance/frustration intolerance (e.g., "I cannot stand when my

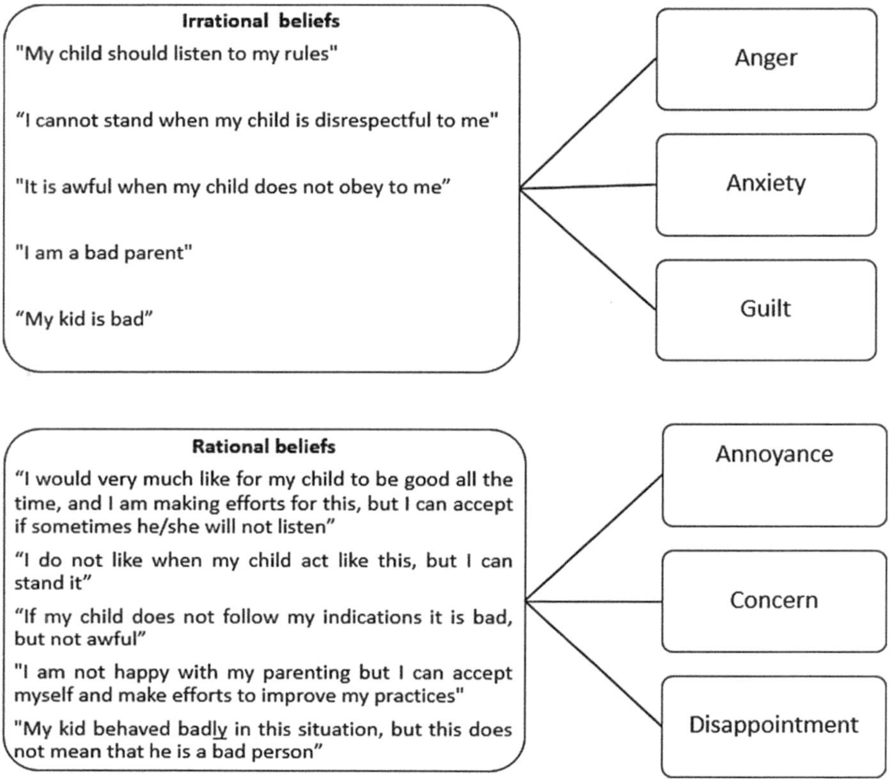

Fig. 15.1 The relationship between irrational/rational beliefs and dysfunctional/functional emotions

child is disrespectful to me"); (4) global evaluation of self, others, or world (e.g., "My kid is very bad"). There are four corresponding categories of rational beliefs, respectively: (1) preferences (e.g., "I would very much like for my child to be good all the time, and I am making efforts for this, but I can accept if sometimes he/she will not be good"); (2) realistic evaluation of badness (e.g., "If my child does not follow my indications it is bad, but not awful"); (3) high frustration tolerance (e.g., "I do not like when my child act like this, but I can stand it"); (4) unconditional acceptance (e.g., "My kid behaved badly in this situation, but this does not mean that he is a bad person"; see Fig. 15.1). It was found (Gavita, DiGiuseppe, & David, 2013) that the most frequent irrational beliefs involved in dysfunctional parent emotions and maladaptive parenting practices are low frustration tolerance and global evaluation, especially in the form of self-downing (e.g., "I am a bad parent"). Therefore, increasing the levels of frustration tolerance and unconditional self-acceptance of parent and other-acceptance regarding the child it is an essential step in REBT parent interventions.

ABCs as Applied to Parenting

In REBT, parents are taught how their beliefs about their children, themselves and life determine how they feel and behave towards their child rather than being caused by their child and his/her behavior. That is, REBT techniques teach parents that their children's behavior is not the cause of their emotional states and behaviors, but the way in which they evaluate the behavior. One of the most used therapeutic tools in REBT for facilitating the awareness and analysis of rational and irrational cognitions as causal factors for parents' functional or dysfunctional emotions is the ABC model. In the parenting context, the ABC model explains that parents' emotions and behaviors (C- consequences) are not directly determined by child- related events (A- activating events), but rather by the way these events are cognitively processed and evaluated (B- beliefs, David, 2015; Ellis, 1994). Thus, one goal in REBT based parenting interventions is to guide parents on how to change their irrational beliefs related to their child's behavior into rational beliefs. Using specific REBT techniques, parents learn how to strengthen their rational beliefs and in this way generate a more adaptive response in different child related situations, and create a positive relationship with their children.

Ellis (Ellis et al., 1966) has underlined that parents can communicate, model and reinforce rational beliefs in their children. He discussed how rational beliefs can be taught by parents to their children:

- Self- and other-Acceptance: Parents need to teach children how to not rate themselves or others globally and judge their behaviors but not their self-worth. This way, they can tech children to accept responsibility for their traits and behavior without judging themselves as good or bad based on them. Parents can use instances when children or they make mistakes to teach them how we do not like all our behaviors or traits but we do not judge ourselves based on them. Children will learn that they and others are capable and likeable in their own unique ways, and their qualities and not lost when bad things happen.
- High Frustration Tolerance: Parents need to teach children that obstacles and frustrations are part of life and that they can stand them. Also, parents need to reinforce the fact that if children want to be successful they sometimes need to do tasks that are not pleasant or exciting in favor of activities that they like at that time.

Types of REBT Parenting Interventions

Based on REBT principles and research, different REBT parent intervention programs have been published and some have empirical data to support them. These programs have different names, but all of them have the goal to educate parents about how to deal with child-related problematic emotions and behavior and how to improve parental practices in order to raise happy and healthy children.

REBT-based parenting programs also focus on assisting parents to overcome their own emotional problems.

In the following section we will describe in detail REBT parent interventions in terms of structure, techniques used, main targets, and their results.

Rational-Emotive Family Therapy

Rational-Emotive Family Therapy (DiGiuseppe & Kelter, 2006; Huber & Baruth, 1989) involves direct intervention with the parents of children with psychopathology (e.g., who are in therapy). DiGiuseppe and Kelter (2006) show that involving parents in therapy is essential in order to generalize therapeutic gains in the ecological environment of the child. Therefore, restructuring parents' irrational beliefs and reducing distress are primary goals that can enable parents to engage in more efficient parenting practices and this way improve child functioning.

DiGiuseppe and Kelter (2006) proposed a general sequence of *Rational-Emotive Family Therapy* consisting of ten stages, each one involving different techniques and strategies, presented below:

1. Assessment: gathering information on the structure of the family, emotions, cognitions, and skills of each member, child behavioral analysis.
2. Engage parents in the therapeutic alliance: motivational interviewing or problem solving.
3. Planning of the behavioral intervention: setting a target behavior and establishing consequences plan to increase child positive behavior or to decrease maladaptive behaviors.
4. Evaluate parents' capacity to implement the intervention: assessment of parents' guilt, anger, anxiety, and underlying of irrational beliefs.
5. Conduct therapy with the parents: cognitive restructuring of the parents' irrational beliefs.
6. Predict resistance: problem-solving techniques.
7. Assess the parents' ability to implement the intervention: evaluation the emotions and the cognitions which can interfere with the results of therapy.
8. Conduct intervention with parents: disputing the irrational beliefs.
9. Assess how the child responds to the plan: repeating the assessment, problem-solving, cognitive restructuring.
10. Conduct individual therapy with the child or adolescent.

Rational-Emotive Behavior Parent Consultation

Rational-Emotive Behavior Parent Consultation (REBPC; Vernon, 1994) is conceptualized as a triadic process, an indirect intervention in which the client is the child but the specialist works with parents to develop specific abilities for dealing with child behavior/problems (Vernon, 1994). The consultation process is characterizing by collaborative problem-solving framework.

REBPC frequently incorporates the ABC model of REBT, teaching the nature of relationships between different beliefs, functional and dysfunctional emotions, and adaptive or maladaptive behaviors (Vernon, 1994, 2006). The sessions involve a directive role of the consultant in prescribing and teaching parenting techniques such as cognitive restructuring, behavioral management strategies, to address the specific concerns of the parent (Vernon, 1994, 2006). Most important topics that are incorporated are self-acceptance, problem-solving, decision-making, and positive discipline (Vernon, 1994, 2006).

Joyce (1990) has documented the positive effects of REBPC in two case studies presenting how to carry out these types of interventions either with individual parents, or in a group format, both for clinical or non- clinical problems. A REBT framework is used for all applications, a special focus being on the relationship between parent irrationality and parent emotional problems, and how the intervention could be applied in a school environment.

REBT-Based Parent Education Programs

Parent education programs based on the REBT framework are using comprehensive curriculums for working with parents in psycho-educational groups, in which parents having similar objectives and/or concerns are learning specific parenting skills in a structured sequence. Several REBT parenting programs have been developed and in the following section we briefly describe them.

Rational-Emotive Parent Education

The Rational-Emotive Parent Education is a non-therapeutic and preventive program which has three main goals (Joyce, 1995, 2006):

1. To teach parents new ways of thinking in order to tackle parenting-related distress;
2. To expose parents to a large range of rational beliefs;
3. To give parents effective strategies for disciplining children;
4. To teach rational-emotive methods for dealing with children's emotional problems.

The key mechanism of change proposed by *Rational-Emotive Parent Education* is the change of parents' irrational beliefs. The main strategies used in order to change irrational beliefs are increasing self-awareness regarding self-statements, identification of the irrational beliefs underlying these self-statements, disputing of irrational beliefs, changing them to rational beliefs, practicing the use of rational beliefs, and the reinforcement of rational beliefs.

Regarding the program's structure, the first step represents psycho-education about emotions and cognitions including the monitoring of levels of different types of emotions, both functional and dysfunctional. The next step is an introduction to *kind and firm* rational parenting styles, including enhancing parental communication with children about emotional processes and developing an emotional management plan for the child. The learning process ends with parents guiding the child through changing beliefs processes and reinforcing rational beliefs and adaptive behaviors.

The efficacy of *Rational-Emotive Parent Education* was demonstrated in a study (Joyce, 1995) with 48 non-clinical participants, randomized in two groups, one which received the intervention and one control group. Results showed that for the experimental group there was a statistically significant decrease in parent irrationality, parent guilt, and parent anger. A ten-month follow-up revealed the maintenance of these results, in addition to a decrease of perceived child behavior problems, and parental self-worth-related irrational beliefs.

The SOS Help for Parents Program

Another REBT-based parenting program is the *SOS Help for Parents* curricula (Clark, 2005). This video program has the goal to teach parents how to better manage their mood and improve their child's behavior; it is and makes use of video modeling vignettes, handouts and self-help books. The core of the program is based on three child-rearing rules recommended for parents and on four major errors that parents are taught how to avoid in the child-management process.

The three golden rules of the *SOS Help for Parents* programs are the following (Clark, 2005):

(a) Reward good behavior;
(b) Do not reward bad behavior;
(c) Correct bad behavior.

In order to implement the first rule, parents are advised to use several positive parenting techniques, including rewards, effective instructions, and grandma's rule. For the second and the third rule, parents learn how to use disciplining techniques, like withholding the rewards, active ignoring, time-out, scolding and disapproval, natural consequences, logic consequences etc. Additional to these core rules, an important part of the program was devoted to help parents to identify the most common mistakes in managing child behaviors and how to avoid these errors. According to this approach, the most common mistakes in child behavior management refer to failing to reward good behavior, accidentally rewarding of bad behavior, accidentally punishing good behavior, or failing to correct bad behavior when mild corrections are needed. The program was recently tested and results document positive effects on both preschool and school age children for a short 6-week format (Khowaja et al., 2016) and a standard format of ten sessions.

The Rational Positive Parenting Program

The Rational Positive Parenting Program (rPPP, David, 2014; David, David, & Dobrean, 2014; David & DiGiuseppe, 2016; Gavița, 2011) is a recent REBT-based parenting program, developed based on the previously mentioned programs (Clark, 2005; Joyce, 1995), but also taking into account empirical and technological advancements in the field of parenting programs.

rPPP aims to help parents manage their emotions, improve their parenting practices and thus child adjustment. rPPP relies on two major principles (David & DiGiuseppe, 2016): (1) emotion-regulation skills of the parents represent a main target of the program, using techniques for changing irrational beliefs and building an unconditional self and child acceptance philosophy; (2) parents learn essential positive parenting strategies based on the "*kind and firm*" parenting style in order to build a healthy relationship with their children and effectively manage child behaviors.

rPPP differs from the standard cognitive-behavioral programs by its focus on helping parents first deal with their dysfunctional emotions and build rational thinking habits. The next sequence is focused on developing a positive parent-child relationship and in the end effective limits and positive discipline. Content of the rPPP is presented in Table 15.1 below together with the sessions focus.

The rPPP can be delivered in three formats: full-length, short version and an online format. The full-length (10 sessions) and short versions (4 sessions) of rPPP are held using a group format. The program is divided in two modules, the first focusing on parent emotion-regulation strategies and the second one on positive parenting, using experiential strategies, forms, video vignettes and monitoring forms. The program uses diverse tools like play, joint activities, coaching regarding the development of emotional and social skills of the child, with the aim to promote a positive relationship between parents and children. Parents are taught how to promote child positive behaviors, how to nurture a secure and positive parent-child relationship, how to effectively set family rules, how to establish a reward and consequences plan, and develop problem-solving abilities. In addition to face-to-face meetings, parents are requested to accomplish specific tasks with the children and family in order to ensure the generalization of the gains outside the program.

An important advantage that is brought by the online version of the rPPP (David, 2014; David, Capris, & Jarda, 2017) is the easy accessibility and the addition of innovative methods. Some examples of such methods are attention bias modification training (Amir, Elias, Klumpp, & Przeworski, 2003) and "psychological pills" (Gavita et al., 2013). Attention bias modification represents a computerized technique which is used to train parents to allocate their attention preferentially to stimuli related to positive emotions and behaviors of children and disengage from allocating attention to the negative behaviors (David & Podină, 2014). In order to change maladaptive emotions of the parents, online rPPP uses several techniques which have the goal to change parents' irrational beliefs and strengthen rational

Table 15.1 *Content of the rPPP program*

Sessions 1–3	Introduction and psycho-education. Managing dysfunctional emotional and behavioral reactions to child misbehavior. Building parent and child unconditional acceptance.
Sessions 4–5	Building positive relationship with the child. Using rewards-based tools and setting effective family rules.
Sessions 6–7	Effective strategies for managing unwanted behavior.
Sessions 7–10	Effective communication and problem-solving skills. Coping with difficult situations. Assessment, maintenance of gains and termination issues.

beliefs in (David, 2012, 2015). These coping statements are called "psychological pills" (e.g., "I can tolerate my feelings, even if they are not pleasant") and are delivered to the parents based on functionality and type of emotion, the cause of emotion, the type of dysfunctional cognition, and the theme of cognitions.

Several studies (David et al., 2017; Gaviţa & Călin, 2013; Gaviţa, David, Bujoreanu, Tiba, & Ionuţiu, 2012; Gavita, David, & DiGiuseppe, 2014), investigated all three formats of rPPP and revealed that these are effective in significantly reducing child externalizing behavior problems and emotional problems. Moreover, follow-up assessments showed even superior results in the favor of rPPP, compared with standard parenting programs. Three randomized clinical trials (David et al., 2017; Gaviţa et al., 2012; Gaviţa & Călin, 2013) with samples of parents with children from all age categories between 2 and 18 years represent a testament for the high efficacy of this program. Also, these trials investigated the mechanism of change of rPPP, suggesting that the most important mediators of the program efficacy were parental distress and parenting behaviors (David, 2014; Gavita et al., 2014).

REBT Parenting Interventions for Parents of Children with Special Problems

An important application of REBT parent education is in the case of children with special problems, even if these problems represent that the child is gifted (McInerney, 1983; McInerney & McInerney, 2006) or if there is a severe disorder involved (Greaves, 1997).

McInerney and McInerney's (2006) approach for working with parents of exceptional children emphasize the role of establishing a strong therapeutic relationship, in which parent could share their emotions and thoughts. It is very important to tackle the misconceptions that most of these parents have about therapy, and to take into account that many of them will be very defensive at the beginning due to their previous negative experience with other professionals from the field. Also, additional to the usual techniques, it is recommended to focus more on encouraging verbal disclosure, using modeling self-disclosure, reinforcing, active listening, or empathetic restatements of parents' emotions and thoughts, in an environment characterized by unconditional acceptance. Moreover, a good and constant communication between parents and school specialist and integration of REBT principles into school-based programs are considered necessary in order to maximize the results of parent education interventions in the case of specially challenged children.

Another example of using REBT parent education for parents of children with special problems is the case of the parents of children with Down syndrome (Greaves, 1997). In this study, 54 mothers were randomly allocated to one of the three groups, Rational-Emotive Parent Education group, Applied Behavior Analysis group, or a control, which did not receive any intervention. Both interventions consisted on 8 sessions. The Rational-Emotive Parent Education intervention focused on core irrationality, and the primary outcome measured was parental distress. Results showed that Rational-Emotive Parent Education was significantly more effective in reducing parental distress than both control groups, reveling that this intervention are useful also in the case of parents of children with more severe disorders.

New Directions in REBT Based Parent Education

In the previous sections of this chapter, we presented how REBT based parenting interventions can successfully improve psychological health of parents, children and adolescents, and can efficiently address youth's misbehaviors. Even though there are studies showing the effectiveness of the programs mentioned above, there are certain aspects that can be improved. After reviewing the state of the art theory and practices in the field of REBT parent education paradigm, it would be helpful to identify strategies in order to facilitate the access to these programs for more parents, to engage parents and prevent drop-out, respectively to maximize intervention efficacy and cost-effectiveness, and to increase evidence-based practices.

Despite the documented success of the newly developed REBT-based parenting programs, at least three significant and interrelated issues remain. First, although there are studies comparing REBT-based parenting programs to standard ones (David, David, & Dobrean, 2014) it is unclear what the relative contributions are of different cognitive and behavioral components commonly included in the REBT packages for parents. Further investigation of significant causative factors among REBT techniques administered into a parent education program could facilitate our knowledge about the mechanisms of REBT-induced change and could thus contribute to further improving the efficacy of the parenting programs. Second, we know very little about how REBT-based parenting programs can be used to successfully address specific risk factors for parenting. A recent qualitative synthesis (Klahr & Burt, 2014) that analyzed the individual differences that can impact the efficacy of parent education programs confirmed that parenting behaviors are multi-determined. Understanding how to develop specific components for REBT-based parenting programs in order to make them suitable for specific vulnerable populations (e.g., parents experiencing couple difficulties etc.) is important if we want to increase their efficacy and to determine the adequate dose-effect relationship between the active ingredients needed and the best outcomes.

Third, even if the efficacy of some REBT based parent programs, like rPPP (Gavița, 2011), is established in terms of both outcomes and REBT based mechanisms (David, 2014; David et al., 2017; Gavița et al., 2012, 2014; Gavița & Călin, 2013), more well-conducted studies are needed to show their efficacy on various parenting and child adjustment outcomes. Until now, we know that rPPP is effective in reducing child externalizing behavior problems and emotional problems, with better results at follow-up than standard cognitive-behavioral parenting programs. Regarding mechanisms of change, studies revealed that parental distress and parenting behaviors are mediating the effects of the intervention on child externalizing symptoms (David, 2014; Gavita et al., 2014). Although these data demonstrate that the rPPP is the most comprehensive and evidence-based REBT parenting program to date, more replication studies are necessary that can offer consistent support in order to consider it a reference parenting intervention.

Another important aspect that must be taken into account in this field is the cost-effectiveness of REBT based parenting programs. To develop people's access to parenting interventions, the cost of such interventions becomes an essential factor. One promising solution for increasing access to evidence-based parenting programs and to decrease the costs of delivering these programs is the use of technology, like web-sites, smartphone-based apps, or therapeutic video games (Luxton, McCann, Bush, Mishkind, & Reger, 2011). The internet has the capacity to increase the access to parenting programs by overcoming barriers common to face-to-face services, de-stigmatizing parenting assistance, and harnessing the power of video-based modeling, interactivity and personalization (Sanders, Baker, & Turner, 2012). The fact that REBT has clear, valid and structured intervention packages for parenting programs is one of the possible reasons why technology can be easily integrated into this paradigm. There are a limited number of studies up to date aiming to investigate the efficacy of online parent education programs. For example, rPPP was developed also as a program that can be accessed online. The online version (David, 2014; David et al., 2017) uses some innovative techniques such as attention bias modification procedures and 'psychological pills' (Gavita et al., 2013). Another REBT e-learning parenting program is the online You Can Do It! Program for Parents (e.g., Bernard, 2004). The aim of the program is (1) to teach parents to help their children to develop positive attitudes, and social and emotional skills, and (2) to help parents to exert a positive influence on the achievement and wellbeing of their children (https://youcandoitparents.com.au).

An increasingly popular option for online interventions is represented by therapeutic computer games (Kearns, 2015), which could be adapted to be used by parents together with their children. Therapeutic computer games capitalize on the general fascination that children and teenagers have for computer games, in order to facilitate the implementation of prevention or intervention programs that address their mental health. Video therapeutic games can be a very suitable media support that can be used as a therapeutic technique by which parents interact with children/adolescents in order to have a common pleasant and educational activity. A new video therapeutic game for children and adolescents, recently developed and tested, is the *RE*Think game (www.rethink.info.ro), developed to promote psychological resilience in children and adolescents. The *RE*Think game can be used for teaching emotional skills in both parents and their children and future studies will need to test its effects on parenting, parent and child adjustment.

In conclusion, based on the state of the art in the field of REBT based parenting interventions we can say that these programs are effective and can be successfully used for both treatment and prevention purposes. For their further development, research in the field must take into account the following directions: (1) The investigation of significant causative ingredients among REBT techniques administered into a parent education program could facilitate our knowledge about the mechanisms of REBT-induced change; (2) There is a need to customize REBT parenting programs based on individual risk factors that can disrupt parenting practices; (3) To develop REBT based parenting interventions as evidence-based programs, there is a need for more studies to show their efficacy on different parents' and children's outcomes; (4) One promising solution for increasing access to evidence-based REBT parenting programs and to decrease the costs of delivering these programs is the use of technology, like online platforms.

References

Amir, N., Elias, J., Klumpp, H., & Przeworski, A. (2003). Attentional bias to threat in social phobia: Facilitated processing of threat or difficulty disengaging attention from threat? *Behaviour Research and Therapy, 41*(11), 1325–1335.

Bernard, M. E. (2004). *The REBT Therapist's pocket companion for working with children and adolescents* (p. 245). New York, NY: Albert Ellis Institute.

Bernard, M. E., Ellis, A., & Terjesen, M. (2006). Rational-emotive behavioral approaches to childhood disorders: History, theory, practice and research. In A. Ellis & M.E. Bernard (Eds.), Rational emotive behavioral approaches to childhood disorders. New York: Springer. (18) (PDF) Albert Ellis and the World of Children.

Clark, L. (Ed.). (2005). *SOS help for parents: A practical guide for handling common everyday behavior problems*. Bowling Green, KY: SOS Programs & Parents Press.

David, D. (2012). *Tratat de psihoterapii cognitive şi comportamentale [handbook of cognitive and behavioral psychotherapies]*. Iaşi, Romania: Polirom.

David, D. (2015). Rational emotive behavior therapy (REBT). In R. L. Cautin & S. O. Lilienfeld (Eds.), *Encyclopedia of clinical psychology*. New Jersey: Wiley-Blackwell.

David, O. A. (2014). The rational positive parenting program for child externalizing behavior: Mechanisms of change analysis. *Journal of Evidence-Based Psychotherapies, 14*(1), 21–38.

David, O. A., Capris, D., & Jarda, A. (2017). Online coaching of emotion-regulation strategies for parents: Efficacy of the online rational positive parenting program and attention Bias modification procedures. *Frontiers in Psychology, 8*, 500. https://doi.org/10.3389/fpsyg.2017.00500

David, O. A., David, D., & Dobrean, A. (2014). Efficacy of the Rational Positive Parenting program for child externalizing behavior: can an emotion-regulation enhanced cognitive-behavioral parent program be more effective than a standard one?. *Journal of Evidence-Based Psychotherapies, 14*(2), 21–38.

David, O. A., & DiGiuseppe, R. (2016). *The rational positive parenting program*. New-York, NY: Springer International Publishing.
David, O. A., & Podină, I. (2014). Positive attentional bias as a resilience factor in parenting. Implications for attention bias modification online parenting interventions. In S. Ionescu, M. Tomita, S. Cace (Eds.), *Volume of the 2nd World Congress on Resilience "From person to society"* (pp. 425–428). Bologna: Medimond International Proceedings.
DiGiuseppe, R., & Kelter, J. (2006). Treating aggressive children: A rational-emotive behavior systems approach. In A. Ellis & M. E. Bernard (Eds.), *Rational emotive behavioral approaches to childhood disorders* (pp. 257–280). New-York, NY: Springer Science & Business Media.
Ellis, A. (Ed.). (1994). *Reason and emotion in psychotherapy*. New-Jersey: Carol Publishing Group.
Ellis, A., Wolfe, J. L., & Moseley, S. (Eds.). (1966). *How to raise an emotionally healthy, happy child*. Carlsbad, CA: Borden Publishing Company.
Gavița, O. (2011). *Evidence-Based Parent Programs for Reducing Disruptive Behavior in Children* (Doctoral dissertation). Koln, Germany: Lap Lambert Academic Publishing.
Gavița, O. A., & Călin, A. (2013). Retman rational stories versus rational parenting program for the treatment of child psychopathology: Efficacy of two formats of rational-emotive behavior therapy. *Journal of Cognitive & Behavioral Psychotherapies, 13*(1), 33–56.
Gavița, O. A., David, D., Bujoreanu, S., Tiba, A., & Ionuțiu, D. R. (2012). The efficacy of a short cognitive–behavioral parent program in the treatment of externalizing behavior disorders in Romanian foster care children: Building parental emotion-regulation through unconditional self-and child-acceptance strategies. *Children and Youth Services Review, 34*(7), 1290–1297. https://doi.org/10.1016/j.childyouth.2012.03.001
Gavita, O. A., David, D., & DiGiuseppe, R. (2014). You are such a bad child! Appraisals as mechanisms of parental negative and positive affect. *The Journal of General Psychology, 141*(2), 113–129. https://doi.org/10.1080/00221309.2013.874971
Gavita, O. A., DiGiuseppe, R., & David, D. (2013). Self-acceptance and the parenting of child. In M. E. Bernard (Ed.), *The Strength of Self-Acceptance* (pp. 193–214). New-York, NY: Springer Science + Business Media.
Greaves, D. (1997). The effect of rational-emotive parent education on the stress of mothers of young children with down syndrome. *Journal of Rational-Emotive and Cognitive-Behavior Therapy, 15*(4), 249–267. https://doi.org/10.1023/A:1025063425172
Hauck, P. A. (1967). *The rational management of children*. New York, NY: Libra Publishers.
Huber, C. H., & Baruth, L. G. (1989). *Rational-emotive family therapy: A systems perspective*. New York, NY: Springer Publishing Company.
Joyce, M. (1994). Rational-emotive parent consultation. In M. E. Bernard & R. DiGiuseppe (Eds.), *Rational emotive consultation in applied settings* (pp. 91–104). New York, NY: Lawrence Erlbaum Associates Publishers.
Joyce, M. R. (1990). Rational-emotive parent consultation. *School Psychology Review, 19*(3), 304–314.
Joyce, M. R. (1995). Emotional relief for parents: Is rational-emotive parent education effective? *Journal of Rational-Emotive and Cognitive-Behavior Therapy, 13*(1), 55–75. https://doi.org/10.1007/BF02354557
Joyce, M. R. (2006). A developmental, rational-emotive behavioral approach for working with parents. In A. Ellis & M. E. Bernard (Eds.), *Rational emotive behavioral approaches to childhood disorders* (pp. 177–211). New York, NY: Springer Science & Business Media.
Kearns, C. (2015). Prescription play: A primer on innovative use of video games technology in healthcare. *Journal of Visual Communication in Medicine, 38*(3–4), 152–163. https://doi.org/10.3109/17453054.2015.1100981
Khowaja, Y., Karmaliani, R., Hirani, S. A., Khowaja, A. R., Rafique, G., & McFarlane, J. (2016). A pilot study of a 6-week parenting program for mothers of pre-school children attending family health centers in Karachi. *Pakistan.. International Journal of Health Policy and Management, 5*(2), 91–97.

Klahr, A. M., & Burt, S. A. (2014). Elucidating the etiology of individual differences in parenting: A meta-analysis of behavioral genetic research. *Psychological Bulletin, 140*(2), 544–586. https://doi.org/10.1037/a0034205

Luxton, D. D., McCann, R. A., Bush, N. E., Mishkind, M. C., & Reger, G. M. (2011). mHealth for mental health: Integrating smartphone technology in behavioral healthcare. *Professional Psychology: Research and Practice, 42*(6), 505.

McInerney, J. F. (1983). A rational-emotive approach to counseling of parents of exceptional preschool children. *New Jersey Journal of School Psychology, 2*, 63–75.

McInerney, J. F., & McInerney, B. C. M. (2006). Working with the parents and teachers of exceptional children. In A. Ellis & M. E. Bernard (Eds.), *Rational emotive behavioral approaches to childhood disorders* (pp. 369–384). New York, NY: Springer Science & Business Media.

Sanders, M. R., Baker, S., & Turner, K. M. (2012). A randomized controlled trial evaluating the efficacy of triple P online with parents of children with early-onset conduct problems. *Behaviour Research and Therapy, 50*(11), 675–684.

Vernon, A. (1994). Rational-emotive consultation: A model for implementing rational emotive education. In M. E. Bernard & R. DiGiuseppe (Eds.), *Rational emotive consultation in applied settings* (pp. 129–147). New York, NY: Lawrence Erlbaum Associates Publishers.

Vernon, A. (2006). *Thinking, feeling, behaving: An emotional education curriculum for children. Grades 1–6*. Champaign, IL: Research Press.

Chapter 16
REBT in the Workplace

Michael E. Bernard

Albert Ellis was always ahead of his time. This is no more in evidence than in the longevity and currency of his theory and practice of REBT in the workplace. Those of us who consult, train and coach in organizations are indebted to his pioneering work best represented in his 1972 book, *Executive Leadership,* where he spelled out the importance of leaders recognizing and overcoming psychological barriers to their effectiveness (e.g., procrastination, indecisiveness) as well as experiencing high levels of mental health and wellbeing. Fifty years ago, Ellis recognized that for leaders to lead effectively and for managers to manage efficiently, *rationality* was a way of viewing their world and responding to problems and challenges that has a positive impact not only on bottom lines (e.g., profit, performance) but also on wellbeing and mental health.

Today, it is becoming recognized that for people to go from good to great, organizations need to invest not only in their technical and social capital, but also in their psychological capital (e.g., Bernard, 2014; Luthans & Youssef, 2004). It was in 2002 that Fred Luthans defined positive organization behaviour as "the study and application of positively oriented human resource strengths and psychological capacities that can be measured, developed, and effectively managed for performance improvement in today's workplace". Developing people's capacity for rationality as propounded by Albert Ellis was one of the earliest forms of modern-day emotional intelligence, resilience and psychological strength-building.

M. E. Bernard (✉)
Melbourne Graduate School of Education, University of Melbourne, Parkville, VIC, Australia

California State University, Long Beach, Long Beach, CA, USA

© Springer Nature Switzerland AG 2019
M. E. Bernard, W. Dryden (eds.), *Advances in REBT*,
https://doi.org/10.1007/978-3-319-93118-0_16

Brief History of REBT at Work

> I started out as a typist and file clerk (who also ran errands and swept the floor) and ended up as the personnel manager (and, unofficially, as the vice president). During this decade, I was probably one of the most efficient men in the business and perhaps the firm's main contributor to its outstanding success: since I did my work beautifully and devised bookkeeping, billing, filing, mail order, and other systems which helped the firm enormously and saved literally thousands of hours of time each year for the president, who was then able to devote his efforts to building up sales. – Albert Ellis

Albert Ellis always had an interest in business and, in particular, making money. In fact, his first university degree was a Bachelor's in Business Administration that he received from the City University of New York. Ellis felt that making money would enable him to achieve sufficient financial independence so that he could pursue his real interest, which was writing. For 10 years, while he was gathering material for some of his future books and while obtaining his doctorate in clinical psychology, Ellis worked for a moderately large gift and novelty wholesale house.

While not a businessman, he was the Executive Director of the Albert Ellis Institute (formerly the Institute for Rational-Emotive Therapy), an operation which employs many professionals and administrative personnel, serves thousands of people and, in the process, takes in and spends hundreds of thousands of dollars each year.

One of the main reasons Ellis' views are good for business is his emphasis on *efficiency*. REBT is directed at helping people overcome inefficient ways of handling their problems at work, the emotional hang-ups they have about these problems (hostility, anxiety, depression), including job-related stress. And REBT is particularly suited to solving one of the main obstacles to success at work; namely, procrastination (e.g., Bernard, 1991a, 1991b; Robb, 1998).

Out of Ellis' personal counselling experiences with countless business people (including leaders of industry and government), have emerged a good many rational ideas and principles. Ellis' earliest writing on applying REBT to work was his article (Ellis & Blum, 1967), 'Rational training: A new method of facilitating management labor relations'.

In the later part of the twentieth century, a brand of REBT emerged in its application to the world of work, *Rational Effectiveness Training* (RET), and involved teaching people without mental health problems how to use the ABC-DE model to increase their personal productivity and manage stress (DiMattia & Mennen, 1990; DiMattia, 1991). Dryden and Gordon (1993) wrote a book on peak performance describing how to become more effective at work using Rational-Emotive Training as did Robert Spillane (1983) in his book "Achieving Peak Performance: A Psychology of Success in the Organisation". Palmer and Burton (1996) provided a manager's guide to dealing with people problems at work on a 'one-to-one' basis by integrating Ellis' ABCDE framework and a seven-step problem-solving model. As distinct from the REBT focus on improving mental health problems, RET's focus was on improving work performance outcomes.

In 1993, two special issues of the *Journal of Rational-Emotive Therapy & Cognitive-Behavior Therapy* were devoted to the theme of "RET in the Workplace" with articles illustrating the breadth of application of REBT to non-clinical problems in helping organizations and employees cope and excel at work. Topics included:

- Teaching REBT in the financial and investment sector (Criddle, 1993)
- A rational-emotive paradigm for organizations (Morris, 1993)
- Integrating RET into management consulting and training (Lange & Grieger, 1993)
- Managing change: A corporate application of rational-emotive therapy (Miller & Yeager, 1993)
- REBT: A powerful tool to turn traumatic job termination into an enlightening career transition (Klarreich, 1993)
- Career counselling: A rational-emotive approach to career development (Reichman, 1993)

And in 1994, Raymond DiGiuseppe and Al Miller described a REBT model of organizational consultation.

In the first two decades of the twenty-first century, REBT was extended into the world of coaching spearheaded by Stephen Palmer in collaboration with colleagues (Neenan & Palmer, 2001) with a strong application to stress management (e.g., Ellis, Gordon, Neenan, & Palmer, 1997). Palmer integrated various aspects of REBT in cognitive behaviour coaching as found in the SPACE model (Edgerton & Palmer, 2005), the PRACTICE model (Palmer, 2007) and in Rational Coaching (Palmer, 2009). Michael Neenan's recent, innovative work on applying REBT at work has been in the area of resilience coaching (e.g., Neenan, 2018a, 2018b, 2018c). During this time, I employed REBT to stress management learning and development (Bernard, 2017) and in 1:1 coaching (e.g., Bernard, 2018a). Today, Rational-Emotive, Cognitive-Behavior coaching has developed into a distinct form of practice with a strong conceptual and empirical base (Bernard & David, 2018).

In 2018, REBT continues to provide REBT organizational and management consultants (Bernard, 2018b, c; Broder, 2012, 2018), counsellors and coaches a robust theory for understanding not only how people's irrational beliefs sabotage personal and organizational goals, exacerbate work stress and contribute to personal problems (e.g., substance abuse) but also how rationality in the form of flexible beliefs and a rational mindset can help everyone perform at their best while enjoying positive mental health.

Table 16.1 Published research: REBT in work settings

Bernard, M. E. (2016). Beliefs and teacher stress. *Journal of Rational-Emotive & Cognitive-Behavior Therapy*, *34*, 209–224. https://doi.org/10.1007/s10942-016-0238-y.
David, A. R., & Szamoskozi, S. (2011). The effectiveness of a Rational Emotive Behavioral Coaching program to reduce irrationality in organizational environment and the mediating effect of modifying irrational cognitions on emotional distress and quality of life. *Transylvanian Journal of Psychology*, 77–93.
David, O. A., Ionicioiu, I., Imbăruş, A. C., & Sava, F. A. (2016). Coaching banking managers through the financial crisis: Effects on stress, resilience, and performance. *Journal of Rational-Emotive & Cognitive-Behavior Therapy, 34*, 267–281.
David, O. A., & Matu, S. A. (2013). How to tell if managers are good coaches and how to help them improve during adversity? The managerialcoaching assesment system and the rational managerial coaching program. *Journal of Cognitive & Behavioral Psychotherapies, 13*, 497–502.
Dryden, W. (1985). Voluntary redundancy and beyond: A counsellor trainer's odyssey. *Counselling: Journal of the British Association for Counselling, 54*, 2–5.
Gyllensten, K., & Palmer, S. (2005). Cancoaching reduce workplacestress: A quasi-experimental study. *International Journal of Evidence Based Coaching and Mentoring, 3*, 75–85.
Klarreich, S. H., DiGiuseppe, R., & DiMattia, D. J. (1987). Cost effectiveness of an employee assistance program with rational-emotive therapy. *Professional Psychology: Research and Practice, 18*, 140–144. https://doi.org/10.1037/0735-7028.18.2.140.
Kushnir, T., & Malkinson, R. (1993). A rational-emotive group intervention for preventing and coping with stress among safety officers. *Journal of Rational-Emotive & Cognitive-Behavior Therapy, 11*, 195–206.
Mahfar, M., & Senin, A. A. (2015, April 5–7). *Managing stress at workplace using rational emotive behavioral therapy (REBT) approach.* Paper presented at the International Conference on Human Resource Development (ICHRD), Johor Bahru, Johor.
Ogbuanya, T. C., Eseadi, C., Orji, C. T., Anyanwu, J. I., Ede, M. O., & Bakare, J· (2018). Effect of Rational Emotive Behavior Therapy on negative career thoughts of students in technical colleges in Nigeria. *Psychological Reports, 121*, 356–374. https://doi.org/10.1177/0033294117724449.
Ogbuanya, T. C., Eseadi, C., Orji, C. T., Ede, M. O., Ohanu, I. B., & Bakare, J. (2017). Effects of rational emotive occupational health therapy intervention on the perceptions of organizational climate and occupational risk management practices among electronics technology employees in Nigeria. *Medicine, 96*. https://doi.org/10.1097/MD.0000000000006765.
Ogbuanya, T. C., Eseadi, C., Orji, C. T., Ohanu, I. B., Bakare, J., & Ede, M. O. (2017). Effects of rational emotive behavior coaching on occupational stress and work ability among electronics workshop instructors in Nigeria. *Medicine, 96*. https://doi.org/10.1097/MD.0000000000006891.
Ogbuanya, T. C., Eseadi, C., Orji, C. T., Omeje, J. C., Anyanwu, J. I., Ugwok, S. C., & Edeh, N. C. (2018). Effect of rational-emotive behavior therapy program on the symptoms of burnout syndrome among undergraduate electronics work students in Nigeria. *Psychological Reports, 1*, 33294117748587. https://doi.org/10.1177/0033294117748587.
Palmer, S., & Gyllensten, K. (2008). How cognitive behavioural, rational emotive behavioural or multimodal coaching could prevent mental health problems, enhance performance and reduce work related stress. *Journal of Rational-Emotive & Cognitive-Behavior Therapy, 26*, 38–52.
Ratiu, L., David, O. A., & Baban, A. (2016). Developing managerial skills through coaching: Efficacy of a cognitive-behavioral coaching program. *Journal of Rational-Emotive and Cognitive-Behavioral Therapy.* https://doi.org/10.1007/s10942-015-0225-8.
Ugwoke, S. C., Eseadi, C., Igbokwe, C. C., Chiaha, G. T. U., Nwaubani, O. O., Orji, C. T., … Abugu, L. I. (2017). Effects of a rational-emotive health education intervention on stress management and irrational beliefs among technical college teachers in Southeast Nigeria. *Medicine, 96*, e7658. https://doi.org/10.1097/MD.0000000000007658.

Research

A thorough analysis of the research in the application of REBT in work settings is beyond the scope of this chapter. Table 16.1 presents a list of many of the published studies in this area that appeared in Daniel David, Cotet, Matu, Mogoase, and Simona (2018) meta-analysis of REBT research supplemented by my independent investigation. The first published research demonstrating the positive impact of REBT in the work setting appears to be Windy Dryden's (1985) case study, an autobiographical account of his voluntary redundancy. The research methodologies employed in these studies makes generalizations of findings problematic. That being said, there is sufficient evidence to assert that irrational beliefs are associated with work-related stress (e.g., Bernard, 2016a, 2016b, 2016c). There is also strong evidence that employee participation in REBT-oriented learning and development, programs produces a beneficial effect as measured by different self-report measures of mental health, wellbeing and stress. As an example of a well designed study, David, Ionicioiu, Imbăruş, and Sava (2016) investigated the effectiveness of a rational management coaching program in enhancing managerial performance and emotion regulation abilities and the specific mechanisms of change that facilitate management of emotional distress. Their results showed that the Rational Management Coaching Program was effective in improving the managerial soft skills, depressive mood, and, marginally, the level of stress. The program was effective in replacing both domain specific and global irrational beliefs with rational beliefs in the managers. Domain-specific rational beliefs were found to be the mechanism of change in the coaching program for lowering levels of work stress, while general irrational beliefs are correlated with improved managerial soft-skills (David, 2018).

Core Rebt Ideas Applied to Work

> "The prelude to controlling organizational processes is exerting a large degree of self-regulation." Albert Ellis, *Executive Leadership,* 1972

There continue to be many excellent books appearing on how to succeed at work. The authors of these books have as their assumption that the main obstacle to success at work can be overcome through helping people acquire practical problem-solving skills such as time-management, goal setting, dealing with difficult people, using the phone effectively, on-the-job assertion, etc. These practical skills are seen as the keys to unlocking the potential for achievement.

Ellis maintained that the experts in the area fail to take into account the inherent limitations of all humans and, in particular, our irrational tendencies, which predispose us to inefficiency. That is, it is not an inconsiderate boss, difficult customers, tedious or hard work, nor the unreasonable demands of the job, which prevent people from working efficiently and achieving goals. Rather, it is the reactions we have to these practical problems, which prevents us from solving them.

REBT's Blueprint for Success

The essential ingredients of Ellis' approach to improving job performance are as follows: First, he helped clarify the value people placed on achieving significant levels of job success. In particular, he showed them how to choose and commit themselves to a long-term level of professional achievement while not limiting themselves by excessive anxieties that may arise from fear of failure. Second, Ellis encouraged people to identify their short-term and long-term professional goals (type of job, level of advancement, professional awards and significant contributions, professional skills and knowledge, financial), which will enable them to realize their chosen level of achievement. Third, Ellis had people focus on their personal obstacles to achieving these goals, including hostility towards others, indecisiveness, self-downing, perfectionism and procrastination to determine which of these they had better overcome. Fourth, Ellis provided them with rational attitudes in order to combat the irrationalities, which are responsible for their problems. And, fifth, Ellis helped people to develop a daily action plan whereby they decided where, when, and how they are going to engage in those actions, which will help them to achieve their various goals.

While REBT also recognizes the importance of practical skills in facilitating goal achievement (communication skills, time management, conflict resolution, etc.) and, frequently, teaches these skills if a person lacks them, it views personal-emotional reactions as the main stumbling blocks to success. Let's look at some examples.

Enhancing Decisiveness

To be a successful leader and manager requires the ability to think through what is required to achieve an objective or to solve a problem and then to act upon one's analysis.

According to Ellis, indecisiveness occurs in situations when you know a decision had better be made for the good of yourself and your work, but you vacillate or avoid the issue because you are afraid that you will make a bad decision and fear other people's reactions. A dire need for approval is at the core of indecisiveness. This problem is created when you irrationally convince yourself that you could not stand to be disapproved of and criticized by others. And further, that such mistakes and disapproval would prove how hopeless you really were. This is especially the case for tough decisions, the ones that entail considerable risk or hardship.

The following exchange between Ellis and a woman who believed the world was exploiting her shows the irrationalities underlying indecisiveness and how REBT can be used to overcome them. Irene, aged 39, is one of two physiotherapists who have an extensive practice. She had the major responsibility for the administration and business side of the operation as well as seeing many patients during the week and on Saturday mornings. Irene is married and mother of two boys. She decided to seek some help for chronic indecisiveness.

A concern she raised with Ellis during the early part of this session is about one of her part-time secretaries whom she believed was being dishonest in the reporting of the number of hours she was working. Additionally, she was concerned about the quality of the work of this secretary. As will be seen, Irene has had a great deal of difficulty being decisive and firm with her secretary and her patients (transcript is from Bernard, 2011).

Irene: I'm going to tell her (the secretary) that I feel she is not happy in this job and that I feel she doesn't provide the kind of work that I need and that I feel that it is more in her interests to find something that she will be happy with in the future. So anyway the upshot is that what's important to me is that this particular incident is repetitive and that I've had other people take advantage of me and I'm kind of victimized a lot I think by my employees. I've got a hard time exerting authority.

Ellis: Because you're afraid of what? Let's suppose you were more authoritative with them and not so friendly, what would you be afraid of?

Irene: I think ultimately I want them to care for me and care for the welfare of my practice and to like me.

Ellis: That's just the point. I think you've got two conflicting views. One, you want them to care for the welfare of your practice because that's what you pay them for. But then two, it sounds like you're demanding in your head that they like *you* and you put their liking you above your making decisions that will add to the welfare of your practice.

Irene: Apparently, and that's not businesslike and with this particular girl it started on the wrong foot from the beginning. We became quite close, it was almost as though we were sisters or mother and daughter or something.

Ellis: Right.

Irene: She asked my advice about a lot of personal things. I know that recently I've been feeling quite unenthusiastic about the prospect of her continuing to work for me because it seems oppressive, there doesn't seem to me to be any future for me in it because I cannot grow professionally and I am so bogged down in my own busy work. Anyway, the upshot is that I see this pattern not only in my office but also with my husband, with my mother, and really, when I think about it, in my childhood I always seemed to have been dominated by someone. And with this secretary I literally can see that she manipulates me in many ways. I ask her to do something and she makes a face and then I say 'Well, what's wrong?' I asked my husband about this and does he think that I make myself a victim all the time. He said 'No', he just thought that I really don't think defensively and that he feels I should run my practice like I drive. You have to drive defensively and not give people too much rope. That really has been true with regard to my employees and even with my patients. Especially, in the beginning when I started practice and because my marriage was unhappy, I tended to get too emotionally involved with patients. And over the years I have toned that down and I've controlled it more and literally I had to start doing it by wearing a facemask. Somehow wearing a facemask kept me from speaking as much and for me personally created distance because I would get so emotionally involved with patients that certainly I think I lost patients over that. I remember even being irritated when they would sort of bring me back to what they came there for. I was so involved in some sort of personal exchange.

Ellis: But again isn't that *neediness, needing* their love, needing their approval?

Irene: Well, that's the thing, I realize that I don't seem to get reinforcement from myself. I constantly *need* to have approval from others, and when I don't get it I think that my day is ruined, or I'm no good. And it's stupid, you know, because so many good things can happen in one day and one bad thing can happen and all that I'll focus on is that one bad thing which shows I'm not liked or a failure.

Ellis: Right.

Irene: So that I'm beginning to understand what you teach is that one has qualities but they don't define what one is. I mean you can do a lousy thing without being necessarily a lousy person.

Ellis: Right, you failed that day but that doesn't make *you* a failure. Or you didn't get the approval of others but that doesn't make *you* unlovable; you've been wrongly concluding that.

Irene: I know. I think I am getting more comfortable with that idea. A few times recently when I realized that I'm depressed or discouraged I tell myself 'Well, this is just this event and this event does not define you'. I'm getting more comfortable with that idea because before I certainly could never separate the two.

Ellis: That's good. Now it's important to keep separating the rating of yourself from the rating of your acts and not liking your failings but accepting you. And you need not like the fact that certain people really don't love you and take advantage of you. You don't have to view yourself as unlovable and rotten because of that. You have been leaning over backward to get even your employees' approval because you think, 'I' *need* it', instead of 'I like it', but I'd like their doing a good job *more.'*

Irene: I guess that I'm uncomfortable with the idea of really demanding excellence from my employees, because then they might leave me.

Ellis: And demand has two meanings. One, 'They absolutely *must* do well' -which is nutty because there's no reason that they must. And, two, a sensible demand or ultimatum, 'If they don't do well then I'll get rid of them because I hired them, I pay them to do reasonably well, they're not going to be perfect but I've a right as an employer to get rid of people who don't do well or to get them to change.' If you decided to keep this woman then it would be better to train her to be more honest and do things better. You have a choice. You do pay them for competence and then you're irrationally saying but I have no right to ask competence. *Why* don't you have a right to ask competence of them, so long as you don't utterly *demand* it?

Irene: The thing is, I suppose I can't understand it, it seems to me that it's obvious that if someone types a letter that they proof read it before sending it out. I don't see why I should be picking up somebody else's errors. And if I have to be repeatedly making that point then there's something very wrong and either they're not paying attention to my authority or there's something wrong with them.

Ellis: Or they know that you're not going to back up your authority. They know that you'll finally do the proof reading. So they can get away with it. Millions of people try to get away with what they can.

Irene: But why in the world do they? What is the point of doing something in a half-assed way?

Ellis: There's a very simple answer to that, and that is called again low frustration tolerance. If they did it in a full-assed way they'd have to devote more time and energy to it and they don't *want* to devote that time and energy, they want to get away with murder. And many of them *do* because of bosses like you. So why shouldn't they try to get away with murder?

Irene: Well that's the thing. Here I'm 39 and I simply don't see the world the way it really is.

Ellis: Right.

Irene: I instantly look for the ideal.

Ellis: You're a romantic. You'd better acknowledge it. I'm not saying that everybody acts poorly. If you have ten employees, about two of them will tum out to be very responsible and on the ball and you don't even have to supervise them. But seven or eight won't. You'd better face that. And either you'd better be prepared to let employees go until you find some good ones or else some to be better. Sometimes you can get an employee who's quite trainable. We find here that when our employees really start goofing it often isn't worth training them. The best thing is, often, to get rid of them and replace them – until you find some good ones- who do exist, but they're rare. I don't think you want to accept that reality. You're saying the world shouldn't be that way, to have so many of these goofers. But it is that way. Now what are you going to do to live more happily in this kind of a world?

Irene: Well obviously I have to tighten up the positions.

Ellis: Right. Supervise more.

Irene: And also be stricter in the beginning.

Ellis: Right. In the case of that woman, you probably let her get away with it. Sometimes you can be very friendly with people and still supervise them closely, but that's difficult. You mainly insisted on the friendship with her and tried very little on the supervision.

Irene: Do you think that I somehow avoid responsibility and avoid making decisions? I don't understand why I'm victimized as much as I am. I think it's because I don't have a clear picture of who I am and what my limitations are. I sometimes can't tell where I end and the other person begins.

Ellis: Let me repeat there are two reasons why you're often, not always, a victim. One, is you have a dire need for approval, rather than go after what *you* want in life. Therefore, as you just said, you just don't see where you end and the other person begins because you think you *need* his or her approval. And two, is your romantic notion, your idealistic notion of the way people *should* be. And you get shocked when you see the facts. But you're not really looking at the facts. You're looking at the ideal and you're letting that ideal obscure the reality.

Ellis helped Irene see the conflict she had between *needing* approval and *wanting* her practice to run more efficiently. By making her more aware of her approval seeking, and less concerned about what others might think of her, Ellis was able to help rid Irene of the major obstacle preventing her from being more efficient and decisive. Disputing her belief that people should be able to do a job conscientiously also helped Irene become less upset about their inefficiencies. This also allowed her to get on with the hiring and/or training of someone who had the work habits she desired.

Poor Self-Esteem

The deleterious effects of low self-esteem are similar in the work environment as they are in one's personal life. When people feel like a failure because of something that has transpired at work, it is very difficult for them to inject the energy necessary to overcome or deal with the presenting set of conditions. And feelings of inferiority and inadequacy are experienced from time to time by most of us -especially when we are confronted by our mistakes and failures as well as with what we perceive as the emotional reactions of others, and, in particular, rejection. These feelings are endemic to the workplace.

Ellis considered the way people think about and evaluate their work performance as often being more of a problem than the event itself. He argued forcefully that because people are human, they are bound to from time to time make mistakes and perform in a sub-standard fashion. In addition, given the irrational, unpredictable nature of market forces as well as the people we work with, occasionally events will conspire against people so that even when one works optimally, one will fail to achieve what we want.

The rational mindset towards setbacks and misfortunes at work is to learn as much as possible about the reason for the problem so that one can, if possible, take steps to rectify the situation. It is quite proper and appropriate to rate one's performance and as a consequence, feel displeased, disappointed, and sad if because of one's own or another's doing, something occurs which prevents one achieving one's work goals. Indeed, such feelings, though negative, may well provide the incentive to continue to improve and do better the next time.

Ellis contended, however, that humans have a propensity, which is reinforced in modern western society, to rate their *self*-worth in terms of their performances, 'I do well, therefore I'm great. I fail at work, therefore I'm a failure'. The irrational equating of self-worth with work performance is at the heart of not only the fear of failure but also the fear of trying for outstanding performances. In the latter case, one may avoid striving for the highest levels of achievement because one views non-achievement or lesser achievement as a sign of one's total worthlessness and are afraid to take the risk. Ellis' main objective was in helping you detach one's ego from one's achievements.

He argued that it is quite right to want to achieve and that it *does* matter if one does not. But it is quite self-defeating and illogical to rate one's self-worth in terms of one's good or bad achievements.

If you want to do something about feeling low and hopeless at work, and especially if anxiety is affecting your concentration and effort, try to identify the activating event. This may be a drop in the performance of your division in comparison with other divisions of your company. Or you may have not achieved a particular objective you set for yourself at work. Or at the very last minute, a big prospective client of yours who up until now was set to sign on the dotted line, drops out.

If you, as a result of these or similar events, feel *overly* down and despondent with yourself and if you find yourself very uptight about dealing with similar situations in the future, you are a self-downer. And it is your own irrational thinking and negative attitudes which are causing your gut to feel bad, not the unfortunate event itself. Rather than evaluating what has happened to you rationally, you blow up the event out of all proportion. You *catastrophize,* 'This is the worst thing that could happen!' and because you see it that way, you experience *low frustration tolerance* ('1 can't stand this!') and *overgeneralize* ('I'll never be able to succeed!'). You crown off your irrational thinking with the harshest *self-rating* of them all: 'Because I failed to achieve, as I *must* I am hopeless and inferior!'

When you find yourself in the emotional doldrums which results from this thinking, you can help yourself out with rational thinking, 'While this happening is unfortunate, it's only 50% or 60% bad, it's certainly not a catastrophe. I can *tolerate* this situation even though I don't *like* it. While I may have performed poorly today, it doesn't mean I can't do better tomorrow. There is much more to me than my work and it is impossible for me or others to judge my worth in terms of what happens at work.'

Perfectionism

Ellis disagreed with the popular sentiment that perfectionism is a good thing. While he encouraged the pursuit of excellence, and, in particular, taking risks to achieve the fullest of people's potential, he steadfastly maintained that if people are perfectionistic, they are not only setting themselves up for a life filled with unnecessary unhappiness, but also for a level of emotional stress which leads to self-defeating work patterns and behavior such as poor concentration, poor organization of ideas, poor public speaking and public performance presentations-or worse, to giving up completely.

The philosophy of perfectionists is quite similar to that of the self-downers. Perfectionists believe' I must perform perfectly at all important things I attempt in life'. The problem with this belief is threefold. First, perfectionists set an extremely high and often unreachable standard to judge their performances ('perfection'). Second, they apply this expectation to many areas of endeavour without taking into account the difficulty of neither the task nor their innate potential and acquired skills to perform this task perfectly. Third, perfectionists take a quite rational preference for high levels of performance in areas of their work life (and, often, personal life), and illogically believe, 'Because I would *prefer* to be totally successful, I *must* be'.

Where the activating event that leads to self-downing is generally something that has already happened, such as making a mistake or failing at a job, the anxiety and stress of a perfectionist rises *in anticipation* of future events, and, in particular, of what might happen. As no doubt you will appreciate, a certain amount of concern about the future can be healthy because it acts as a motivator to get you to put in the extra effort necessary to perform at a high level. Unfortunately, too much anxiety or panic interferes with planning and concerted effort. Ellis showed how perfectionists' preoccupation with the possibility of not succeeding and of what people will think of them actually predisposes them to over-estimate the probability of some stressful or threatening event happening (example, being asked to do something they haven't had a chance to prepare adequately for), underestimating the likelihood they will be able to perform perfectly, and, to cap it all off, to put themselves down when they fail to perform.

There are two main work patterns associated with perfectionism: the 'giving up' pattern and the 'stress' pattern. 'Giving up'is perhaps the more self-defeating of the two and, also, the harder of the two to detect. Perfectionists who 'give up' do so because they believe that if they can't perform perfectly, there's no point in trying at all. By not trying, perfectionists protect their 'egos' by never risking failure. Indeed, 'giving up' perfectionists rationalize their 'lack of effort by saying they really would have succeeded had they tried. If you want to identify 'giving up' perfectionists, look for people who are frittering away their talent by not attempting new challenges, nor specializing in what they do best and who remark, 'I'm not really interested in getting to the top'. 'Giving up' is the best way for perfectionists to protect themselves from bad feelings. 'Giving up' perfectionists believe that they cannot stand pressure and anxiety and that they *must* always be comfortable.

The ‘stress pattern‘is characterized by perfectionists who desperately demand success but who put so much pressure on themselves for ideal performances that they worry themselves sick as they prepare to act and then experience extreme anxiety while performing. Before having to hand in a report, or make a public presentation, ‘stressed’ perfectionists feel extreme discomfort in anticipation of what they have to do because they are obsessed with the irrational thoughts, ‘What if I don’t perform perfectly, what will people think of me?’ Their mental preparation and effort is not what it could be without those distracting thoughts. Additionally, the ‘anticipatory’ discomfort can be so great that perfectionists have to resort to alcohol or drugs to take away the pain of their anxiety. And at these times, when they have to make public presentations these types of perfectionists may be so uptight that they completely fluff the performance.

Ellis’ approach to treating perfectionism involved a number of steps. First, he encouraged the perfectionist to acknowledge he or she is stressed or anxious and not to deny it. Second, he showed the perfectionist that stress and anxiety are part of the human condition. All of us experience it because we’re human. Third, guiding perfectionists along REBT lines, Ellis taught them to accept responsibility for making themselves anxious and stressed and stop blaming their parents or their environment. Fourth, perfectionists are shown that although anxiety and stress is bad (because it is uncomfortable), it is not terrible and it can be tolerated. Fifth, Ellis taught perfectionists self-acceptance by showing them that just because their anxiety and stress is bad, it doesn’t follow that *they* are bad. And sixth, Ellis disputed with perfectionists their demands for perfect performance and encourages them to give up unrealistic standards as well as their demanding that their standards are always achieved.

Procrastination

Perhaps, the biggest obstacle to realizing your potential at work is what appears to be the irrational human tendency to put off till tomorrow that that preferably should be done today. There is little question that top achievers in all professions have the ability to put in sustained effort, especially on the hard or unpleasant tasks that have to be done in order for them to reach their goals.

REBT, perhaps, more so than any other approach provides insights as to why you procrastinate and, more importantly, how you can overcome the problem. Indeed, Ellis’ book ‘Overcoming Procrastination’ (co-author, William J. Knaus) has helped over 250,000 people do something about improving their efficiency at work or in other areas of their life.

Why do people procrastinate? According to Ellis, the cause of procrastination is the way they view hard, unpleasant or boring events, rather than the events themselves. Achievers in life react differently than non-achievers to paperwork, deadlines, repetitious work, long hours, ‘demeaning’ activities and the general drudgery of work. The difference can be found in the rational ways achievers evaluate having to perform these various activities.

In tackling procrastination, Ellis focused on three different emotional reactions. First, he looked for people's tendency to put themselves down for their procrastination. Chronic procrastinators often view themselves as total failures because of their excuse making and goofing. As Ellis counselled, however, what are the chances a *total failure* can do anything successful to overcome any problems? So the first step in modifying procrastination is for people to accept themselves while hating and working hard to change their self-indulgent, inefficient behavior.

Once people stop putting yourself down, they can then work on the main cause of procrastination: low frustration tolerance and the associated irrational attitudes, which underlie this condition.

Now most people, when thinking about having to do paper work, making follow-up 'phone calls or writing reports, experience some degree of discomfort, tension, and frustration. What differentiates procrastinators from self-disciplined workers is their relative inability to tolerate the discomfort they experience in anticipation of performing the tasks and the enormous feelings of frustration they experience about having to do the work. And their different reactions to unpleasant boring, and hard work are reflected in their attitudes and thinking. The self-disciplined worker rationally thinks: 'While it's hard to do this work, it's not too hard, and it's harder if I don't.

While it may be unfair to do these boring tasks and give up my free time, that's the way it is. Life wasn't meant to be fair or easy. I know if I want to achieve tomorrow, I'd better put in today.' This mental approach enables people to tolerate discomfort and reduce frustration by not blowing the unpleasantness of the tasks out of proportion and not demanding that they shouldn't have to do them. The procrastinator, unfortunately, brings to work a different set of attitudes and assumptions.

Some of the faulty assumptions and irrational beliefs which Ellis has identified as being against the procrastinator's desire to work more efficiently and which lead to the constant rationalization as to why the work hasn't been done are: 'It's easier to avoid facing many of life's difficulties and self-responsibilities, than to take on more rewarding forms of self-discipline', 'I don't believe I can discipline myself' ('It's too hard'), 'I shouldn't have to do unpleasant things in order to get pleasant results', 'I need to be comfortable all the time', and 'I must have what I want (short-term pleasures) when I want it, and not what I don't want (discomfort)'.

When faced with having to do unpleasant activities procrastinators, through irrational self-talk, literally make the activities and their feelings about them so horrible, that it is impossible for them to self-motivate: 'This work is not only hard and boring, but it is *too* hard. I *can't stand* it! Life should be easier, fun and more exciting. This is really unfair. It's awful, horrible and terrible!'

Low frustration tolerance is one of the most difficult tendencies for you to overcome. Ellis recognized that in many instances it is not sufficient simply to dispute the irrationality of one's beliefs. Indeed, it is not uncommon for people to intellectually understand their irrationalities, but to be unable to feel or act any differently.

So Ellis advised the use of thinking, feeling, and behavioral methods to encourage change. He employed logical and scientific methods to try to modify people's attitudes as well as encouraging them to write down a list of all the *disadvantages* of procrastinating and the *advantages* of getting it done. Emotionally he encouraged people to forcefully and vigorously shout rational self-statements and also to use rational-emotive imagery in order to change how they feel about their work. Behaviorally, he gave homework assignments which involved them specifying some minimal work behavior they agreed to perform and got them to reward or punish themselves depending on the degree you follow of their own prescriptions.

A final problem that sometimes resides at the core of the procrastinators' belief system is perfectionism. That is, even after you stop putting yourself down because of your procrastination and significantly changes your attitude towards hard and unpleasant work and become more tolerant of frustration, you still may not perform the work because of your demands for perfect performance at these times, and your fear of receiving criticism and disapproval from others. Is it any wonder, then, that procrastination is such an intractable condition? A final step to overcoming procrastination to be taken in cases of perfectionism is to dispute the irrational demands for perfect performance and the need for approval.

Current Applications of REBT in the Workplace

In 2016, the founder of Rational Effectiveness Training, Dominic DiMattia enumerated the following applications of REBT and cognitive-behavior coaching (CBC) in organizations (David, 2016):

1. Sales training – an effective sales person must have high frustration tolerance and a low need for approval. CBC can help a person to work on their perfectionistic attitudes and realize they will not make a sale with every person. We can also help them be less sensitive to rejection since they will be constantly rejected.
2. Stress management – everyone in organizations is always complaining about the excessive demands place on them. CBC can teach them that feelings of stress come from internal dialogues of perfectionism, need for approval and low frustration tolerance. Once an individual realizes the pressure come from them and not external demands they handle the pressure much better.
3. Decision making – individuals are often paralyzed to make decision because they believe they must make the correct decision all the time, which is often impossible. Need to always be right make decision making very difficult.
4. Risk taking – again the need to be successful all the time is impossible. Successful innovators often fail many times before they succeed. Success requires perseverance and learning for mistakes rather than criticizing self for failing. Success comes from trying and learning from our failures.
5. Employee relations/management skills – by helping mangers to realize employees are human and make mistakes they will be more supportive managers rather than critical/punishing bosses.
6. Annual reviews – many managers do not give honest reviews because they are anxious about how the employee will react and feel guilty because they blame themselves for not managing the employee on a day to day basis. The study that Cayer and I did (Cayer, et al. 1988) at JC Penny bore this out. I believe helping

managers and employees to be more rational will increase productivity. Everyone will be focused on getting the job done rather than constantly covering their "asses".

Training and Development

While debate continues on the return on investment of training and development programs, world-wide, companies spend annually in excess of one billion dollars and those that spend more seem to demonstrate higher profit and shareholder return (http://businesstrainingexperts.com/knowledge-center/training-roi/profiting-from-learning/).

There appears to be two ways in which REBT is introduced in organizations (business; not-for-profits). First, consultants who already offer training programs can incorporate REBT into already existing training programs to increase their effectiveness or by offering stand-alone REBT/Rational Effectiveness Training in areas of personal development (e.g., stress management, resilience).

Taking an existing program and introducing REBT concepts periodically can increase the probability that the new behaviour or skill being taught will be maintained and transferred on the job (e.g., DiMattia, Yeager, & Dube, 1989). Examples of such training programs include: performance appraisal, communication skills, sale's effectiveness, conflict management, negotiation skills and time management.

As an example, Cayer, DiMattia and Wingrove (1988) reported that a high percentage of managers who have been trained in well-developed performance appraisal systems are not effective because managers have high needs for approval, avoid unpleasant reactions of workers by giving higher-than-earned ratings and often put themselves down for not regularly managing their employees. Therefore, at the time of a formal performance appraisal, they avoid giving accurate feedback to employees, and the result is a perpetuation of the problem of employee ineffectiveness. These consultants recommended that all supervisors who are expected to give formal appraisals be trained to dispute self-defeating ideas that interfere with their effectiveness. When it is demonstrated that using REBT will strengthen their performance reviews and in the long run reduce problems, supervisors are more willing to learn REBT techniques.

Another example of how REBT can be integrated in a training and development package is *Sales Stars* (Bernard, Quarry, & Ash, 1991) which can be offered as a stand alone program (4 × 2 ½ h sessions) conducted in small groups by a course leader or as part of a wider sales training course. The course was based on the premise that sales stars not only have well-developed sales skills (prospecting, building rapport, presenting, handling objections, closing, after sales service), they also have high levels of 'confidence' and 'persistence' due, in part, to not having different negative sales beliefs (e.g., self-blaming, generalizing, needing immediate results, exaggerating, approval seeking). The program teachers participants the ABCs, how to dispute and change negative sales beliefs and how to deal with difficult sales situations by, in part, increasing their discomfort tolerance.

A prime example of training and development where REBT is the means to the end is stress management training for teachers (e.g., Bernard, Joyce, & Rosewarne, 1983; Forman & Forman, 1978, 1980; Ugwoke et al., 2017). As one of the earliest types of REBT being applied to a work setting, these programs applied Ellis' ideas from therapy such as the ABCs, disputing and IBs/RBs and from Ellis book, *Executive Leadership* (1972). It is possible to introduce REBT in 10–12 sessions of 1 ½ to 2 h with the following as possible session content (from Forman & Forman, 1980): Session 1. The nature of RET and REE, Session 2. The ABCs of Emotions, Session 3. What is Rational? Session 4. Rational Self-Study, Sessions 5 and 6. Common Irrational Ideas, Session 7. Dealing with Anger and Hostility, Session 8. Dealing with Fear and Anxiety, Session 9. Dealing with Guilt and Session 10. Building New Thought Habits. Over the years, I have taught REBT to groups of teachers retired from teaching due to stress in one, full-day workshop (Bernard, 1990, 1991a, 1991b). Ruth Malkinson and her colleague Talma Kushnir reported on the positive effects of a rational-emotive group intervention for preventing and coping with stress among safety officers (Kushnir & Malkinson, 1993).

With the establishment in 1986 of the IRET Corporate Services Division at the Institute for Rational Emotive Therapy (New York), and *Rational Effectiveness Training: Increasing Personal Productivity at Work* (DiMattia & Mennen, 1990) formally announced that REBT was open to business and organizations. Topics covered in *Mind Over Myths* audio program included: A Model for Self-Management (ABCs), Finding Your Own Self-Defeating Behaviors, Managing Your Own Procrastination, Achieving Worker Compatibility, Managing Being Managed and Dealing with Performance Review. A decade later, *Reaching their Minds. A Trainer's Manual for Rational Effectiveness Training* (DiMattia & Ijzermans, 1996), equipped consultants and trainers with the tools needed for conducting training and development in REBT for employees at all levels of the organization. During this time, the greatest success and popularity of rational effectiveness training and development programs was found at the training and consulting company in the Netherlands, Schouten and Nelissen, exemplified in the work of Theo IJzerman, their clinical psychologist and corporate trainer. Current-day REBT training programs are described in the appendix of Dom DiMattia's *CBT in Action. Applications in the Workplace*.

Management and Leadership Development

Effective managers and leaders are individuals who have flexible attitudes and do not let their biases interfere with effective decision-making and who respond to change in an adaptive manner rather than sabotage new programs and ideas (DiMattia, 1991). Over the years, management and leadership programs that have included using REBT helping participants becoming aware of, re-examining and changing non-productive beliefs have helped ensure that decision making is maximized. Additionally, great managers have well-developed relationship skills covering leading teams, conducting performance appraisals and coaching.

Rational Emotive Behavior Coaching (RECBC)

In recent years we have seen a proliferation of organizations offering training in coaching and even programs to certify coaches. Managers have been coached to become better managers and executives have been coached to increase their effectiveness. REBC as an exemplar of cognitive-behaviour coaching has been described in the literature over the past 20 years or more (e.g., Bernard & David, 2018; Criddle, 2007a; Palmer & Gyllensten, 2008; Sherin & Caiger, 2004) and researched (e.g., David, et al., 2016; Ogbuanya, et al., 2018). Here's how Dom DiMattia describes the RECB brand of cognitive-behaviour coaching (DiMattia & Ijzermans, 1996).

> When individuals ask for assistance from coaches they are often burdened with a whole host of emotional issues, which interfere with goal attainment. For example many individuals seek coaching when they are unemployed. It would be foolish to think that they only need to focus on getting a new job without examining their anger, anxiety and depression, which often accompanies unemployment. Supporting the client and keeping them on task is often not enough.
>
> Their anger and or anxiety often keeps them from completing the necessary task to achieve a successful job search. Rigid dysfunctional beliefs are at the root of these sabotaging emotions. Effective coaching requires that we help the client become aware of the thoughts and beliefs that cause these debilitating emotions and teach them to change these thoughts and beliefs so they can stay on task.
>
> Let's look at Luke. He has sought out coaching because his new promotion requires that he give presentations to customers on a regular basis. He has little experience in public speaking. As a coach we can certainly help him find the necessary training to improve his skills but he also reports severe anxiety when in front of a group. He goes blank and cannot remember anything he has been taught. Using REBC we discover that he is very perfectionistic and has high need for approval. These dysfunctional beliefs and self talk "that it would be terrible if he made a mistake and couldn't face the group if they thought he was incompetent." These ruminations and anxiety prevent him from achieving his goal of making a successful presentation. REBC focuses on helping clients identify these dysfunctional cognitions and learn to challenge and replace them with more functional thoughts. It would certainly be unpleasant if he made a mistake but would it really be the end of the world and would he be a failure because he made a mistake? Does he need the approval of every person all the time? These questions posed by a REB coach will help Luke re-examine his perfectionism and need for approval. He would then arrive at the conclusion that most people make mistakes when they are learning a new task and if keeps practicing he will get better at public speaking. Also he will realize it is unrealistic it is unrealistic to expect everyone to approve of his presentation and he has no control over other people's opinions. Now let's examine how a REB coaching session would be conducted.
>
> Step 1: Establish a working alliance with the client. Listen attentively to his/her concerns.
> Step 2: Work with the client to establish specific measurable goals.

Step 3: Determine Specific skills required to achieve these goals.
Step 4: Determine the emotional barriers to working toward these goals.
Step 5: Teach the client that it is not the task that causes the emotions but their beliefs and thoughts.
Step 6: Find the specific beliefs and self-defeating thoughts that they have.
Step 7: Challenge the rigid and catastrophic beliefs and dysfunctional thoughts.
Step 8: Replace dysfunctional thoughts with more adaptive thoughts.
Step 9: Give specific behavioral and cognitive homework to reinforce new behaviors.
Step 10: Summarize and determine if client clearly understands the process.

It would appear that using a Rational Emotive Behavior Coaching approach can only enhance any coaching process and improve the probability that the behavior changes will last. In addition you will be teaching clients a process that can be applied to future situations, which they might encounter.

Coaches must first identify the disturbed emotions that a client is experiencing which would interfere with their goals. Once an emotion is identified the coach must teach the client that the emotion is cause by the dysfunctional beliefs and then challenge those beliefs. Only then can they focus on achieving the goal. It is too simplistic to believe that with support alone the client will achieve their goal.

REBT Managerial and Executive Coaching

Managerial coaching is a process whereby a supervisor/manager facilitates the learning and development processes of his/her subordinates, by strengthening their resources, such as behaviors and professional skills. Since managers are in charge of their team's performance, managerial coaching is an ongoing informal activity based on conversations between the managers, their team and individuals (Ellinger, Beattie, & Hamlin, 2010).

Executive coaching is the term used to describe the process by which a professional trained in one or more models or types of coaching applies various methods and techniques to help an executive who occupies at least a middle management position (although sometimes the beneficiaries could be employees in junior roles, who show high potential) accomplish a set of mutually defined objectives regarding client's skills, performance or development. The principles and methods of Albert Ellis' rational emotive behavioral therapy (REBT) have been described and used as a guide to executive coaching (e.g., Anderson, 2002; Criddle, 2007b; Grieger & Fralick, 2007; Morris, 1988).

Executives are individuals who generally seek coaching to help them develop skills that improve different aspects of work performance (productivity, relations with co-workers, ecision making, leadership etc.) rather than to overcome some emotional disturbances or existential crises – as it happens with many therapy clients. They can reach that goal by learning new strategies of controlling more efficiently own thinking and emotions and acquiring rational philosophies of life. REBC philosophy taps into the mechanisms that explain human reactions across multiple situations. It is, therefore, helpful not only in getting a handle on deficits, but also in enhancing strengths. Thus, REB coaches are well-equipped to assist executives properly, regardless of the specific scope of intervention (Dudău, Salagean, & Sava, 2018).

When coaching executives, REBC methods involve the use of psycho-educational methods in order to teach executives how to assess their beliefs, emotions and behaviors, differentiate between what is rational vs. irrational, healthy vs. unhealthy and adaptive vs. maladaptive, challenge their absolutistic thinking and build a more rational perspective that would help them attain their work goals. In addition, REB executive coaches often focus their intervention not only on present, but also on future, so that executives can grasp what they need to ultimately become own coaches (Palmer & Gyllensten, 2008). This instructional-didactic style is what distinguishes REBEC from more traditional, non-directive coaching. The REBC leadership philosophy can be harnessed to help executives gain control over their internal processes (beliefs, emotions) and behaviors, so that they can control more effectively the external aspects that shape the success of their leadership style and job performance, and, implicitly, influence the success of organization (Dudău et al., 2018).

A series of instruments are available for assessment of rational leadership and managerial coaching behaviors and skills including: *The Managerial Coaching Assessment System* (David & Matu, 2013), *The Freeman-Gavita Prescriptive Executive Coaching Multi-RaterAssessment* (Gavita, Freeman, & Sava, 2012), and *The Manager Rational and Irrational Beliefs Scale* (David, 2013).

Four Promising, REBT Programs at Work

In my review for this chapter, four programs stand out for their excellence in taking the best of REBT and rational effectiveness training and integrating it within the context and realities of conducting learning and development programs as well as coaching in organizations. (The last program described I have developed and has been evaluated by my peers as worthy of being listed here).

Emotionally Intelligent Leadership

Ed Nottingham, a consulting and clinical psychologist, leadership and executive coach and author of "It's Not as Bad as It Seems: A Thinking Straight Approach to Happiness" – revised and expanded edition (2000), is a leading REBT scholar-practitioner, who works in a Fortune 500, Learning and Development area within Human Resource. He has over the past two decades applied the principles of REBT and rational effectiveness training to coaching as well as in leadership and management training. He often introduces that rationale for his work to those he works with using the vehicle of emotional intelligence identifying self-management as a key EQ skill of effective leadership.

> From my experience, I believe leaders too often do not know themselves and, perhaps, more importantly fail to recognize the critical nature of self-management. When there are failures in self-awareness and self-management, other leadership skills such as strategic

> planning, team building, coaching, communication, and other competencies will also fail. I believe leaders require self-awareness and self-management before attempting to lead others. (Nottingham, 2012)

He has created online courses in which he ties REBT to EQ with a specific focus on the relationship "attitude" issues and poor self-management and how rational attitudes help people move from 'good to great' (personal communication). In his coaching of leaders, he sells attitude as a key to having 'emotional muscle.'

According to Nottingham, leader coaches cannot ignore *attitude*; CBC (cognitive-behavior coaching), RET (rational effectiveness training), REBT (rational emotive behavior therapy), CT (cognitive therapy), can provide a solid foundation and may even be the missing link to improving the EI competencies of self-awareness and self-management. Coaching for "emotional muscle" seems to be working with at least some of our leaders. He is orthodox in teaching those he is training and coaching the ABCs and how to change irrational beliefs (he terms 'sharks') that lead to common self-defeating emotional reactions through disputing helping people take the 'high road' through the skill of self-questioning (Nottingham, 2012): "Am I really telling myself the truth? "Can I prove this belief?" "Is the belief helping me?" Is what I believe logical?" "Is there any universal law that supports my belief?" "Why must?" "Is it true I can't stand it?" "Is it really awful, a 100% bad?" He explains that attacking irrational sharks and replacing them with rational ones leads to better emotional self-management and the achievement of one's goals ("Good thinking gets good results and helps us achieve our SMART goals"). As a coach, he teaches disputing through targeted questions: "How's that philosophy (idea, notion, belief, assumption, etc.) helping?" "So, you keep thinking what a jerk your co-worker is, and what does that do for you?" "I know you want your team members to be as dedicated to this project as you are, but do they have to?" "What's another way of looking at this?" "It is disappointing that X happened (e.g., not getting the promotion), but on a scale from 0 to 100, how bad is it?" "You mentioned that (insert name here) was one of your mentors. How would she think about this?" Effective leadership beliefs he counters with include: "Desiring rather than requiring beliefs (wish rather than demanding, musts)," "Events, "things," etc. really are bad but not awful (100%) – hassle not a horror!", "I don't like it, that's OK, I CAN STAND IT anyway!", "USA: Unconditional Self Acceptance" and "UOA: Unconditional Other Acceptance." The effectiveness of his work and REBT is also seen in equipping leaders who coach with skills they can impact those they are coaching (direct reports).

Grieger's Model of Organizational Change

In 1993, Russell Grieger along with Dominic DiMattia edited two special issues of the *Journal of Rational-Emotive & Cognitive-Behavior Therapy*, "RET in the Workplace." In these issues, Grieger continued his life-long interest in REBT and its uses eloquently captured in his 1980 book authored with John Boyd, titled,

"Rational-Emotive Therapy: A Skills: Based Approach." Today, Grieger has harvested the fruits of his earlier labors (e.g., Grieger, 2007; Grieger & Fralick, 2007) by showing how to integrate REBT at work when consulting with organizations and coaching individuals seeking ways to improve work performance (e.g., Grieger, 2017).

Grieger (2018) indicates that whenever he is invited to consult with an organization, his first challenge is to figure out at which of four levels the core problem or need exists: cultural, leadership, interpersonal and personal. Once he understands this, he delves into the human component. Grieger describes a 'Tree of Personal Effectiveness' where the foliage represents the results of work efforts (e.g., profit), the trunk representing the means – work performance skills- that determine the results and the roots of the tree – an individual's personality and character- that is the foundational source that determines the quality of work performance skills and ultimate results. Grieger's divides work skills (the means to the ends) as consisting of technical skills, interpersonal (e.g., communication, conflict resolution, empathy) and personal (e.g., time management, creative thinking, problem solving, emotional self-management).

Grieger writes that he has frequently worked with employees who processed all the necessary skills, but still do not produce their intended results. Most often it's because, at their roots, they are deficient or defective in some aspect of their personality or character. He has identified six core traits that he believes are critical in order for a person to use one's skills to their utmost in order to produce extraordinary performance and results. They are (Grieger & Fralick, 2007):

1. *Mental Muscle* – rational thinking, which provides a person the ability to operate free of the contaminating effects of stress, low frustration tolerance, and anger, and to thereby remain clearheaded, stay focused on personal and organizational goals, use good judgment, function cooperatively with others, and persist until results are produced;
2. *Unconditional Personal Responsibility* – the conviction that one's commitments are sacred, such that a person habitually does what's necessary to produce promised results, despite any and all adverse circumstances;
3. *Courage* – rational thinking that frees one to act without fear of failure, disapproval, and discomfort, so as to boldly and unabashedly strive to meet one's responsibilities and produce committed results;
4. *Passionate Purpose* – holding a clear conceptualization of one's purpose in life, then passionately expressing that purpose through one's work, provides profound motivation to act with integrity and do one's best, persist through stress and other roadblocks, and provides fulfilment through and satisfaction with one's work;
5. *Interpersonal Intelligence* – the endorsement of those beliefs that prompt compassion, generosity, and empathy in all interpersonal relationships as a matter of course; and,
6. *Personal Vitality* – holding the conviction to keep physically, emotionally, and interpersonally refreshed and energetic.

When Grieger assesses that the lack of results and strong personal and interpersonal skills is due to problems at the source, the personality and character of leadership and management, here is when as part his leadership and management training and individual coaching he calls on REBT.

> I delve into the ABCs of the people with whom I am to work. I first use my clinical skills to make explicit any defective or deficient emotional or behavioral reactions that may be present (the C), any activating events (the A), that may exist, and, especially, the key irrational beliefs (at B) that drive these feelings and behaviors. As we REBTers know, if there are character or personality issues in play, it is irrational thinking that most often drive these reactions. Accordingly, some of the key questions I ask are the following. What irrational beliefs – perfectionistic self, other, or situation demanding? catastrophizing? low frustration tolerance? self-damning? – drive these character and/or personality problems? What is the best format to remediate them – seminar? workshop? individual coaching? What would be the best method to communicate the REBT process of cognitive-emotive re-education? (Grieger, 2018)

The Rational Managerial Coaching Program

Developed by Oana David and colleagues (e.g., David & Matu, 2013; David, 2018), this program that teaches "rational thinking mindset and emotion-regulation skills" has received empirical support recently for building managerial coaching skills and leadership. The program consists of a workshop focused on discussing the mindset of rational leadership and models of rational managerial coaching. Experiential exercises, case studies and role plays are used. The training workshop has the following sections: (a) understanding managerial coaching and a solution-focused model for managerial coaching, (b) efficient communication and feedback skills, (c) motivating and empowering employees, and (d) rational leadership.

Each participant formulates his or her own short-term, medium-term and long-term development goals. Also, action plans are created that specify the steps a manager needs to take in order to achieve their goals.

Two or three individual coaching sessions following the training workshop to help support managers' implementation of rational leadership and managerial coaching skills. The sessions are aimed to facilitate the application of the skills gained from the first group session. Each session addresses the progress in achieving one's goals, identifying resources, as well as obstacles faced during the process. Between the individual coaching sessions, there is a shadowing session consisting of observing a typical coaching interaction between the manager and a subordinate related to a current issue. For the rest of the session, feedback is provided regarding the interaction and regarding other concerns related to the implementation of the new, managerial skills. Afterwards, managers receive feedback for improvements and another step in the action plan is followed.

The final session of the Rational Managerial Coaching Program has a group-coaching format and lasts an hour and half. The aim of this session is for participants to share experiences regarding the skills that were practiced over the course of the coaching program, as well as difficulties they met. Also, post-intervention assessments were conducted to evaluate the overall effectiveness of the coaching program (see for details David et al., 2016).

The Manager Rational and Irrational Beliefs Scale (David & Matu, 2013). This is a measure of rational and irrational beliefs that assess flexible or rigid appraisals related to three content areas relevant for managers: (1) appreciation and performance, (2) control, and (3) comfort. Each of these content areas is assessed by 10 items, 5 rational belief items and 5 irrational belief items. Each item is answered on a 4 points Likert format, strongly disagree (1) to strongly agree (4). It was particularized to managers' activity, built on the basis of REBT/C theory. The instrument assesses four principal processes (bi-dimensional: rational and irrational), as follows (irrational vs. rational counterpart): Demandingness vs. Preference, Low Frustration Tolerance vs. Frustration Tolerance, Awfulizing vs. Badness, and Global Evaluation vs. Unconditional Acceptance. General evaluation and unconditional acceptance are assessed with two items each, one referring to employees (other) and one referring to the manager evaluation/acceptance (self). It has adequate reliabilities and concurrent validity. Performance is measured by one open question asking about average target attainment in the last 6 months, if this indicator was applicable for their job.

The High Performance Mindset at Work

Over the past several years (e.g., Bernard, 2013, 2016a, 2016b, 2016c), I have researched the fields of positive psychology, cognitive-behaviorism, emotional intelligence and neuro-science that focuses on peak performance in adults with the goal of isolating the diverse range of psychological strengths (psychological capital) that contribute to what I have called a *high performance mindset*. Here's what I discovered.

> People who excel at work have three highly developed commitments. *Commitment to Success* means they regularly put into practice self-direction, optimism, growth mindset, creativity and high frustration tolerance. *Commitment to Others* means they are very accepting of others, empathic, respectful, supportive and genuine in providing feedback. *Commitment to Self* means they have highly developed self-regard, self-acceptance, authenticity, positive focus and adopt a healthy life style.

Additionally, I (Bernard, 2018b) have identified a range of common, psychological blockers (not mental health disorders) that frequently interfere with work performance in tough situations including: anxiety, feeling down, anger and procrastination.

As a result of this analysis, I have developed a number of learning and development programs, self-assessment tools as well as coaching programs (e.g., Bernard, 2017; visit: www.youcandoiteducation.com.au/work) designed for leaders, managers and employees to make them aware of and to strengthen their own mindset of high performance as well as others (teams; individual performance support) and to help people overcome psychological blockers. REBT methods occupy an central place in these programs as participants learn about the ABCs, how to dispute and change irrational beliefs that contribute to psychological blockers, use rational self-statements and learn about the importance of self-acceptance, other acceptance and high frustration tolerance.

HPMW programs include:

1. HPMW E-learning (leadership, management, employees): six module, e-learning course
2. HPMW Blended Learning (leadership, management, employees): six module, e-learning course combined with interactive weekly group coaching
3. HPMW Intensive Learning (leadership/management): Six module, e-learning course (in-house group training also available); interactive weekly group coaching introductory/concluding group presentations in-house and/or on-line; 1:1 coaching post e-learning course; pre-post quantitative survey data on HPMW and tough work situations
4. HPMW Coaching (leadership, management): six to eight session 1:1 coaching covering basics of high performance mindset, strengthening self-awareness, further development of individual strengths, tackling tough work situations
5. HPMW Consultation (leadership): HPMW consultant meets on a regular basis with leadership, management and human resource personnel to discuss ways in which the high performance mindset can be implemented throughout organisational culture and leadership/management practice

In order to describe the process of HPMW in coaching, I developed the four-step *Grape Model*:

Step 1: **G**OALS – in which the coachee is assisted in identifying professional work goals for coaching sessions;
Step 2: **R**EFLECTION – in which the coachee is assisted in reflecting on different areas of their current approach to their work;
Step 3: **A**CTION **P**LANNING – in which the coachee is assisted to develop an action plan to activate beliefs to strengthen commitments, use behavioral strengths, and remove work performance blockers;
Step 4. **E**VALUATION – in which the coachee is assisted to evaluate and revise the action plan.

Effectiveness of the HPMW program was investigated as an eight-week course presented to 28 school leaders and followed by coaching sessions. Results showed reduction in stress and increase in effectiveness when responding to tough work.

Final Comment

It seems to me that the future of REBT at work is bright – providing we can transform our promising programs into best practices through the conduct of well-designed empirical studies.

Albert Ellis would be the first to agree – as he once said to me and those attending a Wednesday night group therapy session after I explained to a client why he was experiencing such a high degree of social anxiety with females: "You know why Dr. Bernard has such a good understanding of issues we have been explaining to you for weeks – and he hardly knows you at all – it is because he has a good theory!" And I think we agree with Ellis and are thankful for his great theory.

We need to do a great job in marketing what we do to different constituencies including what our distinctive value proposition is compared to our competition. An example of successful networking is Windy Dryden's work at the Henley Business School (University of Reading) where he offered a two-day training program to 40 students in cognitive-emotive-behavioural coaching (Dryden, 2018).

I also think a new door is opening with organizations thinking about the benefits of investing in wellbeing and stress management programs – not only because of the downward, spiralling effects negative employees at all levels have on work performance, the performance of colleagues and teams and on organizational performance. It would be naive to expect given the variety of forces that impact work performance (e.g., culture, leadership, team and individual) that REBT will always be found to have a direct impact on job performance. Moreover, the investment of an organization in REBT-oriented training and coaching is dependent on the mindset of key decision makers in HR, organizational development and the executive leadership team. Enabling key personnel to commit to REBT and maintaining interest and investment over time is most challenging and can be problematic.

What we can say with some assurance is that given the turbulent, ever-changing and time-workload pressures of today's workplace, too many leaders, managers and employees are excessively stressed with such stress having negative ramifications for their emotional and physical health, their relationships with colleagues and family. By strengthening the psychological strength of rationality, we know that people change their thinking, feeling and behaviour leading to less stress – resulting in positive effects on their own work performance as well as their organizations.

References

Anderson, J. A. (2002). Executive coaching and REBT: Some comments from the field. *Journal of Rational-Emotive & Cognitive Behavior Therapy, 20*, 222–223.

Bernard, M.E. (1990). Taking the stress out of teaching. Melbourne, VIC: Collins-Dove, 1990, pp. 336.

Bernard, M. E. (1991a). *Procrastinate later!* (p. 210). Melbourne, VIC: Schwartz-Wilkinson.

Bernard, M. E. (1991b). Taking the stress out of teaching. *Primary Education, 22*, 2–8.

Bernard, M. E. (2011). *Rationality and the pursuit of happiness. The legacy of Albert Ellis* (p. 305). London, UK: Wiley-Blackwell.

Bernard, M. E. (2013). *The high performance mindset at work* (2nd ed., p. 140). Southbank, VIC: The Bernard Group.

Bernard, M. E. (2014). Mindset matters most. *The CEO Magazine*, December Issue, 82–83.

Bernard, M. E. (2016a). Beliefs and teacher stress. *Journal of Rational-Emotive & Cognitive-Behavior Therapy., 34*, 209–224. https://doi.org/10.1007/s10942-016-0238-y

Bernard, M. E. (2016b, June). *High performance mindset at work*. Invited workshop presented at the 2nd International Congress of Cognitive Behavioral Coaching, Athens, Greece.

Bernard, M. E. (2016c). *Coaching the high performance mindset at work*. East Melbourne, VIC: The Bernard Group.

Bernard, M. E. (2017). *Stress management for teachers and school principals*. Oakleigh, VIC: Australian Scholarships Group.

Bernard, M. E. (2018a). Stress management coaching. In M. E. Bernard & O. David (Eds.), *Coaching for rational living. Theory, techniques and applications*. New York, NY: Springer Press.

Bernard, M. E. (2018b). Psychological blockers to successful coaching outcomes. In M. E. Bernard & O. David (Eds.), *Coaching for rational living. Theory, techniques and applications*. New York, NY: Springer Press.

Bernard, M. E. (2018c). Coaching high workplace performance. In M. E. Bernard & O. David (Eds.), *Coaching for rational living. Theory, techniques and applications*. New York, NY: Springer Press.

Bernard, M. E. (2018d). Rationality in coaching. In M. E. Bernard & O. David (Eds.), *Coaching for rational living. Theory, techniques and applications*. New York, NY: Springer Press.

Bernard, M. E., & David, O. (Eds.). (2018). *Coaching for rational living*. New York, NY: Springer Press.

Bernard, M. E., Joyce, M., & Rosewarne, P. M. (1983). Helping teachers cope with stress. In A. Ellis & M. E. Bernard (Eds.), *Rational-emotive approaches to the problems of childhood*. New York, NY: Plenum Press.

Bernard, M. E., Quarry, P., & Ash, E. (1991). *Sales stars (training and development program)*. Middle Park, VIC: Seven Dimensions.

Broder, M. (2012). *Stage climbing: The shortest path to your highest potential*. Philadelphia, PA: MPA Publications.

Broder, M. (2018). Motivational coaching. In M. E. Bernard & O. David (Eds.), *Coaching for rational living. Theory, techniques and applications*. New York, NY: Springer.

Cayer, M., DiMattia, D. J., & Wingrove, J. (1988). Conquering evaluation fear. *Personnel Administrator, 33*(6), 97–107.

Criddle, W. D. (1993). Teaching RET in the financial and investment sector. *Journal of Rational-Emotive & Cognitive Behavior Therapy, 11*, 19–32.

Criddle, W. D. (2007a). Adapting REBT to the world of business. *Journal of Rational-Emotive & Cognitive Behavior Therapy, 25*, 87–105.

Criddle, W. D. (2007b). The transition from therapist to executive coach. *Journal of Rational-Emotive & Cognitive Behavior Therapy, 25*, 121–141.

David, D., Cotet, C., Matu, S., Mogoase, C., & Simona, S. (2018). 50 years of rational-emotive and cognitive-behavioral therapy: A systematic review and meta-analysis. *Journal of Clinical Psychology, 74*, 304–318. https://doi.org/10.1002/jclp.22514

David, O. (2016). The foundations and evolution of cognitive behavioral coaching in organizations: An interview with Dominic DiMattia. *Journal of Rational-Emotive & Cognitive-Behavior Therapy, 34*, 282–288.

David, O. (2018). Managerial coaching and rational leadership. In M. E. Bernard & O. David (Eds.), *Coaching for rational living. Theory, techniques and applications*. New York, NY: Springer.

David, O. A. (2013). The online Prescriptive Index platform for the assessment of managerial competencies and coaching needs: Development and initial validation of the experience sampling Mood Wheel and the Manager-Rational and Irrational Beliefs Scale. *Romanian Journal of Applied Psychology, 15*(2), 41–50.

David, O. A., Ionicioiu, I., Imbăruş, A. C., & Sava, F. A. (2016). Coaching banking managers through the financial crisis: Effects on stress, resilience, and performance. *Journal of Rational-Emotive & Cognitive-Behavior Therapy, 34*, 267–281.

David, O. A., & Matu, S. A. (2013). How to tell if managers are good coaches and how to help them improve during adversity? The managerialcoaching assesment system and the rational managerial coaching program. *Journal of Cognitive & Behavioral Psychotherapies, 13*, 497–502.

DiGiuseppe, R., & Miller, A. R. (1994). A rational-emotive model of organizational consultation. In M. E. Bernard & R. DiGiuseppe (Eds.), *Rational-emotive consultation in applied settings*. Hillsdale, NJ: Lawrence Erlbaum.

DiMattia, D. (1991). RET in the workplace. In M. E. Bernard (Ed.), *Using rational-emotive therapy effectively: A practitioner's guide*. New York, NY: Plenum Press.

DiMattia, D., & Mennen, S. (1990). *Rational effectiveness training: Increasing personal productivity at work*. New York, NY: Institute for Rational-Emotive Therapy.

DiMattia, D., & Ijzermans, T. (1996). *Reaching their minds: A trainers manual to rational effectiveness training*. New York: Albert Ellis Institute.

Dimattia, D. J., Yeager, R. J., & Dube, I. (1989). Emotional barriers to learning. *Personnel Journal, 68*, 86–89.

Dryden, W. (1985). Voluntary redundancy and beyond: A counsellor trainer's odyssey. Counselling. *Journal of the British Association for Counselling, 54*, 2–5.

Dryden, W. (2018). *Cognitive-emotive-behavioural coaching: A flexible and pluralistic approach*. London, UK: Routledge.

Dryden, W., & Gordon, J. (1993). *Peak performance: Become more effective at work*. Didcot, Oxfordshire: Mercury.

Dudău, D. P., Salagean, N., & Sava, F. A. (2018). Executive coaching. In M. E. Bernard & O. David (Eds.), *Coaching for rational living. Theory, techniques and applications*. New York, NY: Springer.

Edgerton, N., & Palmer, S. (2005). SPACE: A psychological model for use within cognitive behavioural coaching, therapy and stress management. *The Coaching Psychologist, 2*, 19–31.

Ellinger, A. D., Beattie, R. S., & Hamlin, R. G. (2010). The 'Manager as Coach'. In E. Cox, T. Bachkirova, & D. Clutterbuck (Eds.), *The complete handbook of coaching* (pp. 257–270). London: Sage.

Ellis, A. (1972). *Executive leadership. A rational approach*. New York, NY: Institute for Rational Living.

Ellis, A., & Blum, M. L. (1967). Rational training: A new method of facilitating management labor relations. *Psychological Reports, 20*, 1267–1284.

Ellis, A., Gordon, J., Neenan, M., & Palmer, S. (1997). *Stress counselling: A rational emotive behaviour approach*. London, UK: Cassell.

Forman, S. G., & Forman, B. D. (1978). A rational-emotive approach to consultation. *Psychology in the Schools, 15*, 400–406.

Forman, S. G., & Forman, B. D. (1980). Rational-emotive staff development. *Psychology in the Schools, 17*, 90–95.

Gavita, O. A., Freeman, A., & Sava, F. A. (2012). The developement and validation of the Freeman-Gavita prescriptive executive coaching (PEC) multirater. *Journal of Cognitive and Behavioral Psychotherapies, 12*(2), 159–174.

Grieger, R. (2007). One REBTers model for business consulting. *Journal of Rational-Emotive & Cognitive Behavior Therapy, 25*, 107–120.

Grieger, R. (2017). *Developing unrelenting drive, dedication, and determination: A cognitive behavior workbook*. New York, NY: Routledge.

Grieger, R. (2018). Coaching for organizational change. In M. E. Bernard & O. David (Eds.), *Coaching for rational living. Theory, techniques and applications*. New York, NY: Springer.

Grieger, R., & Fralick, F. (2007). The use of REBT principles and practices in leadership training and development. *Journal of Rational-Emotive & Cognitive-Behavior Therapy, 25*, 143–157. https://doi.org/10.1007/s10942-006-0038-x

Klarreich, S. (1993). RET: A powerful tool to turn traumatic job termination into an enlightening career transition. *Journal of Rational-Emotive & Cognitive-Behavior Therapy, 11*, 77–90.

Kushnir, T., & Malkinson, R. (1993). A rational-emotive group intervention for preventing and coping with stress among safety officers. *Journal of Rational-Emotive & Cognitive-Behavior Therapy, 11*, 195–206.

Lange, A., & Grieger, R. (1993). Integrating RET into management consulting and training. *Journal of Rational-Emotive & Cognitive-Behavior Therapy, 11*, 51–57.

Luthans, F. (2002). Positive organizational behavior: Developing and managing psychological strengths. *Academy of Management Executive, 16*, 57–72.
Luthans, F., & Youssef, C. M. (2004). Human, social, and now psychological capital management: Investing in people for competitive advantage. *Organizational Dynamics, 33*, 143–160.
Miller, A. R., & Yeager, R. J. (1993). Managing change: A corporate application of rational-emotive therapy. *Journal of Rational-Emotive & Cognitive-Behavior Therapy, 11*, 65–76.
Morris, G. B. (1988). The executive: A pathfinder. *Organizational Dynamics, 16*, 62–77.
Morris, G. B. (1993). A rational-emotive paradigm for organizations. *Journal of Rational-Emotive & Cognitive-Behavior Therapy, 11*, 33–50.
Neenan, M. (2018a). *Developing resilience: A cognitive-behavioural approach* (2nd ed.). London, UK: Routledge.
Neenan, M. (2018b). *Resilience as a framework for coaching*. London, UK: Routledge.
Neenan, M. (2018c). Coaching for rational living. In M. E. Bernard & O. David (Eds.), *Resilience coaching*. New York, NY: Springer.
Neenan, M., & Palmer, S. (2001). Rational emotive behaviour coaching. *Rational Emotive Behaviour Therapist, 9*, 34–41.
Nottingham, E. (2000). *It's not as bad as it seems: A thinking straight approach to happiness* – revised and expanded edition. New York, NY: Writer's Showcase.
Nottingham, E. (2012). *Coaching for emotional muscle*. Society of Consulting Psychology, Mid-Winter Conference, February 10.
Ogbuanya, T. C., Eseadi, C., Orji, C. T., Omeje, J. C., Anyanwu, J. I., Ugwok, S. C., & Edeh, N. C. (2018). Effect of rational-emotive behavior therapy program on the symptoms of burnout syndrome among undergraduate electronics work students in Nigeria. *Psychological Reports, 1*, 33294117748587. https://doi.org/10.1177/0033294117748587
Palmer, S. (2007). PRACTICE: A model suitable for coaching, counselling, psychotherapy and stress management. *The Coaching Psychologist, 3*, 71–77.
Palmer, S. (2009). Rational coaching: A cognitive behavioural approach. *The Coaching Psychologist, 5*, 12–18.
Palmer, S., & Burton, T. (1996). *Dealing with people problems at work*. Maidenhead, UK: McGraw-Hill.
Palmer, S., & Gyllensten, K. (2008). How cognitive behavioural, rational emotive behavioural or multimodal coaching could prevent mental health problems, enhance performance and reduce work related stress. *Journal of Rational-Emotive & Cognitive-Behavior Therapy, 26*, 38–52. https://doi.org/10.1007/s10942-007-0069-y
Reichman, D. R. (1993). Career counselling: A rational-emotive approach to career development. *Journal of Rational-Emotive & Cognitive-Behavior Therapy, 11*, 91–108.
Robb, H. (1998). Reducing procrastination in the workplace. In S. Clerech (Ed.), *Handbook of organization health psychology* (pp. 55–77). Toronto, Canada: Psychosocial Press.
Sherin, J., & Caiger, L. (2004). Rational-emotive behavior therapy: A behavioral change model for executive coaching? *Consulting Psychology Journal: Practice and Research, 56*, 225–233. https://doi.org/10.1037/1065-9293.56.4.225
Spillane, R. (1983). *Achieving peak performance: A psychology of success in the organisation*. New York, NY: Harper Row.
Ugwoke, S. C., Eseadi, C., Igbokwe, C. C., Chiaha, G. T. U., Nwaubani, O. O., Orji, C. T., … Abugu, L. I. (2017). Effects of a rational-emotive health education intervention on stress management and irrational beliefs among technical college teachers in Southeast Nigeria. *Medicine, 96*(31), e7658. https://doi.org/10.1097/MD.0000000000007658

Index

© Springer Nature Switzerland AG 2019
M. E. Bernard, W. Dryden (eds.), *Advances in REBT*,
https://doi.org/10.1007/978-3-319-93118-0

R

FSC
www.fsc.org
MIX
Papier | Fördert
gute Waldnutzung
FSC® C083411

Kolibri 360 GmbH
Ferdinand-Jühlke-Straße 7
99095 Erfurt, Deutschland
produktsicherheit@kolibri360.de